Arts in Health
Designing and Researching Interventions

By Daisy Fancourt

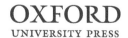

OXFORD
UNIVERSITY PRESS

OXFORD
UNIVERSITY PRESS

Great Clarendon Street, Oxford, OX2 6DP,
United Kingdom

Oxford University Press is a department of the University of Oxford.
It furthers the University's objective of excellence in research, scholarship,
and education by publishing worldwide. Oxford is a registered trade mark of
Oxford University Press in the UK and in certain other countries

© Oxford University Press 2017

The moral rights of the authors have been asserted

First Edition published in 2017

Published in the United States of America by Oxford University Press
198 Madison Avenue, New York, NY 10016, United States of America

British Library Cataloguing in Publication Data

Data available

Library of Congress Control Number: 2017935042

ISBN 978-0-19-879207-9

Acknowledgements

I should like to thank Martin Baum from Oxford University Press for commissioning this book and Charlotte Holloway for her support during its writing. I would also like to acknowledge Aaron Williamon for encouraging me to write this book in the first place and Rosie Perkins who has been my closest collaborator over the last few years in carrying out research in this field.

My own involvement in arts in health was sparked by Singing Medicine; a programme run by Ex Cathedra bringing music interventions to children at Birmingham Children's Hospital. I'm profoundly grateful for the training and experience of working on their programme all those years ago and to Oxford University for working with Ex Cathedra to make the experience possible. Since then, I've been fortunate to work with many inspiring hospitals, universities and arts organizations. There are too many to name them all, but I'd particularly like to acknowledge Action for Young Carers and the Carers Federation, Arts Council England, Breathe Arts Health Research, Chelsea and Westminster NHS Foundation Trust, CW+, Imperial College London, the Royal College of Music, Tenovus Cancer Care, and University College London.

I am grateful to the following people for their expert advice on chapters of the book and their support with proofreading: Michael Brown, Paul Camic, Helen Chatterjee, Yvonne Farquharson, Adam Ockelford, Tim Osborn, Rosie Perkins, and George Waddell. I'd also like to acknowledge the support of Annabelle Lucas who helped in compiling the resources for the fact file in Part IV. I'm delighted that the front cover of this book features the beautiful artwork of Klari Reis. From her series 'A Daily Dish', the image is a photograph of paint in a petri dish and is inspired by work Reis carried out in London hospitals observing the way that blood responds to different pharmaceuticals in petri dishes: an epitome of the fusion of art and health. This book and the research I have been involved in over the last few years would not have been possible without the generous support of Clive Marks. I am privileged to have worked with him. In writing this book, I've also been fortunate to be able to draw on so many wonderful examples of research and practice. I'd like to thank the people involved in these projects and to credit their work, which has helped to build this field.

Finally, I would like to thank my parents Howard and Val, my sister Millie and my partner Tom for their support through all my years of involvement in this field of work.

Daisy Fancourt
London, 2016

Contents

Introduction

Over the past few decades, the use of the arts in health has blossomed. What, for many centuries, was seen as a fringe activity is now being recognized as a field that has enormous potential for having a positive impact on both individuals and societies. However, despite this surge in interest and activity, there is still limited support available for people working in the field. Although the number of practical training courses for artists is growing and more universities are establishing research groups, most training activity occurs in either practice or research; there are relatively few opportunities to gain parallel experience in both. Yet arts in health is an inherently inter-disciplinary field. Researchers are often involved in the conceptualization and implementation of the interventions they are researching, and practitioners are increasingly becoming involved in research. Consequently, the aim of this book is to provide a complete overview of how to go about designing and researching arts in health interventions.

Part I explores the context for arts in health interventions. In Chapter 1, we trace the origins of the use of arts in health, considering the place of the arts in medicine and medical philosophy across the last 40,000 years and the evolution of theory and practice in the field. Chapter 2 looks back at developments over the past 200 years in the concepts of health and medicine, exploring the emergence of models of health such as the biomedical model and biopsychosocial model, and identifying myriad ways in which the arts have been shown to impact on health and wellbeing in relation to these models. Chapter 3 identifies recent health policies and national arts agendas that have made space for arts in health and considers the opportunities these have presented for research and practice. In Chapter 4, we consider what arts in health today actually is: which activities are included within the field, how they have developed, and how the field as a whole relates to other fields such as medical humanities. Each area of activity is illustrated with case studies of projects and sources of further information.

Part II looks more closely at how to go about designing and delivering arts in health interventions. In Chapter 5, we look at how to conceptualize and plan an intervention, moving through a step-by-step process assisted by reputable business models and other healthcare frameworks that are being implemented in healthcare systems around the world to help develop targeted and effective health innovations. In Chapter 6, we move onto the practicalities of implementing an intervention, evaluating its success and planning for its long-term sustainability. Chapter 7 discusses how to identify suitable partners for a project, develop a project brief, draw up contracts, and deliver induction and training programmes. It also covers a topic at the heart of arts in health: how to fund projects. Chapter 8 then outlines some of the essential information for working in healthcare settings, including issues around patient safeguarding, occupational health, and suggestions for how to engage patients and staff in projects.

In Part III, we explore how to research arts in health interventions. Chapter 9 examines the differences between evaluation and research and considers when each is more appropriate. It explores some of the myths that surround arts in health research as well as providing recommendations for new researchers and sources of research findings. Chapter 10 then outlines a step-by-step approach to the research process, introducing different study designs and research methods and advising on how to select outcome measures. Chapter 11 provides a template research protocol, demonstrating how research ideas can be mapped into a research plan and raising some of the key practical points of consideration when designing a research project. Chapter 12 focuses on research ethics, discussing ethical practice and providing template information sheets and consent forms for participants involved in studies.

Finally, Part IV contains a fact file of arts in health research and practice. An overview of 13 of the most common areas of medicine is provided along with five key research findings for each area, some project ideas, and a wealth of further reading and resources designed to inspire future projects.

Naturally, different sections of the book will appeal to different people depending on their backgrounds. For example, for researchers or research students, discussions of research in Part III may already be well known, whereas the steps involved in establishing an intervention outlined in Part II may be new territory. Similarly, for project managers or healthcare professionals, issues such as how to identify arts partners discussed in Chapter 7 may be of particular interest, but details of working in healthcare settings in Chapter 8 may be part of day-to-day practice already. Whereas for artists and arts organizations, this may be the reverse. For those who are simply seeking to find out more about the field, the context described in Part I and the key research findings in Part IV may provide the most engaging information. Overall, the book as a whole aims to provide a full picture of arts in health research and practice and is structured to map onto the lifecycle of an arts in health project. Reading it from cover to cover will hopefully provide a framework for all readers on which previous knowledge can be hung and new information can be contextualized. In keeping with this, each chapter also contains suggestions for further reading for those who want to explore particular topics in more detail. Further reading is highlighted using the symbol 🔍 . However, the book can also be approached as a reference text, with specific chapters used to guide aspects of research and practice. In particular, the fact file in Part IV is intended as a resource that can be revisited as new projects are planned.

Overall, as the title suggests, this book focuses on arts in health interventions: practical projects involving participants. As outlined in Chapter 4, this can include a wide range of activities including participatory arts programmes for specific patient groups, general arts activities in everyday life, arts in psychotherapy programmes, arts in healthcare technology, and arts-based training programmes for staff. But that is not to say the book will be of relevance only to those working on such practical projects. The historical, theoretical, and political background covered in Part I, for example, is relevant to the entire field of arts in health, including, for example, the use of the arts in the design of healthcare environments. Furthermore, increasingly, other types of areas of arts in health activity that might not have historically always been participatory, such as the arts in healthcare environments and the arts to translate health education messages, are now being conceptualized and designed with participatory strands. As such, it is anticipated that the more practical guidance given in Parts II, III, and IV may also be of interest to research and practice across the entire field of arts in health.

In compiling a book such as this, there are far more examples of research, policy and practice around the world than can be captured in a single volume. A difficult decision was what there was not space to include. Consequently, this book takes a particular focus on activity in English-speaking countries, including the UK, Ireland, USA, Australia, Canada, and New Zealand. Nevertheless, particularly special case studies and examples from other parts of the world are drawn in across the book in reference to arts in health being very much a global phenomenon.

As the field continues to progress, it is hoped that research and practice will continue to have the close relationship that they currently have. Through their interaction, clear healthcare needs can be identified, effective interventions designed, tested and honed, impact measured, and successful programmes rolled out to benefit more people. It is through this close relationship that the worlds of arts and health will bring the most to one another and provide the greatest value to individuals and societies globally.

Part I

The context for arts in health interventions

Chapter 1

A history of the use of arts in health

The birth of the arts

The story of art is generally thought to start in the Palaeolithic era: the prehistoric period of human history. Coined by John Lubbock, an English Baron and scientist in 1865, the term 'Palaeolithic' comes from the Greek 'paleo' (meaning old) and 'lithos' (meaning stone).(1) The term is sometimes used alongside the 'Stone Age', although the Stone Age continued long after the end of the Palaeolithic era, encompassing too the Mesolithic and Neolithic eras. Exact dates for these periods vary enormously, but broadly, the Palaeolithic era is thought to extend from the earliest known use of stone tools by *homo habilis* around 2.6 million years ago through the emergence of *homo sapiens* around 195,000 years ago to the end of the latest Pleistocene (glaciation) period around 10,000 years ago.(2) The breadth of history encompassed within this span means that it is commonly split into three subperiods: the early or lower Palaeolithic (from the start of the Palaeolithic period until around 250,000 years ago), the middle Palaeolithic (from around 250,000 to 30,000 years ago), and the late or upper Palaeolithic (from around 40,000 years ago until around 10,000 years ago).

The earliest evidence of art is somewhat disputed. There are some early artefacts, including small sculptures such as the 'Venus of Tan Tan', an alleged artefact that appears to show the female figure found in Morocco, dated to around 300,000-500,000 years ago.(3) However, experts are divided as to whether this (and other very early artefacts) are actual evidence of art, or the result of rock erosion and other natural processes over the ages. Moving beyond these contested early findings, the first uncontested pieces of artwork come from slightly later: the late middle Palaeolithic era and into the upper Palaeolithic era. Archaeologist Steven Mithen argues that art began being produced around this time because of neurological developments in *homo sapiens*. He argues that there are three cognitive processes critical to art making: the mental conception of an image, the intentional communication of this image, and the attribution of meaning to the image. Although some of these processes were present in earlier humans, Mithen explains that it was only with *homo sapiens* that these three elements could be combined in a way that produced art.(4)

The most famous examples of late middle/upper Palaeolithic art are cave paintings. These were generally worked with stone (such as flint and obsidian) or wood or bone tools, and painted in red, black, and ochre through combinations of iron oxide, manganese oxide, and clay. Some of the most beautifully painted caves include Chauvet in France, dating from around 31,000 BC, Altamira in Spain, dating from around 14,000 to 12,000 BC, and Lascaux in France from around 15,000 to 10,000 BC. Images depicted include wild animals and birds alongside human hunters. The cave walls are also not just canvases for the artwork, but become part of the art itself, with a myriad of examples of rock formations woven into artwork designs, such as protruding rocks forming the heads of animals, animals emerging from crevices, or bone objects such as spearheads and teeth jammed into the rock surfaces to add extra texture.(5)

In addition to these cave paintings, a number of sculptures have been found dating from the same middle/upper Palaeolithic period. Many of these take the form of female figures, like the alleged Venus of Tan Tan, but are more deliberate artworks, with clear carvings. A defining feature of these 'Venus figurines', as they have been dubbed, is their anatomical exaggeration of the female figure, leading to theories that they were carved for use in fertility rituals.(6) Two famous examples of Venus figurines are the Venus of Willendorf, a 4 ¼ inch limestone carving discovered in the early twentieth century in caves in Austria and dated to around 28,000-25,000 BC; and the Venus of Hohle Fels, discovered nearly a hundred years later in caves near Ulm and the Danube source and dated to around 36,000 years ago. Support for the theory of these carvings' use in fertility rituals is the parallel discovery of a number of other sexual carvings, such as vulvar symbols carved on a limestone block from La Ferrassie rock shelter in southwest France, dated to around 35,000 years ago; and a phallus carved from the horn of a bison discovered in the Blanchard rock shelter nearby and dated to around the same time.(7) What is remarkable about these discoveries is that they suggest that some of the earliest sculptures ever made were created specifically to support rituals around fertility and health. In other words, arts and health were very much interwoven from the beginning.

It has been suggested that these fertility rituals were a part of expressions of religious ecstasy practised by shamans (healers seen to form an intermediary between humans and gods) in the Palaeolithic period. Shamanism is believed to have been ubiquitous among hunter-gatherer societies, with shamans entering altered states of consciousness to converse with spirits, welcome new life, heal the sick, and send the dead on their way.(8) Experts have suggested that cave paintings were recreations by shamans of the hallucinations they experienced during their states of consciousness, with the journeys between life and the spirit world, consciousness and unconsciousness, also epitomized in and facilitated by the networks of caves descending deep underground where these pieces of artwork and sculptures have been found.(5) The trance-like nature of many of the cave paintings, including blends of abstract and representational imagery, overlapping scenes, and sometimes surreal combinations of animals and humans has been seen to attest to their creation during the climax of ecstatic rituals.

Furthermore, it is not just paintings and sculpture that appear to have been involved in these shamanic health and healing rituals. In 2009, a series of flutes made from bird bones were discovered dating back to around 35,000 years ago, just feet away from the Venus of Hohle Fels.(9) Similar discoveries have been made of musical instruments carved from the radial bones of swans and griffon vultures and from mammoth ivory. Remains found in upper Palaeolithic graves also show that animal skin drums were in use at the time, and an archaeologist working in 2002 made the discovery that stalactites in some of the caves where these discoveries have been made also produce deep booming sounds when struck.(5) All of these elements suggest that music as well as sculpture and wall art may have played a part in cave rituals. Other scholars have theorized that dance was involved: findings from the Le Tuc D'Audoubert caves in France show children's heel prints dated to the upper Palaeolithic time embedded in the soft clay floor next to some sculptures believed to be indicative of sexual initiation rituals; rare and important physical evidence of the involvement of movement. (8) There are also theories around the use of animal head dresses and costumes, as well as literature exploring the theatrical aspects of shaman rituals, suggesting that the rituals were a rich composite of a range of art forms. Consequently, it appears that Palaeolithic health and healing rituals were expressed in early examples of art, sculpture, music, dance, and theatre.

However, the associations between arts and health go further than this. Humans have evolved to engage with rituals that are selectively advantageous. Some scholars have speculated that the shamanic rituals helped to reduce anxiety, with the calming and repetitive behaviours helping to assert control over stressful situations, such as coming to terms with death, and helping to regulate emotions, thereby functioning in themselves not just as symbolic rituals but as health-promoting activities.(10) Another theory is that the rituals led to enhanced group bonding, leading to the release of social bonding hormones such as oxytocin and neuropeptides such as beta-endorphin. Indeed, this ties in with other theories suggesting that singing in particular helped to bond social groups, taking over from grooming as humans evolved to be part of larger social networks.(11,12) Social bonding was vital to health by encouraging early humans to stay located within communities where they could protect one another, such as through defence against dangers and care of the sick. It has even been hypothesized that this social bonding was one of the factors that facilitated the territorial and demographic expansion of modern humans relative to culturally more conservative and isolated Neanderthal populations.(9) This suggests that ritual behaviours, whether in cave painting during rituals, the sculptures produced to assist them, the music played, the costumes worn, the dancing that took place, or the theatrical presentations, may have been seen as valuable in maintaining group cohesion and supporting the health of both individuals and communities.

This picture of the birth of art may come as a surprise: it appears the arts were not separated into component parts but woven together in layers of combined artistic practice. Of course, evidence of certain art forms such as dance is harder to trace as the evidence is more circumspect than sculpture, say, where specific artefacts can be preserved. So it is possible that certain strands of art have an even longer history. Furthermore, it may be that the arts had further uses in society beyond the rituals identified by archaeologists. Nevertheless, the upper Palaeolithic period seems to be an exciting point in history during which the arts as a group began to flourish. Most tantalizingly, the evidence around the birth of the arts in early human rituals also points to the intertwining of art, health, and healing: it would seem the birth of art was also the birth of arts in health.

Q For further information about early cave art, Gregory Curtis' *The Cave Painters* provides an accessible introduction.(13) For more on shamanism, *The Shamans of Prehistory* by Jean Clottes and David Lewis-Williams explores how trance and magic were interlinked with early art.(8)

Myths of the Ancient world

Naturally, a criticism that could be levelled against such theories is that some of the evidence is circumspect: shamanic healing rituals are widely discussed by archaeologists and historians and certainly seem to fit well with the evidence available, but we are limited by the lack of written records from the time so the reliance is on physical objects excavated from caves and anatomical understandings of early *homo sapiens*. However, if we move forwards in history, an interesting pattern is noted: the arts appear in the early written records of major medical tradition from across the Ancient world, many of them with practices that appear very similar to those hypothesized for the upper Palaeolithic *homo sapiens*.

Let us take an example from the Ancient Egyptians. The earliest written sources on Egyptian medicine come from papyrus manuscripts from around 2000 BC, which depict the role of Pharaohs in maintaining the health of their subjects and the role of priests in undertaking healing practices. These practices constituted a theatre of healing, with patients giving formal ceremonial announcements of their medical problems and priests responding. Sometimes these responses consisted of incantations, coaxing or threatening the malady to disappear. At other times, priests would put on disguises and appear to the patient as the god of the body part affected and use voice, gesture, and relics such as amulets (engraved gems, drawings, bone statues, or pendants) to chase away evil spirits.(14) The very spaces used for these healing rituals may also have been designed to enhance the effect of the arts. On the west bank of the Nile opposite the city of Luxor in Egypt there is a complex of mortuary temples including the healing chapel dedicated to the priest Amenhotep. As well as being a deified healing saint himself, Amenhotep was closely associated with Imhotep, who is widely considered the earliest physician in history, living around 2650-2600 BC. Amenhotep and Imhotep were often worshipped together in Egyptian healing temples. Recent acoustics research of the chapels and burial chambers has shown that the architectural design maximized reverberation.(15) This may have enhanced the immersive experience of healing ceremonies.

Egypt is just one example of where these theatrical healing practices occurred, but they can be traced across a wide geographical area. For example, the indigenous Indian medical system of Ayurveda placed therapeutic importance on magico-religious incantations: mantras. The *Atharvaveda*, a medical text from Northern India compiled around 1200-1000 BC, contains 6,000 mantras and 730 hymns, including magico-religious rites. The therapeutic value of the arts is also mentioned in one of the most renowned medical texts of Ayurveda, the *Sushruta Samhita*. For example, this text states that people should 'enjoy soft sounds, pleasant sights and tastes' after eating 'since such pleasurable sensations greatly help the process of digestion'.(16) Similarly, theatrical healing practices are found in ancient Greek medical traditions too. In Northern Greece, the cult of Dionysus arose around 1500-1100 BC, and by 600 BC was practised annually throughout Greece. Celebrating the god of fertility, theatre, and wine, it involved ecstatic and hysterical outpourings of emotions as part of group rituals such as the 'dithyramb', which was a choral ode to Dionysus supported by music, costume, and dancing.(17) As the dithyramb evolved, it began to take on a more theatrical style involving storytelling, eventually evolving into Greek theatre. Although the style of the celebrations evolved, the main purpose stayed the same: catharsis. Through witnessing the outpourings of emotions during the dithyramb and later theatre performances, audiences vicariously experienced a broad range of emotions, which was seen as a purging experience. Aristotle, in his work on dramatic theory *Poetics*, compared the effects of theatre on the mind to a cleanser on the body, describing the purpose of theatre as the 'purging of the spirit of morbid and base ideas or emotions by witnessing the playing out of such emotions or ideas on stage'.(18) Through this process, Aristotle believed that passions could be moderated and balance restored to the heart. Catharsis in theatre had direct parallels to contemporary Greek medicine, where Hippocrates had proposed that processes such as vomiting helped to purify the body. Furthermore, over 2,000 years later, Aristotle's ideas on catharsis influenced a number of psychotherapy models including Freudian psychoanalysis and Jacob L. Moreno's theories of psychodrama, which will be discussed more in Chapter 4.

Theatre was not the only way that the arts were used to support health. Indeed, individual art forms began to be examined on their own. This particularly began to be seen with poetry, dance, and music, which all became the object of a significant amount of theoretical debate. Continuing with the example of the Ancient Greeks, the mathematician and philosopher Pythagoras from the sixth century BC is credited with teaching about the benefits of music for health. Although none of Pythagoras' own writings survive, the philosopher Aristoxenus wrote that Pythagoreans (the school founded by Pythagoras) 'used medicine for purifying the body, music for purifying the soul'. This was also discussed in other cultures. For example, in the Roman philosopher Porphyry's *Life of Pythagoras*, he discusses 'rhythms, melodies and incantations' being used to charm away 'psychic and somatic afflictions…He had healing songs also for illnesses of the body which he would sing over the sick and cure them'.(19) The influence of these ideas is also shown in their reference in ancient Islamic texts. (20) However, it is difficult to know whether these accounts were accurate or not, given that many of them were written some time after Pythagoras.

Other writers afterwards continued to reference the healing effects of music and literature. For example, the medical writer Rufus of Ephesus (c. AD 100) recommended music and listening to poetry for the relief of lovesickness. Greek physician Galen of Pergamon noted in the second century AD that people's ethos, and consequently their health, could be corrupted by the words and music to which they listened. And the Alexandrian physician Herophilus found relationships between the pulse and different musical and poetic rhythms. But perhaps these theories were best brought together by the philosopher Boethius. In *De institutione musica*, written in the early sixth century AD, he combined anecdotes and theories from the Greeks and Romans. For example, he discussed neo-Platonic theories that harmonic vibrations were a microcosmic reflection of the vibrations of the universe; he drew on the ancient theory of humourism, developed by Hippocrates, which suggested that both mental and physical health are maintained through a balance between the fluids or 'humours', tracing the influence of music on this balance; he explored the ethos doctrine that suggested that the different modes in music had specific properties that could influence the mind; and he discussed whether music, through its influence on the mind, could lead to changes in health.(21)

A testament to the prominence of the arts in health and healing in the Ancient world, both in practice and theory, is the number of references to them in religion and popular culture. For example, in religion, a number of gods stood as symbols of both healing and the arts, such as the Gaelic goddess Brigit, goddess of poetry and healing; Mycenaean god Pajawo of 2000 BC who reportedly used holy song to cure disease; the Greek and Roman God Apollo (father of Asclepius, the god of medicine) who combined roles as healer, musician, and poet; and the Etruscan goddess Menrva of art and health. Even among mere mortals, references in literature to the healing capacity of the arts abound. For example, *The Odyssey* from the eighth century BC, describes the bleeding of Odysseus's wounds from a wild boar only being stopped with an incantation.(22) The tragic poet Pratinas in the sixth century BC recorded a plague in Sparta that was quelled by the paean composer Thaletas through music.(23) And in the bible, in Samuel 16:23 it says that 'when the evil spirit from God was upon Saul...David took an harp, and played with his hand: so Saul was refreshed, and was well'.(24)

However, despite these many references to the use of arts in health and theoretical discussions of their value across the Ancient world, it is important to note that most of these writings and ideas came from philosophers. Although physicians did engage with the arts and they are found in medical texts, in general across the Ancient world, the arts in health were sustained primarily through philosophy and artistic practice. However, moving into the Middle Ages, this began to change.

Q For more on ancient theatre and its influence on modern medicine, Thomas Scheff explores the concept of catharsis in *Catharsis in Healing, Ritual and Drama*.(25) For richer histories of music in the Ancient world, Martin West's chapter in *Music as Medicine: The History of Music Therapy Since Antiquity* is recommended.(26)

Theories of the Middle Ages

The Middle Ages in Europe began with the fall of the Roman Empire in the fifth century and spanned the next 1,000 years, until the start of the Renaissance period of cultural 'rebirth'. As the Romans withdrew, medical practice in Europe fell into decline. Many of the old Greek and Roman writings were lost to Europe. However, medicine was supported by the growth of monasteries and monastic communities. As a result of their remote and self-sufficient design, monks had to have among themselves the skills necessary to treat one another. Much care provided was palliative rather than curative, drawing on folk remedies and local healing practices that had survived through oral history, but as the cultivated expertise of monks blossomed, they became centres for supporting healing in pilgrims and the surrounding communities.(27) This led to a more disciplined study of medicine between monasteries and monastic orders, the sharing of ideas from further afield such as the Far East through travel and trade, and, importantly, the chronicling of monastic medical theories and advances. Far from remaining an insular practice, the work of the monks and nuns began to influence medicine outside of Europe.

A defining feature of monastic medicine was the dual emphasis on healing people physically and spiritually. One of the most famous leaders of monastic medicine was the German Benedictine abbess Hildegard of Bingen (1098-1179), who embodied the holistic attitude towards health that was common to the period. During her lifetime, she wrote two medical major works (*Physica*, a nine-volume description of the scientific and medicinal properties of animals, plants, and stones; and *Causae et Curae*, a catalogue of medical practices and remedies), wrote three volumes of visionary theology, and composed over 70 pieces of music including one of the first known forms of opera. Hildegard described her compositions as 'celestial harmony' and believed that 'every creature had a tone' within it, locating the arts (in this case, music) within medicine by embedding it directly within an individual's spiritual health.(28) This view of the essential value of music to health and healing became interwoven with beliefs about the purpose of music within religion, with miraculous legends spreading across European churches. For example, in one legend from southern France, a cripple was restored with the ability to walk while listening to the antiphon 'Homo iste fecit mirabilia in vita sua' (translated as 'This man performed wonders in his life') for the Feast of St Vivian.(28)

Music was not the only art form to be interwoven with health. Monasteries themselves came to function as patrons of the arts, encouraging (and undertaking themselves) reading, needlework, sculpture, and painting. Art existed comfortably alongside health, such as in beautifully illustrated medical texts and carved monumental tombs to honour the dead.(29) And partly in attempts to harness the perceived power of the arts, a number of hospitals were founded between AD 1000 and 1300 with richly decorated chapels attached, many of which remain as music venues, such as Spitalfields (from the word 'hospital') in London. Some hospitals even had explicit statutes dictating the amount of music provision required, such as the Hotel-Dieu in Pontoise whose members were required to sing at all the canonical hours.

However, this close proximity among arts, health, and religion did not last. As just one example, Medieval church councils were held within the Diocese of Clermont-Ferrand in the modern-day Auvergne in France. At the Council of Clermont in 1130 there were concerns that monks should be dedicating themselves to sacred rather than secular study, such as spirituality and church doctrine, and the first steps were taken to reduce the involvement of church with subjects such as medicine and law.(27). Further religious developments widened the gap between religion and medicine yet more, and in England with the dissolution of the monasteries in the 16th century by King Henry VIII, the church ceased to support hospitals. Instead, hospitals such as St Bartholomew's and Bethlehem hospitals in London were transferred to the City of London, new hospitals were established by City officials, and medicine began to receive more direct secular support. However, the separation of medicine from the monasteries did not mark the breaking of the bridge between medicine and religion altogether. Chapels remained an integral part of hospital design and many hospitals continued to be named after saints. Furthermore, new hospitals continued to be beautifully decorated. Consequently, the arts lived on among the changing landscape of medicine.

Given the centrality of the arts, especially paintings and music, to monastic and more general religious life, it could of course be argued that the arts were only included within healing because they were simply 'there'; as a part of daily monastic practice they could easily be drawn into healing practices, whether or not they actually had any perceived benefit. However, during the Middle Ages it was not just in European religious practices that the arts were being drawn into medicine. Physicians further afield were also advocating the health benefits they could offer. During the Middle Ages, a number of key writings from ancient Indian, Greek, Roman, and Byzantine medical practices, such as 129 of the works of Galen, were translated into Arabic by scientists such as ninth-century physician Hunayn Ibn Ishaq and the learning from these spread rapidly across the Arab world and became a template for important medical advances. What is intriguing is that the arts retained their place within medicine even as these advances took place. One of the most famous books to come out of this period was *The Canon of Medicine*, a five-volume encyclopaedia of medicine that drew together developments from the previous 500 years, compiled by Persian philosopher Avicenna (Ibn Sina) around 1025. The book covers basic medical and physiological principles, medical substances, essays on the diagnosis and treatment of illnesses and diseases, and a formulary of compound remedies. So influential was this book that it remained a standard medical textbook until the eighteenth century and is still used in branches of Perso-Arabic traditional medicine. What is rarely discussed is that this book actually contains over 150 mentions of the arts, specifically 74 references to dance, 56 references to music, 10 to poetry, five to painting, three to arts and crafts, two to sculpture, and one each to dramatic art and literary art.(30) Another eleventh-century Arabic example was the *Taqwīm as-siḥḥah* ('Maintenance of Health'). Written by the physician Ibn Butlan of Baghdad, the book was originally written as a lay guide to health, probably for upper aristocracy. However, in the thirteenth century it was translated into Latin, *Tacuinum sanitatis*, enabling its influence to be extended into Europe. It contains over 200 miniatures, each focusing on the role of a different food, drink, season, sensation, or activity for both physical and mental health. Several of these pertain to the arts. For example, one miniature focuses on the health benefits of storytellers and is accompanied by text discussing their role as 'one of the causes of sleep' as well as in improving 'digestion, senses and spirit'. These examples of arts practice are a further demonstration of how well embedded the arts were within health and medicine. In fact, the popularity and influence of this book in Western Europe is evinced through the fact that the word 'taccuino' (from its name *Tacuinum sanitatis*) developed to mean any kind of pocket handbook or guide.(31)

The examples in this section have shown how, during the Middle Ages, the arts found a place in two very different approaches to medicine: European folk and monastic traditions of care, and Islamic physician-led developments charted in treatises. However, by the later part of the Middle Ages, further developments in the history of medicine were under way that would eventually reconcile these different traditions. With the twelfth century renaissance and a period of economic and population growth in Europe, new translations of books from Muslim and Jewish sources in Spain began to circulate; universities began to be established in a number of major European cities such as Paris (1150), Bologna (1158), Oxford (1167), and Padua (1222); and in the fifteenth century, following the fall of Constantinople, a new wave of learning was brought into the West. These developments not only furthered the development of medicine but also led to a cultural enrichment and increase in both theory and practice relating to the arts.

Consequently, the Middle Ages not only saw enormous cross-fertilization of ideas from across different Empires, but it also saw a shift in the balance between medicine as a spiritual versus a secular practice, and a readjustment of the way people thought about the natural and the supernatural; the body and the spirit in healing practices. This shift would become a defining feature of the next era.

Q For more information on the rise of art in hospitals, Richard Cork's *The Healing Presence of Art* provides a beautifully illustrated history.(32) For more about the rise of medicine in non-Western cultures, Helaine Selin's edited book *Medicine Across Cultures* provides a rich overview.(33)

Enlightenment rationalization

Between the end of the Middle Ages and the start of the Enlightenment period, advances in thinking and practice of arts in health predominantly followed on from previous thought, with Platonic and Arabic texts continuing to hold sway. As many of the key theoretical writings to be preserved pertained to music, this became one of the art forms that drew the most attention. For example, humoural medicine (blood, phlegm, choler, and melancholy) remained popular, based on the principles of Hippocratic and Galenic medicine. The Italian music theorist and composer Gioseffo Zarlino theorized in his *Istitutioni harmoniche* of 1558 that the four musical modes corresponded to the four humours of the body and the four elements of the Earth. In addition, the Florentine philosopher Marsilio Ficino's *De vita* (1480-1489) explored the associations between music and melancholy, suggesting that music was linked to the *spiritus mundi*; a channel of influence between the heavenly bodies and the sublunar world.(34) This theory was widely disseminated in popular literature and also taken up in some seventeenth-century texts, including Robert Burton's *Anatomy of Melancholy* (1620) and Athanasius Kircher's *Musurgia universalis* (1650). But many of the prevailing beliefs about the healing value of the arts were still steeped in mysticism and magic from the Middle Ages and Ancient world.

However, with the beginning of the Enlightenment period in the late seventeenth century, physicians and philosophers began to break away from previous ways of conceptualizing the arts in health. This did not, at first, lead to a decrease in the number of sources citing the arts. Indeed, the sheer quantity of medical treatise that included references to the arts increased in the late seventeenth and eighteenth centuries. However, it did affect the tone of writing and the way that past theories were cited. One of the most influential examples of this new tone is Richard Brocklesby's *Reflections on the power of musick* from 1749. Brocklesby was a physician and Surgeon General of the British Army. Brocklesby was enthusiastic about music's therapeutic potential for illnesses that 'have hitherto too frequently eluded the ordinary powers of medicine' and was keen to show its widespread practice in America, Africa, Asia, and Europe. But Brocklesby was also wary of previous theories. Indeed, he warned against 'superstitious and fabulous accounts' of music's effects, explaining that the tales passed down from ancient times 'partly consist in an elegant exaggeration of physical truths'. He also took a critical view of society for being so gullible, labelling it a 'surprising readiness … to deceive [itself], and be imposed on, with the grossest improbabilities, and silliest delusions that folly could entertain or craft could devise'.(35) Brocklesby wanted arts in health not just to be debated theoretically but researched scientifically.

It was not only physicians who wanted to break from the previous mythical tales of music and the other arts. Artists, musicians, and historians too were keen to separate fact from fiction. Historian Charles Burney's *A General History of Music* (1776) discussed with excitement the possible applications of music within medicine, but complained about how 'men delight in the marvellous, and many bigoted admirers of antiquity … have given way to credulity to so far as to believe, or pretend to believe, these fabulous accounts'. This is not to say that physicians stopped believing in the use of the arts within health; indeed, the more scientific and rational approach to the arts (in particular music) and health encouraged more physicians to engage in what began to be taken seriously as a means of treatment.(36)

However, at the same time that scientific appreciation of the arts was growing, there were two developments that presented challenges. First, the efforts of people such as Brockelsby and Burney were insufficient to turn the tide of superstition and mysticism surrounding arts in health entirely. For example, in the 1750s, a centuries-old theory that the sound from rubbing glasses filled with liquids could produce healing effects on the listener was given a new lease of life, when scientist and founding father of the United States, Benjamin Franklin, invented his own version of the glass armonica. Franklin himself is purported to have cured listeners by playing the armonica, including Princess Izabella Czartoryska of Poland, who heard it on her deathbed in 1772 and then went on to live another 60 years. And the German physician Franz Mesmer, caused a scandal by playing the armonica at his séances to heal patients, leading to claims that the armonica's music could wake the dead. Over 300 bespoke compositions were written for the instrument, including by Wolfgang Amadeus Mozart.(37)

The second development was the parallel advancement in modern medicine. Since the sixteenth century, there had begun to be countermovements to the Ancient theories. For example, physicians Andreas Vesalius and William Harvey produced detailed anatomical depictions and descriptions of the circulation of the blood that ran counter to prevailing Ancient thought.(38) Initially, these countermovements were simply seen as corrections on Ancient thought. However, as discovery into the anatomical make-up of the body, its 'biology' (coined around 1800), its chemistry (including discovering carbon dioxide and its role in respiration), and later the pathological factors of disease developed, it became clear that medicine was entering a new chapter, less concerned with a holistic understanding of disease and more focused on an anatomical one. The development of laboratory medicine, microscopy, and experimental medicine furthered this thinking. To begin with, these early developments in modern medicine were of help to the field of arts in health, providing fresh ideas to apply to how the arts could be supporting health. But as the modern medicine movement gathered momentum, the core biomedical pursuit began to outpace other aspects of care.

This is not to say that the arts ceased to be practised. Indeed, the nineteenth century saw the development of some exciting new movements within arts in health. As just one example, the Guild of St. Cecilia was formed 'for the purpose of supplying trained musicians who may promptly obey the summons of physicians desiring to use their services'.(39) The group built up a reputation in medical circles, appearing several times in the *Lancet* and *British Medical Journal* where they set forth ideas about how to provide calming music to patients through music boxes so it could be on demand, reported case studies of impact, were credited with helping patients during a scarlet fever epidemic in 1892, and proposed research ideas around topics such as music and pain.(40) The Guild is just one example; other individuals and organizations continued to have sustained success in delivering arts interventions within hospitals and for health. However, within mainstream medical documents, the growing scientific understanding and increasing number of options for treating patients essentially served as competition for the use of the arts in health.

Nevertheless, the nineteenth century also afforded new opportunities for the use of the arts in health, in particular in what was to become the field of psychiatry. In medieval and pre-modern times, people regarded as 'mad' were labelled as 'lunatics' or 'spiritually afflicted' and looked after (or locked up) at home or in monasteries.(41) However, in the eighteenth and nineteenth centuries throughout Europe and the Eastern side of North America, 'madhouses' or 'lunatic asylums', as they were labelled, began to open. Treatments initially involved attempting to control people through drugs or restraints, often with barbaric techniques. However, 'madness' gradually came to be seen not just as a physical disease but as a product of bad habits and personal afflictions. As the nineteenth century moved on, madness became more prominent as suggestions were made that cases were developing in response to modern living with the new industrial pace of life leading to mental strain; an idea that became a precursor to the work of Sigmund Freud in the early twentieth century. Instead of asylums being seen as places to lock people up, their segregated environments came to be seen as an advantage as they offered the opportunity to reshape the mind and behaviour of people affected. Although some, such as Foucault, have questioned whether this new approach was in fact more humane than the previous, or whether it merely replaced one form of control with another (one that isolated patients and focused on their 'correction'), this new approach did provide an opportunity for the arts.(42)

In Germany, one of the leading asylums was the Cure and Nursing Home Illenau. Notably, Illenau was renowned for promoting sensory stimulation over pharmaceutics or restraints, not only employing the arts, but positively depending on them. It maintained a house choir, marching band, chamber orchestra, concert series featuring 140 performances a year, and a full-time music instructor who worked closely with the physicians. The team at Illenau believed that only certain music was appropriate for its patients, so each piece to be performed had to receive medical approval, and any that were deemed too aesthetically demanding were rewritten. In fact, the asylum published the *Illenauer Liederbuch*, which featured specially composed hymns that became standard in asylums throughout Germany. Illenau also had its own gymnastics hall and gymnastics instructor, and classes were accompanied by guitar. Within these classes, choreographed dance sequences were developed to aid patients in synchronizing with others around them.(43) In addition, in England, Ticehurst Private Asylum had a list of permitted recreational activities which included writing, drawing, spinning, sewing, and playing the violin or harpsichord. Worcester City and County Lunatic Asylum employed English composer Edward Elgar as bandmaster to compose dance sets for patients. While in France, the psychiatrist Wilhelm Horn reported that the bath house of an asylum which contained eight stone baths had also been fitted with a loud organ, drum, and cymbals in an unusual form of shock therapy. In other asylums and hospitals, the visual and fine arts were actively encouraged. For example, at Crichton Royal Hospital in Scotland, doctor William Browne appointed artists to work with patients in 1847. He found that patients who engaged in drawing experienced improvements in their condition. Similarly, in 1901 Royal Montrose Mental Hospital in Scotland gave an art studio to one of its patients, Adam Christie, where he worked making over 200 pieces of sculpture using broken bottles rather than conventional tools and carving wood with a nail.(44)

However, the arts were not always seen as positive for health. Madness was considered in some quarters to be the result of an overindulgence of the imagination exacerbated by the arts. For example, the Romantic author Alexander Sternberg reported that when the pianist Franz Liszt performed in public, women were overtaken by an 'insane stupor', referring to them as 'die Electrisierten' (the mesmerized ones).(34) And women themselves were portrayed as victims of madness in nineteenth-century opera, with their madness attributed to a weakness of their gender and their inability to process dramatic emotional events; Donizetti's *Lucia di Lammermoor* of 1835 is one example, in which a mad turn from the protagonist Lucia leads her to kill her own bridegroom. But men were not exempt. The poetry of British poet Alfred, Lord Tennyson, epitomizes the obsessive intrigue with madness yet fear of its encroachment on society. And the Romantic British poet John Clare became famous for suffering delusions which eventually led to him being committed to an asylum, which only furthered concerns around excessive engagement with the arts.(45)

Nevertheless, the eighteenth and nineteenth centuries marked turning points in the history of the arts in health. Not only did these two centuries see the rise of a more scientific and rational approach to the field, but they also saw the arts become a core part of the new field of psychiatry, paving the way for the emergence of new areas of arts in health practice in the following century.

Q Mary De Young's *Encyclopedia of Asylum Therapeutics*, 1750-1950s explores a wide range of expressive therapies that were used to treat people with mental health conditions including photography therapy.(43) Penelope Gouk's *Musical Healing in Cultural Contexts* provides more on the theoretical attitudes to the arts and science during the Enlightenment.(46)

Twentieth century exploration

The start of the twentieth century saw divided opinion on arts in health. The horrors of World War I led to two schools of thought. One of these saw even the most reverential artworks in hospitals as a waste of public money. Instead, simpler and cleaner designs were adopted in some hospitals and the 'clinical' emphasized. This move was reinforced by a number of factors. A growing awareness of infection and the focus on cleanliness and hygiene encouraged white hospitals so that dirt could be spotted more easily. Second, there were moves in architecture towards functionalism and rationalism at the start of the twentieth century that foregrounded the purpose of a building and saw decoration as unnecessary.(47) This had a profound impact on the design of some hospitals, with a prime example being the starkly functional Baťa's Hospital in the town of Zlin in what was Czechoslovakia in 1927.(48) Third, in the 1920s there arose a professional opinion that Greek temples and Romanesque and Gothic cathedrals had been all white; a belief that persisted until the 1960s when further evidence came out showing their rich colourful decorations. It has been hypothesized that these architectural moves were instrumental in the shift away from artistic hospitals to more clinical designs.

However, the war also provided an outpouring of art.(49) Some artworks arose directly in response to the war as people struggled to represent the unprecedented and epoch-defining events. Artists such as Gilbert Rogers graphically depicted the scenes they had witnessed. Others shrank from the energy and violence towards a more abstract and less raw depiction, such as English painter Percy Wyndham Lewis. For others still, art was used for escapism, with nostalgic impressions of landscapes, such as in the work of British painter Gilbert Spencer. Not just visual art, but also performing arts became a mode of escapism, with plays, books, poetry, and music flourishing both during and after the war. This attitude seeped into hospitals and healthcare too. In contrast to the simpler, functional hospitals preferred by some, others looked for beauty. So alongside clinical designs, increasingly elaborate hospitals were also built, and a range of countries, including Norway, the Netherlands, the USA, Canada, France, and Italy also introduced 'percentage laws', by which the expenditure of a certain percentage of the building cost for major new public buildings (including hospitals) had to be spent on art. One of the beautiful hospitals to emerge from this scheme is the Academisch Ziekenhuis at the University of Amsterdam built in 1974, which has a separate unit for each of the post-war movements in the arts in the Netherlands, from Zero to Neo-Expressionism, totalling 5,000 pictures. Alongside visual arts, performing arts were reinvigorated within healthcare, with entertainments services that had provided support for people during the war, such as the Entertainments National Services Association (ENSA), which had brought live music to wounded servicemen in military hospitals, transitioning their efforts into healthcare and leading new movements to provide holistic support to patients (see Chapter 4).

However, what this divided approach highlighted was that the relative significance and prominence of arts in health was very much dependent on factors such as individual opinion and societal fashions. Arts in health had relatively little autonomy or authority in its own right. But by the mid-twentieth century, this was all changing. Inspired by specific medical traditions or theories, off-shoots of arts in health activity began to emerge, taking root in different countries and developing into the leading fields of activity within arts in health that are active today, including arts therapies, arts-based learning, and targeted patient programmes. In Chapter 4, we will explore how this development occurred and how the first national and international organizations formed. However, underpinning these practical developments was a broader shift in mind-set regarding how medicine was viewed, which has provided further opportunities for the arts.

Discussions about the 'art' of medicine are traced throughout history. But the prominence of these discussions has varied, with core advances in science often temporarily casting aside discussions about the 'art'. However, in the twentieth century, the 'art' of medicine has been brought back into the mainstream as a concept. Sir William Osler, a Canadian physician widely considered to be the Father Modern Medicine, wrote in an essay entitled *Aequanimitas*, 'The practice of medicine is an art, based on science',(50) highlighting distinctions between the 'science' of knowing medical facts and the 'art' of drawing on individual observations, experience, and personal judgement in putting this knowledge into practice. The 'art' of medicine is also used to describe other aspects of patient care, such as treating people with respect, compassion, empathy, and humanity as well as trying to optimize patient experience, which is now seen as a priority within many healthcare systems.(51) Although this might seem peripheral to the more important prescription of medications or undertaking of procedures, research suggests that patients who feel personally involved in their own care are more likely to following treatment guidelines and lead the lifestyles needed to ensure their own health. This will be discussed more in Chapter 2. There are also specific areas of medicine in which aesthetics are recognized as integral to the medicine itself, broadening further discussions around the 'art' of medicine. For example, cosmetic surgery and some branches of plastic surgery centre around artistic principles of beauty.

Of course, 'art' in relation to the 'art of medicine' is very different to the application of the arts in health. But what the rising prominence of the 'art' of medicine is doing is normalizing discussions around creativity alongside discussions of medicine, bringing theoretical considerations of the worlds of 'art' and 'science' closer together and emphasizing the importance of a holistic approach to health. This all helps to foster a more receptive mind-set among healthcare professionals, funders, and policy-makers for proposals of arts in health interventions. Indeed, it is probably no coincidence that the greatest flourishing of arts in health over the last 100 years has occurred alongside the rise again of the acceptance that medicine is both an art and a science.

Q For a further discussion and history covering 2,000 years on the topic of the art of medicine, the illustrated book by Julie Anderson, Emma Shackleton, and Emm Barnes is a wonderful resource.(52)

Summary

In this chapter, we have explored the use of the arts in health across the past 40,000 years. The understanding and scientific accuracy of accounts of the health benefits of the arts has evolved dramatically in this time, but so too has the understanding and scientific accuracy of theories of medicine. We have seen how the relationship between arts and health has shifted over the centuries, brought closer or pushed further away by developments in theories around health and medicine. In the next chapter we will focus specifically on some of the most influential models of health of the last 200 years and consider how current thinking is providing opportunities for the arts in health and paving the way for the expansion of the field.

References

1. **Lubbock J.** Prehistoric times, as illustrated by ancient remains, and the manners and customs of modern savages [Internet]. London: Williams and Norgate; 1872 [cited 2016 Nov 16]. 660 pp. Available from: http://archive.org/details/7edprehistorictimelubbuoft.

2. **Hardt T.** Handbook of Paleoanthropology: Principles, Methods and Approaches v. 1-3. 2007 edition. Henke W, Tattersall I, editors. New York: Springer; 2007. 2069 pp.

3. **Bednarik R.** A Figurine from the African Acheulian. Curr Anthropol. 2003;44(3):405–13.

4. **Mithen PS.** The Prehistory Of The Mind: A Search for the Origins of Art, Religion and Science. New Ed edition. London: W&N; 1998. 480 pp.

5. **Lewis-Williams D.** The Mind in the Cave: Consciousness and the Origins of Art. Reprint edition. London: Thames & Hudson; 2004. 320 pp.

6. **Cunningham LS, Reich JJ, Fichner-Rathus L.** Culture and Values: A Survey of the Humanities. 8 edition. Boston, MA: Cengage Learning; 2013. 976 pp.

7. **Mellars P.** Archaeology: Origins of the female image. Nature. 2009 May 14;459(7244):176–7.

8. **Clottes J, Lewis-Williams D.** The Shamans of Prehistory: Trance and Magic in the Painted Caves. New York: Harry N. Abrams; 1998. 120 pp.

9. **Conard NJ, Malina M, Münzel SC.** New flutes document the earliest musical tradition in southwestern Germany. Nature. 2009 Aug 6;460(7256):737–40.

10. **Dissanayake E.** Homo Aestheticus: Where Art Comes from and Why. Reprint. Seattle: University of Washington Press; 1992. 320 pp.

11. **Mithen PS.** The Singing Neanderthals: The Origins of Music, Language, Mind and Body. New Ed edition. London: W&N; 2006. 384 pp.

12. **Pearce E, Launay J, Dunbar RIM.** The ice-breaker effect: singing mediates fast social bonding. R Soc Open Sci. 2015 Oct 1;2(10):150221.

13. **Curtis G.** The Cave Painters: Probing the Mysteries of the World's First Artists. Reprint. New York: Anchor; 2007. 288 pp.

14. **Jayne WA.** The Healing Gods of Ancient Civilizations. Kessinger Publishing, LLC; 2010. 586 pp.

15. **Alford AF.** Pyramid of Secrets: The Architecture of the Great Pyramid Reconsidered in the Light of Creational Mythology. Walsall, England: Eridu Books; 2003. 446 pp.

16. **Bhishagratna KK.** The Sushruta Samhita: An English Translation Based on Original Texts. New Delhi: Cosmo Publications; 2006. 2000 pp.

17. **Hamilton E.** The Greek Way. Revised ed. edition. New York: W. W. Norton & Company; 1993. 272 pp.

18. **Aristotle.** The Basic Works of Aristotle. Reprint edition. McKeon R, editor. New York: Modern Library; 2001. 1520 pp.

19. Horden P, editor. Music As Medicine: The History of Music Therapy Since Antiquity. 1 edition. Aldershot ; Brookfield, USA: Routledge; 2000. 416 pp.

20. **Burgel JC.** The Feather of Simurgh: The 'Licit' Magic of the Arts in Medieval Islam. Illustrated edition. New York: New York University Press; 1988. 200 pp.

21. **Kleisiaris CF, Sfakianakis C, Papathanasiou IV.** Health care practices in ancient Greece: The Hippocratic ideal. J Med Ethics Hist Med [Internet]. 2014 Mar 15 [cited 2016 Nov 5];7. Available from: http://www.ncbi.nlm.nih.gov/pmc/articles/PMC4263393/.

22. **Homer, Rouse WHD.** The Odyssey: The Story of Odysseus. New York: New American Library; 1999. 308 pp.

23. **West ML.** Ancient Greek Music. New York: Clarendon Press; 1992. 452 pp.

24. The Old Testament: The Authorized Or King James Version of 1611. Everyman Publisher; 1996. 1382 pp.

25. **Scheff T.** Catharsis in Healing, Ritual, and Drama. Lincoln, NE: iUniverse; 2001. 252 pp.

26. **West M.** Music Therapy in Antiquity. In: Horden P, editor. Music as Medicine: The History of Music Therapy Since Antiquity. Aldershot, Hants: Ashgate; 2000. pp. 51–68.

27. **Prioreschi P.** Medieval Medicine. Omaha: Horatius Press; 2003. 795 pp.

28. Medieval Music: Chant as Cure and Miracle [Internet]. Gresham College; 2015 [cited 2016 Nov 5]. Available from: http://www.gresham.ac.uk/lectures-and-events/medieval-music-chant-as-cure-and-miracle.

29. **Nees L.** Early Medieval Art. Oxford University Press; 2002. 276 pp.

30. **Abu-Asab M, Amri H, Micozzi MS.** Avicenna's Medicine: A New Translation of the 11th-Century Canon with Practical Applications for Integrative Health Care. Rochester Vermont, Toronto, Canada: Inner Traditions/Bear & Co; 2013. 426 pp.

31. **Bovey A.** Tacuinum sanitatis: an early renaissance guide to health. Sam Fogg; 2005. 92 pp.

32. **Cork R.** The Healing Presence of Art: A History of Western Art in Hospitals. 1 edition. New Haven Conn.; London: Yale University Press; 2012. 496 pp.

33. **Selin H.** Medicine Across Cultures: History and Practice of Medicine in Non-Western Cultures. Springer Science & Business Media; 2006. 428 pp.

34. **Horden P.** Music as medicine: the history of music therapy since antiquity. Aldershot, Hants: Ashgate; 2000. 424 pp.

35. **Brocklesby R.** Reflections on the power of musick. London: M Cooper; 1749.

36. **Burney C.** A General History of Music, from the Earliest Ages to the Present Period: Volume the First. Author; 1789. 716 pp.

37. **Gallo DA, Finger S.** The power of a musical instrument: Franklin, the Mozarts, Mesmer, and the glass armonica. Hist Psychol. 2000 Nov;3(4):326–43.

38. **Barber N.** Renaissance Medicine. Raintree; 2013. 50 pp.

39. **Harford FK.** The Guild of St. Cecilia. Br Med J. 1891 Sep 5;2(1601):574.

40. **Harford FK.** The St. Cecilia Guild. Br Med J. 1892 Jun 4;1(1640):1228.

41. **Porter R.** The Cambridge Illustrated History of Medicine. Cambridge University Press; 2001. 404 pp.

42. **Foucault M.** Madness and Civilization 1st (first) edition Text Only. Vintage; 1988.

43. **Young MD.** Encyclopedia of Asylum Therapeutics, 1750-1950s. Jefferson, North Carolina: McFarland; 2015. 377 pp.

44. **Hogan S.** Healing Arts: The History of Art Therapy. London and Philadelphia: Jessica Kingsley Publishers; 2001. 338 pp.

45. **Burwick F.** Poetic Madness and the Romantic Imagination. Pennsylvania: Penn State Press; 2010. 317 pp.

46. Gouk P, editor. Musical Healing in Cultural Contexts. 1 edition. Aldershot ; Brookfield, USA: Routledge; 2000. 240 pp.

47. **Collins P.** Changing Ideals in Modern Architecture, 1750-1950. McGill-Queen's Press—MQUP; 1998. 370 pp.

48. Haldane D, Loppert S, editors. The Arts in Health Care: Learning from Experience. London: King's Fund; 1999.

49. **Brandon L.** Art and War. London and New York: I.B.Tauris; 2012. 193 pp.

50. **Osler SW.** Aequanimitas. Philadelphia, Pennsylvania: P. Blakiston's Sons & Company; 1904. 406 pp.

51. **Goldman L, Schafer AI.** Goldman-Cecil Medicine, 2-Volume Set, 25e. 25 edition. Philadelphia, PA: Elsevier; 2015. 3024 pp.

52. **Anderson J, Shackleton E, Barnes E.** The Art of Medicine: Over 2,000 Years of Images and Imagination. University of Chicago Press; 2011. 255 pp.

Chapter 2

The theoretical background to arts in health

Theoretical developments in health

What is health?

Arguably the most famous definition of health was published in a preamble to the Constitution of the World Health Organization (WHO) at the International Health Conference in New York in 1946, entering into force on 7 April 1948. Signed by representatives of 61 states, showing the largest-scale agreement on a definition seen to date, health was described as 'a state of complete physical, mental and social wellbeing and not merely the absence of disease or infirmity'.(1) This definition has now been in use for nearly 70 years, which could on the surface suggest that our understanding and conceptualization of health has enjoyed a period of relative stability. However, not only was the WHO definition a contrast to the views of just a few decades earlier, but 'health' has since become one of the most debated concepts within science.

A biomedical model of health

As discussed in Chapter 1, the eighteenth and nineteenth centuries saw huge advances in the theory and practice of medicine across Europe. As just one example, in the early nineteenth century, Italian scientist Agostino Bassi showed for the first time that disease could be caused by microorganisms.(2) This came to be known as 'germ theory' and was famously further advanced by chemist and microbiologist Louis Pasteur.(3) Germ theory was revolutionary for laboratory science, hospital medicine, and surgery, leading to more accurate diagnoses and safer surgical conditions. Germ theory also focused people's attention onto individuals and specifically onto the aetiology of disease and its immediate cause. Microorganisms, germ theory, and the seemingly unending capabilities of other new medical techniques led to a shift in attitude towards illness and disease that came to be known as the biomedical model.(4)

According to the biomedical model, disease was seen as an externality, either as an invader of the body or the result of involuntary internal physical changes.

Treatment for these conditions resided with medical professionals, with patients seen as victims; out of control of what was happening inside them. Health was, as a consequence, seen as the absence of disease, and was often categorized as a binary: well or ill. The role of the mind was little considered within this model of health. So although illness was seen as capable of having psychological consequences, it was not seen as having psychological causes.(5)

There were many positives to the rise of this model of health in terms of the development of medicine. First, by placing responsibility on the physician to cure illness, it encouraged yet more research, leading to a wave of scientific advances. Alongside this, more regulations came into force, the discipline of medicine was further professionalized and there was a rise of professional bodies.(6) For example, in the UK, the Provincial Medical and Surgical Association (later renamed the British Medical Association) was founded in 1832 and the General Medical Council established in 1858. It also led to more support for people with health conditions, especially certain health conditions that had previously been dismissed as moral weakness or sin, such as alcoholism, but were now taken more seriously and considered as something that could be treated.(7)

However, there were also many issues that arose under the biomedical model that were not fully addressed. For example, by placing responsibility for health and illness in the hands of professionals, it diminished some of the responsibility among individuals. The development of a larger scientific vocabulary also increased the mystification around medicine and decreased public accessibility, further distancing people from their own health. Furthermore, while scientific advances under the biomedical model did reduce mortality associated with surgery, there was limited immediate impact on reducing mortality from disease and many conditions remained chronic or incurable.(8) As a result, alternative therapies continued to hold thrall, and, unsurprisingly, other areas of medicine also grew in prominence.

 For more information about the biomedical model the *Encyclopedia of Health Psychology* contains an entry that can be read alongside other models of health.(9)

Public health

One of the fields of research and practice in health that developed alongside the biomedical model was public health. We have evidence that public health was considered thousands of years ago. For example, the Babylonians in Mesopotamia embraced regulatory hygiene customs. Although primarily to encourage spirituality, these customs simultaneously reduced the occurrence and spread of disease.(10) The Romans built elaborate sewage systems, baths, and fresh water aqueducts in their cities across their empire. However, in the Middle Ages, there was a spate of diseases including leprosy, smallpox, measles, tuberculosis, and the bubonic plague in towns and cities. With growing urbanization and industrialization in the 1800s, overcrowding became a major issue in cities in Europe, with London and New York providing potent case studies. Denser living arrangements provided greater opportunity for pestilence, epidemics, and disease, which in turn provided the catalyst for the introduction of formal public health measures. In 1842, Edwin Chadwick published a report entitled *The Sanitary Conditions of the Labouring Population*. This highlighted the discrepancy in disease between the working class and the upper class, concluding that unsanitary environments were responsible for poor health.(11) Chadwick championed sanitary reform, which became the basis for public health activities in Great Britain and the United States. In 1848 the first Public Health Act was passed in England which created a general board of health. However, just 5 years later in 1854, parliament refused to renew it because of the perceived imposition and economic cost of improving drainage and water systems.

In the same year there was a major cholera outbreak in London. The cause of this outbreak initially mystified doctors, until doctor John Snow mapped the geographical location of the outbreak and traced its origins back to a water pump in Soho, which he suggested was contaminated. Despite initial opposition, the removal of the water pump led the outbreak to subside, with the recognition that it was a combination of social and biomedical factors that were influencing people's health. This helped pave the way for new infrastructure projects providing clean water, rubbish removal, and improved sewerage systems in urban areas, as well as new legislation on standards of housing and overcrowding and a second compulsory Public Health Act in 1875.(12)

Consequently, public health, like the biomedical model, also focused on disease and was strengthened by similar developments such as germ theory. However, public health looked beyond the individual at the wider social environment that could be causing its development and spread, highlighting the importance of sanitation and other social and living conditions in the control of communicable diseases. Public health programmes today also focus on the prevention of non-communicable disease and health promotion. They set standards of health within societies and monitor their implementation; assess health hazards and plan for potential problems and emergencies; monitor health trends to shape research agendas; clarify the causes of health problems and inform health policy and strategies; and identify and implement the most appropriate interventions.

Q The History of Public Health and the Modern State explores in more detail how public health developed in countries around the world.(13)

Psychosomatic medicine

Another particularly influential field that arose alongside the biomedical model was psychosomatic medicine. This came to prominence in the early twentieth century in response to psychoanalytic theories such as those of Sigmund Freud on the relationship between mind and physical illness. Freud examined patients coming to him experiencing loss of mobility in their limbs but was unable to identify any anatomical reason for this paralysis. Instead, he hypothesized that such paralysis was caused by hysteria set in motion by repressed experiences and feelings.(14) This not only suggested that the mind and body interacted, but that the mind could actually cause illness.

Interestingly, this idea was not new. Indeed, the genesis of theories on this combined mind-body approach to medicine can be traced through every major ancient tradition of medicine. One example lies in the Islamic tradition, made famous by the Persian physician Abu Sayd Ahmed ibn Sahl Balkhi (Al-Balkhi). Born in Khorasan (modern-day northern Afghanistan) in AD 850, Al-Balkhi became renowned for criticizing the medical doctors of his day for concentrating solely on physical illnesses and neglecting the psychological and mental health of their patients. He developed the concept of 'mental hygiene', coining the phrases 'al-Tibb al-Ruhani' (spiritual and psychological health) and 'Tibb al-Qalb' (mental medicine), and in his famous book Masalih al-Abdan wa al-Anfus (Sustenance for Body and Soul), he argued that the two concepts were interwoven.(15) Far from claiming that this was a new concept, he traced his own ideas on mental health to verses of the Qur'an and hadiths attributed to the prophet Muhammad. Al-Balkhi's ideas were echoed in the work of other esteemed Islamic scientists, including Yaqoob al-Kindi (801-873) and Acivenna (Ibn Sina) (980-1037).

However, despite this and other traditions of a combined mind and body approach to medicine, in the seventeenth century, philosopher René Descartes proposed that in fact the mind and body were different substances, with the mind existing outside the body. Although this idea had been considered before and can be traced back to the Ancient Greeks, it gained particular ground following the writings of Descartes and came to be known as Cartesian dualism ('Cartesian' meaning 'pertaining to Descartes'). Descartes' theories had immediate opponents: Dutch philosopher Baruch Spinoza, for example, responded by hypothesizing that the mind and body were in fact identical, with events in one mirrored by events in the other; a concept he referred to as psychophysiological parallelism. And in the eighteenth and nineteenth centuries these opponents gained in force, supported by the developing interest in mental illness and materalist models of the mind. For example, eighteenth-century German reformer Johann Christian Reil argued that psychiatry (a term he is credited with being the to use) and the study of the brain and psyche should be a mainstream part of medicine. In 1812, Benjamin Rush's *Medical Inquiries and Observations Upon the Diseases of the Mind* further helped to define psychiatry as a medical discipline. And in 1818, the medical term 'psychosomatic' (referring to the interaction of mind and body) was first used in conjunction with mind-body medicine by the German physician Johann Christian Heinroth.(16)

The work of Freud and his colleagues mentioned above meant that the early approaches in psychosomatic medicine were predominantly psychoanalytic and psychodynamic. However, through the influence of other individuals, the field broadened. Psychosomatic medicine now explores a range of topics, including the potential psychiatric contributions to medically unexplained symptoms, functional disorders, diseases, and pain management. It also focuses on the psychological implications of chronic conditions, including identifying predictors of mental health conditions. The psychological focus is not just on the individual but also on the social aspects of disease, such as social support networks and social resilience. Other major strands of research include psychophysiological manifestations and consequences of acute and chronic stress, the role of placebo, and the effects of complementary and alternative medicines. This psychosocial focus in many ways marked a theoretical challenge to the biomedical model by broadening considerations away from pure laboratory science and surgical techniques and demonstrating the role of the mind and social environment in both the development and treatment of illness.

Q For more information, the book *Psychosomatic Medicine* by Michael Blumenfield and James J Strain covers the history alongside core research findings that have helped to define the field.(16)

Behavioural medicine

Another field that has arisen alongside the biomedical model is behavioural medicine. The term 'behavioural medicine' is thought to date back to 1973 in the title of a book by scientist Lee Birk entitled *Biofeedback: Behavioral Medicine*. The field had such a fast rise that just 3 years later, the National Institute of Health in the US created the Behavioural Medicine Study Section to support collaborative research, and in 1977 the Yale Conference on Behavioural

Medicine and a meeting of the National Academy of Sciences were organized to define and further the field.

Behavioural medicine focuses on how risk factors such as smoking, poor diet, alcohol consumption, and physical inactivity impact health. The statistics behind behavioural medicine are striking: approximately 75% of all deaths from cancer are related to behaviour. From the 10 leading causes of death, 50% of mortality is related to behaviour. And 90% of all lung cancer deaths are attributable to cigarettes.(17) These behaviours are closely linked to the environment: the environment itself can impact directly on health (such as through air pollution); certain behaviours can be encouraged by an environment (such as an urban area with lots of fast food restaurants promoting unhealthy eating); and individuals within an environment can be influenced by environmental norms (such as family behaviours or community pressures).

An important aspect of behavioural medicine is identifying potential barriers to behaviour change. These can include socioeconomic factors, local and national policies, and individual factors such as psychological state. Barriers to behavioural change can be closely linked with health inequalities, with healthy behaviours often less common among disadvantaged communities. Behaviours and their barriers are not just limited to potential illness-provoking behaviours, but also to the controlling of illness, such as treatment adherence and compliance. Aspects of doctor-patient relationships and patient monitoring have been shown to be important in supporting recovery. Further developments in behavioural medicine have focused on biological and genetic influences. For example, behavioural medicine has intersected with recent work in epigenetics: the study of changes in organisms caused by modification of gene expression rather than alteration of the genetic code itself. Behavioural epigenetics has shown that behaviours and our environment can modify the expression of genes.(18) Consequently, our behaviours can have long-lasting and deep-seated effects on our health.

Behavioural medicine proposes a different view to the biomedical model by suggesting that individuals have a duty of care to themselves, arguably shifting some of the responsibility away from doctors onto patients. However, under the framework of behavioural medicine, policy-makers also have a responsibility to develop health prevention and promotion strategies to encourage healthy behaviours and counteract unhealthy lifestyle recommendations by commercial organizations such as the marketing of alcohol, cigarettes, and unhealthy foods. Overall, behavioural medicine is gradually being recognized as a critical way of increasing life expectancy and improving quality of life. Indeed, in 2010, the Annual Status Report of the National Prevention, Health Promotion and Public Health Council in the US stated 'the most effective approach to address the leading causes of death is to reduce and prevent underlying risk factors including physical inactivity, poor nutrition, tobacco use, and underage and excessive alcohol use'.(19)

Q The *Encyclopedia of Behavioral Medicine* explores behavioural issues and care for a comprehensive range of health conditions to support research and practice among those working in and studying health.(20)

A biopsychosocial model of health

Aspects of public health, psychosomatic medicine, and behavioural medicine as well as other related fields such as health psychology are brought together in the 'biopsychosocial' model, first articulated by American psychiatrist George Engel as a challenge to the biomedical model in a paper published in the journal *Science* in April 1977.(21) Engel proposed that the traditional bio-medical model did not operate in isolation but was actually integrated with psychological factors and social factors with direct and indirect pathways to health.

As with psychosomatic medicine, the concept of the biopsychosocial model was not new. It can be traced back to the very origins of the Western med-ical tradition in the Hippocratic school of medicine, which placed an emphasis on environmental factors such as personal hygiene, sanitation, and nutrition. Furthermore, during the Middle Ages, when mortality rates were high with few cures available, there was a strong emphasis given to mental, social, and spir-itual dimensions of health. It was only with the strides forwards made within medicine in the eighteenth and nineteenth centuries that the biopsychosocial model waned. In 2004, the prominent medical historian Theodore Brown was interviewed at the University of Rochester.(22) He explained that this move away from the biopsychosocial towards the biomedical in the nineteenth cen-tury was not surprising:

'That's actually a recurrent phenomenon that I see in medical history. When you have a new discovery, whether it be Pasteur in the 19th century or recent discoveries of peni-cillin, there's such a desire for them and they play so well, they're so sexy, and they're so easy to market, both figuratively and literally, that they just overwhelm the rest of the field.'

Indeed, some have seen the biomedical model as a temporary impediment to a broader definition of health: it appeared to provide so many answers that at the turn of the twentieth century it was believed that all disease would be conquered in a short space of time. By reintroducing the biopsychosocial model, Engel aimed to revitalize the previous approach to health. The term itself—biopsychosocial—had actually been coined by the neurologist and psychiatrist Roy Grinker in 1954 as a way of emphasizing the 'bio-' within psychoanalytics. But Engel changed the meaning, instead emphasizing the 'psychosocial' within biomedical. Engel called the model a 'blueprint for research, a framework for teaching, and a design for action in the real world of healthcare'. (21) In essence, Engel tried to bring the biopsychosocial back, not just as a theory or a concept, but as something practical.

Engel was not alone in his views, and in many ways encapsulated the thoughts of other scientists of the time.(23) However, worthy though the aims of those proponents of the biopsychosocial model were, there has been debate as to whether the biopsychosocial model was properly adopted. Indeed, the World Health Organization (WHO) definition of health, which encompasses a biopsychosocial approach, was, for a long time, considered an idealistic view of health, but not a practical definition. Psychologist Robert Ader, in the same interview with Theodore Brown in 2004 said he felt there was 'more lip service to than actual implementation of the biopsychosocial model' in clinical practice. However, Ader himself has arguably been credited with changing this through leading a new field of scientific research coined in the 1970s: psychoneuroimmunology. Brown explained:

> 'In my view as a historian, psychoneuroimmunology came as a great shock because there, in the midst of the biomedical approach were unmistakably rigorous investigations and undeniably powerful evidence that seemed to question some of the foundations of the biomedical approach from a research point of view rather than a clinical one, and from hard data rather than from rhetorical pronouncements.'

Psychoneuroimmunology demonstrated that the mind and immune system were connected bi-directionally, with psychological thoughts not only capable of altering immune activity, but the immune system itself also capable of feeding back and leading to alterations in psychological state. The importance of this research was that it provided further weight to the biopsychosocial model by showing that incorporating psychological and environmental factors into the clinical practice of medicine was not just an idealist position but was fundamental to understanding and treating diseases. Certainly, there remain debates such as around how comprehensively the biopsychosocial model is implemented in practice, but it is still generally recognized as the dominant theoretical model of health.

Q For more information on psychoneuroimmunology, Jorge H Daruna's *Introduction to Psychoneuroimmunology* provides an accessible overview of different aspects of the field.(24)

Mental health

In tandem with the shift from biomedical to biopsychosocial models of health and the rise of psychosomatic research, another major move has been the increasing focus on mental health. In the first half of the twentieth century, the dominance of psychoanalytics had led to a focus on mental illness, with recovery associated with the absence of symptoms. However, among certain psychologists, this absence of mental illness in itself was not enough to constitute mental health, and this led to the rise of a new kind of psychology: humanistic psychology.(25) This movement returned to ideas of the ancient Greeks and Renaissance, which had advocated the importance of happiness, fulfilling one's potential and expressing oneself through creativity. Socrates, for example, had cited self-knowledge as key to happiness. Happiness became a central theme of different philosophical movements, including Epicureanism and Stoicism, and religions, including Judaism and Christianity, which draw on the Divine command theory of happiness (that happiness comes from following the commands of the Divine). Building on some of these earlier ideas, humanists took a holistic view of life, believing that as well as our biochemistry and environments affecting our health, we are also influenced and motivated internally to fulfil our human potential.

One of these humanist psychologists was Abraham Maslow. Maslow said of the humanist movement 'it is as if Freud supplied us the sick half of psychology and we must now fill it out with the healthy half'.(26) Maslow built on the work of his colleagues to study 'self-actualization': the motive to realize one's full potential through the pursuit of knowledge, giving to society, a quest for spiritual enlightenment, and expressing oneself creatively. Maslow proposed that there was a 'hierarchy of needs' among humans. On a basic level, we require physiological things, such as food, water, and sleep. Beyond this, our next priorities are for safety and a sense of love and belonging. Once we have these things, we then require esteem, including feeling confident and respected. If we achieve these things, we can then enjoy self-actualization and peak experiences of euphoria: feeling in perfect harmony with ourselves and our surroundings (see Figure 2.1).

In 1954, Maslow coined the term 'positive psychology', and in 1996, the newly elected President of the American Psychological Association, Martin Seligman, picked up on this term and chose it as the central theme for his term of presidency. This was an important step for positive psychology as it helped move the field away from humanism and into a scientific and epistemological domain. Seligman, in collaboration with his colleague Mihaly Csikszentmihalyi, defined positive psychology as 'the scientific study of

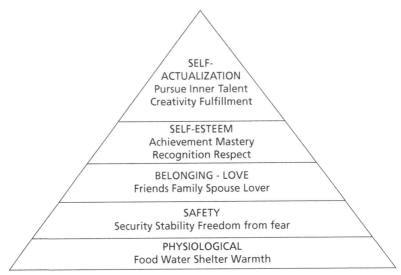

Figure 2.1 Abraham Maslow's Hierarchy of Needs. Reproduced from Maslow, Abraham H., Frager, Robert D. Faidman, James, *Motivation and Personality*, 3rd Ed., ©1987. Reprinted by permission of Pearson Education, Inc., New York, New York.

positive human functioning and flourishing on multiple levels that include the biological, personal, relational, institutional, cultural, and global dimensions of life'.(27) Seligman followed on from Maslow in wanting to shift the focus away from just mental illness into positive aspects of health. So the new positive psychology focused on positive experiences, relationships, institutions, and psychological traits.

In 1999, the first Positive Psychology Summit took place, followed shortly afterwards by the First International Conference on Positive Psychology in 2002. In 2006, a course at Harvard University used the positive psychology framework, which led to greater attention among the general public. And in 2009 the First World Congress on Positive Psychology took place at the University of Pennsylvania. As the field has evolved, positive psychology has arguably shifted in direction. In 2011, Seligman published his book *Flourish*, in which he wrote 'I used to think the topic of positive psychology was happiness … I now think the topic of positive psychology is wellbeing'.(28) Wellbeing, like health, has proved difficult to define, although it is often split into different dimensions such as hedonic wellbeing, which includes happiness and positive affect; eudaimonic wellbeing, which includes feeling a sense of purpose and meaning in life; and evaluative wellbeing, which includes general satisfaction with life.(29) Broadly, it is now widely recognised that good mental health is about both the absence of mental illness and the presence of wellbeing.(30)

Not only have wellbeing and wider positive psychology research broadened the way we approach mental health, but research has demonstrated that these positive states can in themselves impact on our wider physical health. For example, even among people who have the same level of exercise, drinking, sleep, and smoking, happier people have longer life expectancies, and positive emotions are associated with greater resistance to colds and flu.(31) In return, healthy behaviours such as eating fruit and vegetables are associated with greater happiness and life satisfaction.(32,33)

This research into mental health returns us to the WHO definition of health from 1946 as 'a state of complete physical, mental and social wellbeing and not merely the absence of disease or infirmity'. In 1946, and for decades afterwards, this definition was viewed in certain circles as idealistic. However, the gradual challenges to the biomedical model of health that was dominant in the nineteenth century, the (re-)rise of the biopsychosocial model and the increasing prominence of wellbeing have turned the ideal into a more tangible concept and one that now lies at the heart of the research and policy agendas of many governments globally.

Arts in health: opportunities within health theory

These theoretical developments over the last 100 years have provided a range of opportunities for the application of the arts in health. In the fact file in Part IV, we will look in more detail at how the arts have been found to affect various dimensions of different health conditions. However, if we take a broader view for now, following the biopsychosocial model, the arts have been shown to have effects at all three levels.

Bio-

The brain

Physiological research into the arts over the past century has demonstrated a variety of effects on different organs. For example, there has been a wealth of research on the impact of the arts on the brain. The multi-sensory aspects of many types of arts engagement, involving hearing, seeing, touching, and moving, mean that a wide range of brain areas have been shown to be involved in arts perception, including the sensory cortex, auditory cortex, visual cortex, and various rhythmic processing centres including the primary sensorimotor areas.(34,35) Furthermore, as many arts activities involve an emotional response, areas critical to memory, reward, and emotion processing also have been found to be affected, such as the amygdala, medial orbitofrontal cortex, and hippocampus.(36)

Not only are different areas of the brain activated by arts engagement, but they have also been shown to be structurally altered. For example, people who learn music from an early age have been shown to have larger motor, auditory, and visual-spatial brain regions and can have enhanced brain plasticity.(37,38) Music listening can also induce structural changes in grey matter (which contains, among other things, the cell bodies of neurons) in people who have experienced a stroke.(39) And children with one-sided paralysis (hemiplegia) who practise magic tricks have been shown to have increased integrity of white matter (which connects different parts of grey matter together) in the brain and greater activation of the part of the brain affected by the hemiplegia.(40)

Other organs

The arts also have been found to impact on other organs. For example, singing has been shown to enhance lung function, including forced vital capacity, forced expiratory volume, and breathing control.(41) Dance has been shown to alter heart rate and oxygen uptake.(42,43) And both listening to and making music have been shown to affect blood pressure and heart rate variability, which suggests that music also alters the activation of the sympathetic and parasympathetic nervous systems (two branches of the nervous system that involve bodily functions including breathing, heartbeat, and digestive processes).(44–46) Indeed, music has been shown to impact on the digestive system, including increasing gastric myoelectrical activity, gastric motility, and gastric emptying, and reducing nausea and vomiting.(47)

Physical function

The arts also have been shown to lead to changes in physical function. For example, magic tricks can enhance hand function and bimanual ability.(48,49) Rhythmic music can support improvements in gait velocity, stride length, cadence, and standing ability in people undergoing physiotherapy.(50,51) Importantly, these changes have not just been seen in healthy participants but also in people affected by strokes, spinal cord injuries, and brain trauma, (52,53) as well as people with chronic conditions such as Parkinson's disease, Huntington's disease, muscular sclerosis, and chronic obstructive pulmonary disease (COPD).(54–56) As another benefit for physical function, dance can lead to increased bone mineral density and reduce falls risk in older adults.(57,58)

Biological markers

The arts also have been shown to affect biological markers of the endocrine and immune systems. For example, music has been shown to affect stress hormones including cortisol and adrenaline, sex hormones involved in stress response, including testosterone and progesterone, a range of different white blood cells, inflammatory proteins, and neuropeptides involved in social bonding and pain response.(59) Similarly, dance has been shown to affect levels of the neuropeptides serotonin and dopamine over several weeks of involvement and reduce blood glucose levels,(60,61) while writing therapy has been shown to reduce stress hormones.(62)

Psycho-

Cognition and development

It is not just physiological aspects of health and illness that are affected by the arts; they also have profound psychological effects. For example, the arts have been shown to have an impact on cognition, including temporal and spatial abilities, language, and memory.(63,64) In healthy individuals, such as infants and young children, this has been shown to lead to improvements in learning and social development.(65) But the arts also have been shown to support cognition in people with neurological conditions such as those with Alzheimer's disease and dementia.(66) And they have been shown to be a source of valuable psychological support for people with neurological conditions and neurodevelopmental disorders. For example, art and music therapy have been found to support development, behavioural adjustment, and emotional regulation in children with autism, and poetry therapy has been found to support grief and empowerment following acquired brain injury, among other examples.(67–69)

Stress, anxiety, and pain

Similarly, in addition to physiological stress, a range of art forms also have been shown to affect psychological stress and anxiety.(70–73) This is an important finding as research has demonstrated that both acute and chronic stress are associated with illness.(74,75) Consequently, ways of reducing stress or buffering its effects, including mindfulness, are currently being recommended as part of a healthy lifestyle. The stress-reducing effects of the arts have been shown in healthy populations as well as those affected by trauma, such as studies showing the benefits of diary-writing for post-traumatic stress,(76,77) art therapy with sexual abuse survivors,(78) play therapy for children in crisis situations,(79) and both art and music therapy for refugees.(80)

Linked in with stress is perceived pain: not only is stress associated with enhanced pain perception, pain has been found to increase negative psychological states such as anxiety and fear,(81,82) with implications for mental health. However, various types of music and arts interventions have been shown to reduce both short-term and chronic pain in different patient groups,(83–85) with demonstrations that certain art forms such as music may evoke activation of the descending analgesia pathway in the brain and lead to a reduced need for sedatives and analgesics.(86–88)

Emotions and mental health

The arts also have been shown to be powerful regulators of emotions. Music, dance, poetry, art, and crafts all have been shown to alter emotional states, sometimes through emotional expression, other times through mastery over and acceptance of emotions.(89,90) Linked in with the alteration of emotion through the arts is their impact on mental health and wellbeing. Studies have shown the value of participating in the arts and more general cultural engagement on both negative symptoms of mental illness, such as anxiety and depression, and positive aspects of mental health, such as wellbeing and quality of life.(91–93) This has been demonstrated in a range of populations from people with mild or moderate symptoms through to people with bipolar disorder and schizophrenia.(94,95) Part of the importance of these positive psychology findings is that, even in the absence of any changes in physical health status, it has been shown that people can have dramatic shifts in their appraisal of their health and, through more positive appraisal and enhanced wellbeing, have a very different quality of life. Therefore, findings of the effects of the arts on positive psychology are hugely important for supporting individuals who are physically healthy and also those with a range of health conditions.

Health behaviours

In addition, there are also a range of benefits associated with the arts that come under the umbrella of health psychology. Many of these have been identified as part of larger studies on the effects of arts involvement or exposure, but their full psychological potential has yet to be ascertained. Some of these effects of the arts are related to people's health beliefs and behaviours. In 1984, American psychologist Joseph Matarazzo separated health behaviours into 'health-impairing' behaviours or 'behavioural pathogens' (such as smoking, drinking, eating unhealthily, etc.) and 'health-protective' or 'behavioural immunogens' (such as attending health checks, exercising, getting enough sleep, etc.).(96) Much health promotion and education work involves encouraging people away from behavioural pathogens and towards behavioural immunogens. However, simple though this sounds, changing behaviour can be very difficult, partly because it is intrinsically linked with people's health beliefs and entrenched patterns of behaviour. Nevertheless, there are a range of models around health beliefs that have been shown to alter people's behaviours, and a number of studies have highlighted how the arts can modulate these beliefs. For example, a key obstacle to people changing their health behaviours is whether they perceive their health to be controllable by them (an internal locus of control) or uncontrollable by them (an external locus of control).(97,98) People who believe themselves to be in control are more capable of changing their behaviours and leading a healthy lifestyle and feel more personally responsible for their own health. Studies involving the arts have shown enhanced mastery from people who take part, which in turn has been shown to lead to an enhanced sense of control in other areas of their lives.(99)

Sense of 'self'

Related to this concept of control are issues relating to selfhood. It has been shown that people are motivated to protect their sense of self-integrity and want to see themselves as morally satisfactory or adequate.(100) If they are presented with information that suggests they are not adequate (e.g. a smoker being presented with warnings about the health dangers of smoking), they behave defensively. However, if they are able to affirm that they are morally satisfactory in another area of their lives, then they become less defensive overall and are more open to changing behaviours that might not be as healthy, as this change is no longer seen as such an assault on their sense of self. Art has been demonstrated to be a way of enhancing self-affirmation, for example through engagement in art as a child,(101) and through arts interventions such as writing.(102)

Another concept relevant to behaviour change is self-efficacy. This was developed by psychologist Albert Bandura in 1977 and describes how capable an individual believes they are of changing their behaviour.(103) If they perceive themselves as incapable, they are unlikely to even try and change their behaviour. However, the arts, including singing and needlework, have been shown to enhance self-belief and self-efficacy in different populations.(104,105)

These concepts all lead on to the issue of self-identity. Individuals tend to carry out behaviours that fit and reinforce their image of themselves.(106) For example, people who perceive themselves to be healthy eaters will want to continue eating healthily. The arts have been shown to help individuals redefine their sense of self at key turning points in their lives.(107) This enhanced sense of self through the arts has been shown to support individuals in their perceptions of what they can achieve.(108) Self-identity is also very much bound up with self-esteem.(109) Again, arts interventions such as arts therapy have been shown to enhance self-esteem and self-worth.(110,111)

Illness cognitions

Still under the umbrella of health psychology, the arts also can help if an individual becomes ill. When people are diagnosed with an illness, they develop 'illness cognitions'; frameworks for understanding and coping with their illness.(112) These include shifting their sense of identity to incorporate their new illness (e.g. becoming a 'patient'), rationalizing the cause of that illness (such as attributing it to a virus or behaviour), setting a timeline for recovery (whether acute or accepting it as long term), considering the physical and emotional consequences, and accepting whether it is curable or controllable by them. These cognitions then lead on to different sets of attitudes and behaviours. Some people learn coping skills.(113) Coping skills include problem-focused coping (including seeking support and taking problem-solving action), emotion-focused coping (such as acceptance, maintaining hope, regulating their moods, and discharging negative emotions such as venting of feelings of anger or despair), and appraisal-focused coping (mental preparation and acceptance of the situation, sometimes avoiding or denying the illness; other times embracing it). Supporting these coping behaviours is important as they can prevent more negative coping styles such as behavioural disengagement, in which people no longer take responsibility for their behaviours, which can lead to non-adherence to medication and unhealthy behaviours such as drinking or substance abuse.(114) A broad range of arts and leisure activities have been shown to support coping, including enhancing adaptations to new physical conditions, supporting psychological coping under abnormal circumstances, and constructing meaning for families in palliative care.(115–117). In addition, creative technologies have been shown to directly affect behavioural engagement. For example, educational apps and other technologies that 'gamify' aspects of health behaviours (turning them into a game in order to motivate participation) have been shown to lead to improved coping, such as increased adherence to medication, enhanced self-efficacy and improved understanding of the medical condition.(118)

Other people can approach illness cognitions with cognitive adaptation. (119) These can include searches for meaning, in which individuals try and find explanations for their illnesses. Social psychologist Bernard Weiner called this 'attribution theory' and explored how searching for this answer can become an important part of cognitive adaptation.(120) Following on from this is the search for mastery, by which people try and undertake behaviours or attitudes that they think will help to put them in control of their condition again. And then there is a process of self-enhancement, by which people try and find ways to improve their self-esteem. Sometimes, these stages result in illusions, such as people believing they understand why something happened to them and how to stop it in the future, when in fact the causes can be genetic and beyond their control. However, these illusions can be helpful in coping and wellbeing. The arts, for example music therapy, have been shown to support cognitive adaptation, helping people to find meaning in their illness, providing an opportunity for people to start a new creative activity that helps them to feel they are taking positive steps in supporting their health and wellbeing, and, through engagement in communal activities with other people experiencing similar health challenges, helping people to normalize their condition.(121,122) Finally, cognitive adaptation also can be linked with benefit finding. People who have undergone illnesses or traumas often report improvements in areas of their lives, such as perceived changes in themselves, closer family relationships, better life philosophies, a better perspective on life, and a strengthened belief system.(123) The arts have been linked in with this benefit finding, with some of the benefits highlighted by different patient groups including taking up new hobbies ranging from reading to lace-making to engaging more with culture.(124)

Social

Social support

There has been a wealth of research into the social benefits of arts engagement, with implications for people's health. 'Social' aspects that have been most linked in with health are loneliness and social isolation, with research over the past two decades in particular highlighting their negative effect on health. For example, people who experience loneliness are two to five times more likely to die prematurely.(125) Unfortunately, estimates suggest loneliness is very common. For example, the UK White Paper *Healthy Lives, Healthy People* (2010) highlighted that around one in 10 older people experience chronic loneliness.(126) In contrast, social support has been shown to support mental health, wellbeing, cardiovascular, neuroendocrine and immune function, and mortality,(127–129) as well as acting as a buffer for psychological stress.(130) The arts have been shown to impact directly on various aspects of social support, including social bonding,(131–133) with enhanced social support itself becoming a mediator to wider health enhancements.(59,133–135)

Social identity and relationships

Moving from this focus on the individual to looking at group effects, the arts have been shown not only to affect self-identity but also to support a sense of collective self in society. The collective self is the idea that individuals' interactions influence one another.(136) Social interaction gives rise to social representations and social identity.(137,138) This social identity can also support group cohesiveness, including solidarity, team spirit, and morale. Some of the most obvious manifestations of culture are made through the arts, as seen in indigenous cultural traditions, dress, and rituals involving dance, art, and music.(139,140) And the arts also have been shown to foster intergroup social cohesion within societies.(141)

This group identity and cohesiveness also has implications for minority groups. Research has shown that minority groups that are disadvantaged either economically, politically or educationally typically have lower self-esteem than non-minority groups.(142) Low self-esteem in itself can lead to people being more vulnerable, more easily persuaded and influenced, and more sceptical socially.(143) But the arts have been shown to be capable of challenging these relationships between groups, leading to improvements in pride and individuals' feelings of self-worth in their own abilities, as well as enhancing the social resilience of those involved, which can provide support to individuals when tackling other social issues in their lives.(144,145)

Social behaviours

Tied in with this, the arts have been shown to affect intergroup behaviour and reduce social unrest, including reducing conflict in communities, promoting prosocial behaviour, furthering social change, and promoting collective action.(146) As well as effects within groups, the arts also have been used to challenge how groups themselves are seen from the outside, in particular reducing prejudice and discrimination and highlighting oppression, such as with refugees and survivors of torture and war.(146) As well as social behaviours, the arts can support social communication. Certainly the arts, in particular music, literature, and fine art, have been shown to be a proxy language both for new babies and for people with developmental delay and autism. (147–149) Moving out further to a society level, the arts have been shown to be a powerful source of social influence, affecting compliance, obedience, and conformity, for example enhancing patriotism or reducing antisocial behaviour in public places.(150)

Consequently, the arts are recognized as having a wide range of benefits for society. Indeed, statements at the European Communities Summit in 2005 described 'effective access to and participation in cultural activities' as 'an essential dimension of promoting an inclusive society'.(151) Furthermore, an interesting point to note regarding the social effects of the arts is that, as the examples above have illustrated, the arts appear to act across all levels of society, influencing people from a broad range of socioeconomic backgrounds. Consequently, the arts can have an impact across social inequalities, which makes them a powerful tool in reaching mixed demographics and minority groups.

Summary

This chapter has considered some of the rich and varied ways in which the arts can support the health and wellbeing of individuals, communities, and societies, and how these effects fit within contemporary models of health. These include both supporting specific health conditions and more generally enhancing wellbeing, health behaviours, and social engagement. We have focused exclusively on evidence of positive effects. However, that is not to say that the arts are not capable of having negative effects. For example, individual arts engagement such as music listening also has been associated with negative psychological states, such as associations found between rock and metal music and suicidal thoughts, acts of deliberate self-harm, depression, delinquency, drug-taking, and family dysfunction.(152) At a society level, the arts also have been appropriated for use in dangerous propaganda.(153,154) Even when the intention is to use the arts to good effect, mismanaged interventions, unethical procedures, or a lack of consideration for the potential psychological and physical consequences of involvement in an intervention can put participants at risk of harm, as will be discussed further in Chapters 8 and 12.

Nevertheless, if the arts are carefully and appropriately applied, they can be powerful tools for supporting health. Indeed, the consideration in this chapter of the biopsychosocial effects of the arts merely scratches the surface in terms of the impact the arts have been shown to have on people's health and wellbeing. What is perhaps most remarkable is the breadth of this impact; a breadth that can sometimes be to the detriment to the field as the myriad of areas of research and practice can be hard for people to draw together (a topic that will be explored more in Chapter 4). Nevertheless, this web of ties between the arts and health is arguably why the field is beginning to be taken so seriously. Indeed, speaking in favour of the theoretical importance of arts and culture, the then-editor of the *British Medical Journal* (BMJ) Richard Smith wrote an editorial in 2002 entitled 'Spend (slightly) less on health and more on the arts'. He suggested that 0.5% of the healthcare budget should be diverted to the arts to support public health. He explained 'if health is about adaptation, understanding, and acceptance, then the arts may be more potent than anything that medicine has to offer'.(156) Although a provocative suggestion, it certainly highlights the potential importance that the arts could have for health; an importance that is highlighted in the way the arts have been foregrounded in policy over the past few decades. In the next chapter, we will explore how the alignment of the arts with health theory has, over the last 50 years, led to its involvement in a number of key policy documents around the world, and consider the implications of this for research and practice.

References

1. **World Health Organization**. Constitution [Internet]. Geneva; 1948 [cited 2015 Dec 7]. Available from: http://www.who.int/about/mission/en/.

2. **Harant H, Theodorides J.** [A pioneer of parasitology and a forerunner of the Pasteur doctrine: Agostino Bassi (1773-1856)]. Montp Med. 1956 Nov;**50**(3):393–9.

3. **Pasteur L.** On the extension of the germ theory to the etiology of certain common diseases [Internet]. France: l'Academie des Sciences; 1880 [cited 2016 Nov 3]. Available from: https://ebooks.adelaide.edu.au/p/pasteur/louis/exgerm/.

4. Medicine's paradigm shift: An opportunity for psychology [Internet]. [cited 2016 Nov 3]. Available from: http://www.apa.org/monitor/2012/09/pc.aspx.

5. **Barry A-M, Yuill C.** Understanding Health: A Sociological Introduction. London, Thousand Oaks, New Delhi: SAGE; 2002. 164 pp.

6. **Brown M.** Performing Medicine: Medical Culture and Identity in Provincial England, C.1760-1850. 1 edition. Manchester : New York: Manchester University Press; 2011. 272 pp.

7. **Tracy SW.** Alcoholism in America: From Reconstruction to Prohibition. Baltimore and London: JHU Press; 2009. 475 pp.

8. Bynum WF, Porter R, editors. Companion Encyclopedia of the History of Medicine. 1 edition. London; New York: Routledge; 1997. 1848 pp.

9. **Christensen AJ, Martin R, Smyth JM.** Encyclopedia of Health Psychology. New York: Springer Science & Business Media; 2014. 355 pp.

10. **Rosen G, Imperato PJ.** A History of Public Health. Baltimore: JHU Press; 2015. 441 pp.

11. **Porter D.** Health, Civilization and the State: A History of Public Health from Ancient to Modern Times. Abingdon: Routledge; 2005. 397 pp.

12. **Bartram J.** Routledge Handbook of Water and Health. London and New York: Routledge; 2015. 1066 pp.

13. **Porter D.** The History of Public Health and the Modern State. Amsterdam: Rodopi; 1994. 452 pp.

14. **Mitchell SA, Black MJ.** Freud and Beyond: A History of Modern Psychoanalytic Thought. New York: Basic Books; 1995. 322 pp.

15. **Deuraseh N, Abu Talib M.** Mental health in Islamic medical tradition. Int Med J. 2005;**4**(2):76–9.

16. Blumenfield M, Strain JJ, editors. Psychosomatic Medicine. 1 Har/DVD edition. Philadelphia, PA: LWW; 2006. 987 pp.

17. **Ogden J.** Health Psychology: a textbook. 4 edition. Maidenhead; New York: Open University Press; 2007. 528 pp.

18. **Moore DS.** The Developing Genome: An Introduction to Behavioral Epigenetics. Oxford University Press; 2015. 321 pp.

19. **National Prevention, Health Promotion and Public Health Council**. 2010 Annual Status Report. US; 2010.

20. **Gellman M, Turner JR.** Encyclopedia of Behavioral Medicine. Springer New York; 2012. 2116 pp.

21. **Engel GL.** The need for a new medical model: a challenge for biomedicine. Science. 1977 Apr 8;**196**(4286):129–36.

22. **Ader R, Brown T.** The biopsychosocial model: interdisciplinarity in science and medicine. J Undergrad Res. 2004;3(1):6–9.

23. **Dubos R.** Mirage of Health: Utopias, Progress, and Biological Change. New Brunswick: Rutgers University Press; 1987. 282 pp.

24. **Daruna JH.** Introduction to Psychoneuroimmunology. London, Waltham, San Diego: Academic Press; 2012. 336 pp.

25. **Schneider KJ, Pierson JF, Bugental JFT.** The Handbook of Humanistic Psychology: Theory, Research, and Practice. Thousand Oaks, California; SAGE Publications; 2014. 832 pp.

26. **Maslow AH.** Toward a Psychology of Being. Simon and Schuster; 2013. 212 pp.

27. **Seligman ME, Csikszentmihalyi M.** Positive psychology. An introduction. Am Psychol. 2000 Jan;55(1):5–14.

28. **Seligman MEP.** Flourish: A Visionary New Understanding of Happiness and Well-being. New York: Simon and Schuster; 2012. 370 p.

29. **Ryan RM, and Deci EL.** On Happiness and Human Potentials: A Review of Research on Hedonic and Eudaimonic Well-Being. Annu Rev Psychol. 2001;52(1):141–66.

30. **Keyes CL.** Mental Illness and/or Mental Health? Investigating Axioms of the Complete State Model of Health. J Consult Clin Psychol. 2005;73(3):539–48.

31. **Chida Y, Steptoe A.** Positive psychological well-being and mortality: a quantitative review of prospective observational studies. Psychosom Med. 2008 Sep;70(7):741–56.

32. **Conner TS, Brookie KL, Richardson AC, Polak MA.** On carrots and curiosity: eating fruit and vegetables is associated with greater flourishing in daily life. Br J Health Psychol. 2015 May;20(2):413–27.

33. **White BA, Horwath CC, Conner TS.** Many apples a day keep the blues away--daily experiences of negative and positive affect and food consumption in young adults. Br J Health Psychol. 2013 Nov;18(4):782–98.

34. **Thaut MH.** Neural Basis of Rhythmic Timing Networks in the Human Brain. Ann N Y Acad Sci. 2003 Nov 1;999(1):364–73.

35. **Levitin DJ, Tirovolas AK.** Current Advances in the Cognitive Neuroscience of Music. Ann N Y Acad Sci. 2009 Mar 1;1156(1):211–31.

36. **Koelsch S.** Towards a neural basis of music-evoked emotions. Trends Cogn Sci. 2010 Mar;14(3):131–7.

37. **Gaser C, Schlaug G.** Brain Structures Differ between Musicians and Non-Musicians. J Neurosci. 2003 Oct 8;23(27):9240–5.

38. **Wan CY, Schlaug G.** Music Making as a Tool for Promoting Brain Plasticity across the Life Span. The Neuroscientist. 2010 Oct 1;16(5):566–77.

39. **Särkämö T, Soto D.** Music listening after stroke: beneficial effects and potential neural mechanisms. Ann N Y Acad Sci. 2012 Apr 1;1252(1):266–81.

40. **Weinstein M, Myers V, Green D, Schertz M, Shiran SI, Geva R,** et al. Brain Plasticity following Intensive Bimanual Therapy in Children with Hemiparesis: Preliminary Evidence. Neural Plast. 2015;2015:798481.

41. **Panigrahi A, Sohani S, Amadi C, Joshi A.** Role of music in the management of chronic obstructive pulmonary disease (COPD): a literature review. Technol Health Care Off J Eur Soc Eng Med. 2014;22(1):53–61.

42. De Angelis M, Vinciguerra G, Gasbarri A, Pacitti C. Oxygen uptake, heart rate and blood lactate concentration during a normal training session of an aerobic dance class. Eur J Appl Physiol. 1998 Jul;78(2):121–7.

43. Bell JM, Bassey EJ. A comparison of the relation between oxygen uptake and heart rate during different styles of aerobic dance and a traditional step test in women. Eur J Appl Physiol. 1994;68(1):20–4.

44. Iwanaga M, Kobayashi A, Kawasaki C. Heart rate variability with repetitive exposure to music. Biol Psychol. 2005 Sep;70(1):61–6.

45. Roque AL, Valenti VE, Guida HL, Campos MF, Knap A, Vanderlei LCM, et al. The effects of auditory stimulation with music on heart rate variability in healthy women. Clinics. 2013 Jul;68(7):960–7.

46. Williamon A, Aufegger L, Wasley D, Looney D, Mandic DP. Complexity of physiological responses decreases in high-stress musical performance. J R Soc Interface. 2013 Dec 6;10(89):20130719.

47. Yamasaki A, Booker A, Kapur V, Tilt A, Niess H, Lillemoe KD, et al. The impact of music on metabolism. Nutrition. 2012 Nov;28(11–12):1075–80.

48. Green D, Farquharson Y. The Magic of Movement: Integrating magic into rehabilitation for children with hemiplegia. Dev Med Child Neurol. 2013;5(S2):19.

49. Green D, Schertz M, Gordon AM, Moore A, Schejter Margalit T, Farquharson Y, et al. A multi-site study of functional outcomes following a themed approach to hand-arm bimanual intensive therapy for children with hemiplegia. Dev Med Child Neurol. 2013 Jun;55(6):527–33.

50. Plante TG, Gustafson C, Brecht C, Imberi J, Sanchez J. Exercising with an iPod, Friend, or Neither: Which is Better for Psychological Benefits? Am J Health Behav. 2011 Mar 1;35(2):199–208.

51. Suh JH, Han SJ, Jeon SY, Kim HJ, Lee JE, Yoon TS, et al. Effect of rhythmic auditory stimulation on gait and balance in hemiplegic stroke patients. NeuroRehabilitation. 2014 Jan 1;34(1):193–9.

52. Hayden R, Clair AA, Johnson G, Otto D. The effect of rhythmic auditory stimulation (RAS) on physical therapy outcomes for patients in gait training following stroke: a feasibility study. Int J Neurosci. 2009 Nov 16;119(12):2183–95.

53. Hurt CP, Rice RR, McIntosh GC, Thaut MH. Rhythmic Auditory Stimulation in Gait Training for Patients with Traumatic Brain Injury. J Music Ther. 1998 Dec 21;35(4):228–41.

54. Conklyn D, Stough D, Novak E, Paczak S, Chemali K, Bethoux F. A Home-Based Walking Program Using Rhythmic Auditory Stimulation Improves Gait Performance in Patients With Multiple Sclerosis: A Pilot Study. Neurorehabil Neural Repair. 2010 Nov 1;24(9):835–42.

55. Ho C-F, Maa S-H, Shyu Y-IL, Lai Y-T, Hung T-C, Chen H-C. Effectiveness of Paced Walking to Music at Home for Patients with COPD. COPD J Chronic Obstr Pulm Dis. 2012 May 29;9(5):447–57.

56. Nombela C, Hughes LE, Owen AM, Grahn JA. Into the groove: Can rhythm influence Parkinson's disease? Neurosci Biobehav Rev. 2013 Dec;37(10, Part 2):2564–70.

57. Kudlacek S, Pietschmann F, Bernecker P, Resch H, Willvonseder R. The impact of a senior dancing program on spinal and peripheral bone mass. Am J Phys Med Rehabil Assoc Acad Physiatr. 1997 Dec;76(6):477–81.

58. **Shigematsu R, Chang M, Yabushita N, Sakai T, Nakagaichi M, Nho H, Tanaka K.** Dance-based aerobic exercise may improve indices of falling risk in older women. Age Ageing 2002;**31**(4):261–66.

59. **Fancourt D, Ockelford A, Belai A.** The psychoneuroimmunological effects of music: A systematic review and a new model. Brain Behav Immun. 2014 Feb;**36**:15–26.

60. **Jeong Y-J, Hong S-C, Lee MS, Park M-C, Kim Y-K, Suh C-M.** Dance Movement Therapy Improves Emotional Responses and Modulates Neurohormones in Adolescents with Mild Depression. Int J Neurosci. 2005 Jan 1;**115**(12):1711–20.

61. **McMurray RG, Hackney AC, Guion WK, Katz VL.** Metabolic and hormonal responses to low-impact aerobic dance during pregnancy: Med Sci Sports Exerc. 1996 Jan;**28**(1):41–6.

62. **Smyth JM, Hockemeyer JR, Tulloch H.** Expressive writing and post-traumatic stress disorder: Effects on trauma symptoms, mood states, and cortisol reactivity. Br J Health Psychol. 2008 Feb 1;**13**(1):85–93.

63. **Zhao TC, Kuhl PK.** Musical intervention enhances infants' neural processing of temporal structure in music and speech. Proc Natl Acad Sci. 2016 May 10;**113**(19):5212–7.

64. **Jansen P, Richter S.** Effects of a One-Hour Creative Dance Training on Mental Rotation Performance in Primary School Aged Children. Int J Learn Teach Educ Res [Internet]. 2015 Nov 18 [cited 2016 Nov 18];13(4). Available from: http://ijlter.org/index.php/ijlter/article/view/502.

65. **Deasy RJ.** Critical Links: Learning in the Arts and Student Academic and Social Development. [Internet]. Washington, DC: Arts Education Partnership, 2002 [cited 2016 Nov 30]. Available from: http://eric.ed.gov/?id=ED466413.

66. **Simmons-Stern NR, Budson AE, Ally BA.** Music as a memory enhancer in patients with Alzheimer's disease. Neuropsychologia. 2010 Aug;**48**(10):3164–7.

67. **Martin N, Lawrence KS.** Art Therapy and Autism: Overview and Recommendations. Art Ther. 2009 Jan 1;**26**(4):187–90.

68. **Kaplan RS, Steele AL.** An Analysis of Music Therapy Program Goals and Outcomes for Clients with Diagnoses on the Autism Spectrum. J Music Ther. 2005 Mar 20;**42**(1):2–19.

69. **Whipple J.** Music in Intervention for Children and Adolescents with Autism: A Meta-Analysis. J Music Ther. 2004 Jun 20;**41**(2):90–106.

70. **Boehm K, Cramer H, Staroszynski T, Ostermann T.** Arts Therapies for Anxiety, Depression, and Quality of Life in Breast Cancer Patients: A Systematic Review and Meta-Analysis. Evid Based Complement Alternat Med. 2014 Feb 26;2014:e103297.

71. **Caine J.** The effects of music on the selected stress behaviors, weight, caloric and formula intake, and length of hospital stay of premature and low birth weight neonates in a newborn intensive care unit. J Music Ther. 1991 Winter;**28**(4):180–92.

72. **Heijden MJE van der, Araghi SO, Dijk M van, Jeekel J, Hunink MGM.** The Effects of Perioperative Music Interventions in Pediatric Surgery: A Systematic Review and Meta-Analysis of Randomized Controlled Trials. PLoS One. 2015 Aug 6;**10**(8):e0133608.

73. **Hole J, Hirsch M, Ball E, Meads C.** Music as an aid for postoperative recovery in adults: a systematic review and meta-analysis. Lancet. 2015 Oct;**386**(10004):1659–71.

74. **Backé E-M, Seidler A, Latza U, Rossnagel K, Schumann B.** The role of psychosocial stress at work for the development of cardiovascular diseases: a systematic review. Int Arch Occup Environ Health. 2011 May 17;**85**(1):67–79.

75. Ginzburg K, Kutz I, Koifman B, Roth A, Kriwisky M, David D, et al. Acute Stress Disorder Symptoms Predict All-Cause Mortality Among Myocardial Infarction Patients: a 15-Year Longitudinal Study. Ann Behav Med. 2015 Oct 27;50(2):177–86.

76. Jones C, Backman C, Griffiths RD. Intensive Care Diaries and Relatives' Symptoms of Posttraumatic Stress Disorder After Critical Illness: A Pilot Study. Am J Crit Care. 2012 May 1;21(3):172–6.

77. Garrouste-Orgeas M, Coquet I, Périer A, Timsit J-F, Pochard F, Lancrin F, et al. Impact of an intensive care unit diary on psychological distress in patients and relatives. Crit Care Med. 2012 Jul;40(7):2033–40.

78. Backos AK, Pagon BE. Finding a Voice: Art Therapy with Female Adolescent Sexual Abuse Survivors. Art Ther. 1999 Jan 1;16(3):126–32.

79. Play therapy with children in crisis: A casebook for practitioners. Vol. xviii. New York, NY, US: Guilford Press; 1991. 460 pp.

80. Dokter D. Arts Therapists, Refugees, and Migrants: Reaching Across Borders. London and Philadelphia: Jessica Kingsley Publishers; 1998. 294 pp.

81. Fordyce W, Steger J. Chronic pain. In: OF Pomerleau and JP Brady (eds). Behavioral medicine: Theory and practice. Williams and Wilkins; 1979. pp. 125–53.

82. Crombez G, Vlaeyen JW, Heuts PH, Lysens R. Pain-related fear is more disabling than pain itself: evidence on the role of pain-related fear in chronic back pain disability. Pain. 1999 Mar 1;80(1–2):329–39.

83. Nainis N, Paice JA, Ratner J, Wirth JH, Lai J, Shott S. Relieving Symptoms in Cancer: Innovative Use of Art Therapy. J Pain Symptom Manage. 2006 Feb;31(2):162–9.

84. Trauger-Querry B, Haghighi KR. Balancing the focus: Art and music therapy for pain control and symptom management in hospice care. Hosp J. 1999;14(1):25–38.

85. Nilsson U. The anxiety- and pain-reducing effects of music interventions: a systematic review. AORN J. 2008 Apr;87(4):780–807.

86. Dobek CE, Beynon ME, Bosma RL, Stroman PW. Music Modulation of Pain Perception and Pain-Related Activity in the Brain, Brain Stem, and Spinal Cord: A Functional Magnetic Resonance Imaging Study. J Pain. 2014 Oct;15(10):1057–68.

87. Koch ME, Kain ZN, Ayoub C, Rosenbaum SH. The sedative and analgesic sparing effect of music. Anesthesiology. 1998 Aug;89(2):300–6.

88. Lepage C, Drolet P, Girard M, Grenier Y, DeGagné R. Music decreases sedative requirements during spinal anesthesia. Anesth Analg. 2001 Oct;93(4):912–6.

89. Juslin PN, Sloboda J. Handbook of Music and Emotion: Theory, Research, Applications. Oxford University Press; 2011. 1389 pp.

90. Hillman J. Emotion: A Comprehensive Phenomenology of Theories and Their Meaning for Therapy. Evanston, Illinois; Northwestern University Press; 1960. 340 pp.

91. Johnson JK, Louhivuori J, Siljander E. Comparison of well-being of older adult choir singers and the general population in Finland: A case-control study. Music Sci. 2016 Apr 20;1029864916644486.

92. Fancourt D, Williamon A. Attending a concert reduces glucocorticoids, progesterone and the cortisol/DHEA ratio. Public Health. 2016 Mar;132:101–4.

93. Cuypers K, Krokstad S, Holmen TL, Knudtsen MS, Bygren LO, Holmen J. Patterns of receptive and creative cultural activities and their association with perceived health, anxiety, depression and satisfaction with life among adults: the HUNT study, Norway. J Epidemiol Community Health. 2011 May 23;jech.2010.113571.

94. **Gold C, Solli HP, Krüger V, Lie SA**. Dose–response relationship in music therapy for people with serious mental disorders: Systematic review and meta-analysis. Clin Psychol Rev. 2009 Apr;**29**(3):193–207.

95. **Maratos A, Gold C, Wang X, Crawford M**. Music therapy for depression. In: Cochrane Database of Systematic Reviews [Internet]. John Wiley & Sons, Ltd; 2008 [cited 2016 Jun 27]. Available from: http://onlinelibrary.wiley.com/doi/10.1002/14651858.CD004517.pub2/abstract.

96. **Matarazzo JD**. Behavioral immunogens and pathogens in health and illness. In: Hammonds BL, Scheirer CJ, editors. Psychology and health. Washington, DC, US: American Psychological Association; 1984. pp. 9–43. (Master lecture series, Vol. **3**.).

97. **Norman P**. Health locus of control and health behaviour: An investigation into the role of health value and behaviour-specific efficacy beliefs. Personal Individ Differ. 1995 Feb 1;**18**(2):213–8.

98. **Norman P, Bennett P, Smith C, Murphy S**. Health Locus of Control and Health Behaviour. J Health Psychol. 1998 Apr 1;**3**(2):171–80.

99. **Cohen G**. Research on Creativity and Aging: The Positive Impact of the Arts on Health and Illness. Generations. 2006 Apr 1;**30**(1):7–15.

100. **Harris PR, Epton T**. The Impact of Self-Affirmation on Health Cognition, Health Behaviour and Other Health-Related Responses: A Narrative Review. Soc Personal Psychol Compass. 2009 Dec 1;**3**(6):962–78.

101. **Lewis HP**. Child Art: The Beginnings of Self-Affirmation. [Internet]. Diablo Press, 1978 [cited 2016 Oct 17]. Available from: http://eric.ed.gov/?id=ED415128.

102. **Crocker J, Niiya Y, Mischkowski D**. Why Does Writing About Important Values Reduce Defensiveness? Self-Affirmation and the Role of Positive Other-Directed Feelings. Psychol Sci. 2008 Jul 1;**19**(7):740–7.

103. **Bandura A**. Self-efficacy: Toward a unifying theory of behavioral change. Psychol Rev. 1977;**84**(2):191–215.

104. **Reynolds F**. Managing depression through needlecraft creative activities: A qualitative study. Arts Psychother. 2000;**27**(2):107–14.

105. **Clift S, Hancox G, Morrison I, Hess B, Kreutz G, Stewart D**. Choral singing and psychological wellbeing: Quantitative and qualitative findings from English choirs in a cross-national survey. J Appl Arts Health. 2010 Jan 1;**1**(1):19–34.

106. **Sparks P, Guthrie CA**. Self-Identity and the Theory of Planned Behavior: A Useful Addition or an Unhelpful Artifice?1. J Appl Soc Psychol. 1998 Aug 1;**28**(15):1393–410.

107. **Hays T, Minichiello V**. The meaning of music in the lives of older people: a qualitative study. Psychol Music. 2005 Oct 1;**33**(4):437–51.

108. **Davidson L, Strauss JS**. Sense of self in recovery from severe mental illness. Br J Med Psychol. 1992 Jun 1;**65**(2):131–45.

109. **Bergami M, Bagozzi RP**. Self-categorization, affective commitment and group self-esteem as distinct aspects of social identity in the organization. Br J Soc Psychol. 2000 Dec 1;**39**(4):555–77.

110. **Franklin M**. Art Therapy and Self-Esteem. Art Ther. 1992 Apr 1;**9**(2):78–84.

111. **Hartz L, Thick L**. Art Therapy Strategies to Raise Self-Esteem in Female Juvenile Offenders: A Comparison of Art Psychotherapy and Art as Therapy Approaches. Art Ther. 2005 Jan 1;**22**(2):70–80.

112. Leventhal H, Meyer D, Nerenz D. The common sense representation of illness danger. In: S Rachman (ed.) Contributions to medical psychology 2. Pergamon Press; 1980. pp. 7–30.

113. Moos RH, Schaefer JA. The Crisis of Physical Illness. In: Moos RH, editor. Coping with Physical Illness [Internet]. Springer US; 1984 [cited 2016 Oct 17]. pp. 3–25. Available from: http://link.springer.com/chapter/10.1007/978-1-4684-4772-9_1.

114. Folkman S, Lazarus RS. The relationship between coping and emotion: Implications for theory and research. Soc Sci Med. 1988 Jan 1;26(3):309–17.

115. Romanoff BD, Thompson BE. Meaning Construction in Palliative Care: The Use of Narrative, Ritual, and the Expressive Arts. Am J Hosp Palliat Med. 2006 Aug 1;23(4):309–16.

116. Hutchinson SL, Loy DP, Kleiber DA, Dattilo J. Leisure as a Coping Resource: Variations in Coping with Traumatic Injury and Illness. Leis Sci. 2003 Apr 1;25(2–3):143–61.

117. Councill T. Art Therapy with Pediatric Cancer Patients: Helping Normal Children Cope with Abnormal Circumstances. Art Ther. 1993 Apr 1;10(2):78–87.

118. Kato PM, Cole SW, Bradlyn AS, Pollock BH. A video game improves behavioral outcomes in adolescents and young adults with cancer: A randomized trial. Pediatrics. 2008 Aug;122(2):e305–17.

119. Taylor SE. Adjustment to threatening events: A theory of cognitive adaptation. Am Psychol. 1983;38(11):1161–73.

120. Weiner B. An attributional theory of achievement motivation and emotion. Psychol Rev. 1985;92(4):548–73.

121. Kydd P. Using music therapy to help a client with Alzheimer's disease adapt to long-term care. Am J Alzheimers Dis Other Demen. 2001 Mar 1;16(2):103–8.

122. Thaut MH, Gardiner JC, Holmberg D, Horwitz J, Kent L, Andrews G, et al. Neurologic Music Therapy Improves Executive Function and Emotional Adjustment in Traumatic Brain Injury Rehabilitation. Ann N Y Acad Sci. 2009 Jul 1;1169(1):406–16.

123. Tedeschi RG, Calhoun LG. TARGET ARTICLE: 'Posttraumatic Growth: Conceptual Foundations and Empirical Evidence'. Psychol Inq. 2004 Jan 1;15(1):1–18.

124. Thambyrajah C, Herold J, Altman K, Llewellyn C. 'Cancer Doesn't Mean Curtains': Benefit Finding in Patients with Head and Neck Cancer in Remission. J Psychosoc Oncol. 2010 Nov 2;28(6):666–82.

125. Marmot MG, Allen J, Goldblatt P, Boyce T, McNeish D, Grady M, et al. Fair society, healthy lives: Strategic review of health inequalities in England post-2010 [Internet]. London UK: The Marmot Review; 2010 Feb [cited 2016 Jun 22]. Available from: http://discovery.ucl.ac.uk/111743/.

126. Healthy Lives, Healthy People: our strategy for public health in England—Publications—GOV.UK [Internet]. [cited 2016 Jun 27]. Available from: http://www.gov.uk/government/publications/healthy-lives-healthy-people-our-strategy-for-public-health-in-england.

127. Cohen S. Social Relationships and Health. Am Psychol. 2004;59(8):676–84.

128. Uchino BN. Social Support and Health: A Review of Physiological Processes Potentially Underlying Links to Disease Outcomes. J Behav Med. 2006 Jun 7;29(4):377–87.

129. Shankar A, McMunn A, Banks J, Steptoe A. Loneliness, social isolation, and behavioral and biological health indicators in older adults. Health Psychol. 2011;30(4):377–85.

130. Cohen S, Wills TA. Stress, social support, and the buffering hypothesis. Psychol Bull. 1985 Sep;98(2):310–57.

131. Tarr B, Launay J, Dunbar RIM. Music and social bonding: 'self-other' merging and neurohormonal mechanisms. Front Psychol [Internet]. 2014 Sep 30 [cited 2015 Apr 28];5. Available from: http://www.ncbi.nlm.nih.gov/pmc/articles/PMC4179700/.

132. Karkou V, Glasman J. Arts, education and society: the role of the arts in promoting the emotional wellbeing and social inclusion of young people. Support Learn. 2004 May 1;19(2):57–65.

133. Murrock CJ, Madigan E. Self-Efficacy and Social Support as Mediators Between Culturally Specific Dance and Lifestyle Physical Activity. Res Theory Nurs Pract. 2008 Aug 1;22(3):192–204.

134. Cohen G, Perlstein S, Chapline J, Kelly J, Firth KM, Simmens S. The Impact of Professionally Conducted Cultural Programs on the Physical Health, Mental Health, and Social Functioning of Older Adults—2-Year Results. J Aging Humanit Arts. 2007 Jun 8;1(1–2):5–22.

135. Crawford P, Lewis L, Brown B, Manning N. Creative practice as mutual recovery in mental health. Ment Health Rev J. 2013 Jun 21;18(2):55–64.

136. McDougall W. The group mind, a sketch of the principles of collective psychology, with some attempt to apply them to the interpretation of national life and character [Internet]. New York, London, G.P. Putnam's Sons; 1920 [cited 2016 Oct 17]. 456 pp. Available from: http://archive.org/details/groupmindsketcho00mcdo.

137. Abrams D, Hogg MA. Comments on the motivational status of self-esteem in social identity and intergroup discrimination. Eur J Soc Psychol. 1988 Aug 1;18(4):317–34.

138. Hogg MA. Social identity theory. In: Burke PJ, editor. Contemporary Social Psychological Theories. Stanford: Stanford University Press; 2006.

139. Leuthold S. Indigenous Aesthetics: Native Art, Media, and Identity. University of Texas Press; 1998. 260 pp.

140. Coleman EB. Aboriginal Art, Identity and Appropriation. Aldershot, England ; Burlington, VT: Routledge; 2005. 206 pp.

141. Lee D. How the Arts Generate Social Capital to Foster Intergroup Social Cohesion. J Arts Manag Law Soc. 2013 Jan 1;43(1):4–17.

142. Vaughan GM. Social change and racial identity: Issues in the use of picture and doll measures. Aust J Psychol. 1986 Dec 1;38(3):359–70.

143. Baumeister RF, Boden JM. Aggression and the self: High self-esteem, low self-control, and ego threat. In: Geen RG, Donnerstein E, editors. Human aggression: Theories, research, and implications for social policy. San Diego, CA, US: Academic Press; 1998. pp. 111–37.

144. Harris R. Singing the Village: Music, Memory and Ritual Among the Sibe of Xinjiang. OUP/British Academy; 2004. 262 pp.

145. Harrison K. 'Singing my Spirit of Identity': Aboriginal Music for Well-being in a Canadian Inner City. MUSICultures [Internet]. 2013 Feb 11 [cited 2016 Oct 17];36(0). Available from: https://journals.lib.unb.ca/index.php/MC/article/view/20244.

146. **Levine E, Levine SK.** Art in Action: Expressive Arts Therapy and Social Change. London and Philadelphia: Jessica Kingsley Publishers; 2011. 244 p.

147. **Ockelford A.** Songs Without Words: Exploring How Music Can Serve as a Proxy Language in Social Interaction with Autistic Children. In: MacDonald R, Kreutz G, Mitchell L, editors. Music, Health, and Wellbeing. OUP Oxford; 2012.

148. **Whitehurst GJ, Falco FL, Lonigan CJ, Caulfield M.** Accelerating language development through picture book reading. Dev Psychol. 1988;**24**(4):552–9.

149. **Falk D.** Prelinguistic evolution in early hominins: whence motherese? Behav Brain Sci. 2004 Aug;**27**(4):491–503–583.

150. **Kertz-Welzel A.** Patriotism and Nationalism in Music Education. Farnham, Surrey: Routledge; 2016. 202 p.

151. The Role of Culture in Preventing and Reducing Poverty and Social Exclusion. European Commission; 2005. 6 pp.

152. **Martin G, Clarke M, Pearce C.** Adolescent Suicide: Music Preference as an Indicator of Vulnerability. J Am Acad Child Adolesc Psychiatry. 1993 May;**32**(3):530–5.

153. **Steinweis AE.** Art, Ideology, and Economics in Nazi Germany: The Reich Chambers of Music, Theater, and the Visual Arts. Univ of North Carolina Press; 1993. 260 pp.

154. **Edmunds N.** 'Lenin is always with us': Societ musical propaganda and its composers during the 1920s. In: Soviet Music and Society Under Lenin and Stalin: The Baton and Sickle. Routledge; 2004.

155. **Smith R.** Spend (slightly) less on health and more on the arts. BMJ. 2002 Dec 21;**325**(7378):1432–3.

Chapter 3

The political background to arts in health

As a result of the increasing evidence base of wide-ranging effects of the arts on biopsychosocial determinants of health, policy-makers have increasingly come to recognize the value of the arts for health. Since the Millennium in particular, there have been a range of papers (from both the arts world and the health world) that discuss arts in health in relation to specific policies or that make recommendations for policy-makers, such as advocating for the integration of the arts within healthcare systems or highlighting the health benefits that the arts can bring. In some instances, this advocacy has come indirectly: for example, the WHO's Quality of Life brief measure (WHOQOL-BREF) explores 24-facets to assess quality of life, one of which one is 'participation in and opportunities for recreation/leisure activities'.(1) However, there have also been policy papers directly relating to arts in health. The impact of these has been significant for the field, including leading to increased funding for research and practice, more developed lines of communication between the arts world and health world, and strategic opportunities for the profiling of arts in health activity, which all have led to increased awareness of how the arts can support health. As many arts in health programmes operate at more local levels and do not directly depend on government or other national endorsement to attract funding, partners, or participants, this political activity is often not well known among the general public. However, for programmes seeking to expand from working at a local level to operating on a larger scale, such policy activity becomes of real significance in providing evidence of high-level support and endorsement for the field.

This chapter outlines some of the key policy activities and papers of relevance to policy relating to arts in health from the past two decades. In many cases, such activities and papers have brought together representatives from arts and from health. However, for the purposes of this chapter to facilitate the tracing of a narrative between different political events, activity and papers have been separated into those that have been led by arts organizations or branches of government and those that have been led by health organizations or branches of government. Three case studies of countries in which there has been significant activity are provided for arts policy: Ireland, the UK, and the USA. Similarly, three case studies are provided for health policy: the UK, Australia, and Nordic countries. The documents referenced are not intended to be an exhaustive list, but rather give a flavour of some of the key policy documents from different countries that have shaped the development of the field internationally.

Arts policy papers

Ireland

The Arts Council of Ireland is the national agency for funding, developing, and promoting the arts in Ireland. It was one of the first major arts bodies globally to strategically promote the arts in health at a national level as a central part of core arts practice. Arts Council Ireland has supported arts in health practice since the late 1990s when it collaborated with the Eastern Health Board (which, in 2005, became the Health Service Executive) on the development of five pilot projects. The findings from this were published in *The Picture of Health*.(2) In 2001, the Arts Council of Ireland commissioned a study to map the levels of artistic activity taking place in healthcare settings: *Mapping the Arts in Healthcare Contexts in the Republic of Ireland*. This identified 150 projects in existence at the time; much higher than had been perceived. Furthermore, it emerged that one-third of the projects were already supported by a local authority (an administrative body in local government), demonstrating political buy-in.(3) In *Partnerships for the arts in practice 2006-2008*, arts in health was outlined as one of the priorities, with new funding programmes established, new initiatives planned to support practice, and a programme of advocacy work set in motion to encourage best practice and 'a higher level of recognition of arts and health as a legitimate area of artistic practice'.(4)

This led on to the appointment in 2008 of a Specialist Adviser in arts in health to develop policy and strategy work, culminating in the 2010 first *Arts and Health Policy and Strategy* document.(5) This summarized research findings to date, explored the values underpinning the Arts Council's approach to arts in health, and made recommendations for how arts in health could be promoted at a national level. Since then, the Waterford Healing Arts Trust (initially set up to support the hospital environment in Waterford Regional Hospital) and Create, the national development agency for collaborative arts in social and community contexts, have developed a website funded by the Arts Council of Ireland dedicated to arts in health: www.artsandhealth.ie. Interestingly, however, despite this volume of previous activity, the Arts Council strategy (2016-2025) did not mention health or wellbeing.(6)

UK

Within the UK, Arts Councils exist for each of the four countries: England, Wales, Scotland, and Northern Ireland. In particular, two of these have been especially active in the development of strategies for arts in health: Arts Council England and the Arts Council of Wales.

Arts Council England

Arts Council England is the national development agency for the arts in England, providing funding for a range of arts activities. In 2004, Arts Council England produced a report entitled *Arts in Health: A Review of the Medical Literature* (later followed up in 2011 as *Arts and Music in Healthcare: An overview of the medical literature 2004-2011*).(7,8) The report explored the effects of the arts on clinical outcomes, staff outcomes, training of arts practitioners, and mental health. It was carried out by Dr Rosalia Staricoff who, a few years earlier, had undertaken out a ground-breaking research study into the effects of visual and performing arts in healthcare at Chelsea and Westminster Hospital in London.(9)

A year later, Sir Nigel Crisp, the former NHS Chief Executive and Permanent Secretary at the Department of Health, set up an Arts and Health Working Group which consulted with over 300 individuals in the health service, local government, Arts Council, and other professional bodies alongside patients and members of the public and produced a report. The report explored previous NHS involvement with the arts, summarized previous research, explored what 'success' looks like in arts in health and identified barriers to wider adoption. The report concluded that 'Arts and health are, and should be firmly recognised as being, integral to health, healthcare provision and healthcare environments, including supporting staff … There are opportunities for the Department of Health and the NHS to use the arts to bring about change in some of the key influencers of health and in the use of the NHS'.(10)

The findings from the 2004 and 2006 documents were brought together in 2007 in a publication jointly issued by Arts Council England and the Department of Health entitled *A Prospectus for Arts and Health*. The prospectus stated:

> 'Some people might dismiss the arts as simply add-on activities, which have little place in a modern, technically-focused healthcare system. But this is far from being the case, as reflected in this prospectus. Those who are involved in the wealth of activity across the country have amply demonstrated the tangible benefits of arts and health. Hundreds of research projects, organisations and individuals are showing that the arts are an integral part of the nature and quality of the services we provide. They reveal the effectiveness and value of arts and health initiatives, and the benefits they bring to patients, service users and their carers, and to communities and healthcare workers in every sector.'

This prospectus celebrated the benefits of the arts in wellbeing, health, and healthcare and was a crucial step in mainstreaming arts in health in the UK.(11)

In 2013, *Towards Plan A: A new political economy for arts and culture* was published in collaboration with the Royal Society of Arts, unveiled in the inaugural lecture of Sir Peter Bazalgette when he became Chair of the Arts Council. (12) Based on a seminar series bringing together business, finance, government, local authorities, and local enterprise partnerships, the report encouraged the arts sector to consider its achievements and potential in relation to the nation's wider social and economic objectives, including the general health of society, as part of a 'holistic' case for investment. Part of the impetus behind the report was to identify whether there was a return on cultural investment. In partnership with health economists from the London School of Economics, it considered complex issues such as how to quantify and monetize improvements in wellbeing as a result of arts engagement. This has paved the way for several key publications since. In 2013, the Centre for Economics and Business Research wrote a paper for Arts Council England entitled *The Contribution of the Arts and Culture to the National Economy*.(13) One of the ways that the arts were identified as supporting national productivity was through improving wellbeing: 'an essential determinant of an individual's productivity'. The value of happiness gained through arts and cultural activities was identified as £2,047 for being an audience member to the arts, £1,500 from participating in the arts, and £3,228 from visiting museums. Specific examples were also given of the impact of the arts on health outcomes. Leading on from this, further wellbeing research was published by Arts Council England in 2015: *Cultural Activities, Artforms and Wellbeing*.(14)

Over the years since, Arts Council England has undertaken a range of other activities to encourage arts in health, including in 2015 announcing a new research grants programme, which aimed to fund pioneering research into the value of the arts across the following 3 years. This policy and advocacy work from Arts Council England has now begun to influence developments within central government too. For example, in March 2016, the Department of Culture, Media and Sport published *The Culture White Paper*; the first culture white paper in more than 50 years. This recognized the role of the cultural sectors in making 'a crucial contribution to the regeneration, health and wellbeing of our regions, cities, towns and villages'. The paper stated 'we are beginning to understand better the profound relationship between culture, health and wellbeing'.(15)

Arts Council of Wales

Arts Council of Wales is the country's official funding and development organization for the arts. Its principal sponsor is the Welsh Government. It funds, supports, and promotes the role of the arts in people's lives across Wales. Like Arts Council England, over the past decade, Arts Council of Wales has produced a series of publications highlighting the important role of the arts in health. For example, in 2005, Arts Council of Wales published a *Review of Arts and Health Activities in Wales*, which provided a snapshot of activity undertaken across 2004-2005. This highlighted a considerable body of work but showed that there was no coordinated approach. Consequently, the report made seven recommendations for developing the field further, including suggesting an All Wales strategic commitment to arts in health.(16)

Following this initial review, *Arts in Health and Well-being: an Action Plan for Wales* published in 2009 was part of a collaborative action between the Welsh Assembly Government and Arts Council of Wales to benefit and enhance the health and creativity of the population of Wales through the arts.(17) The document overviewed action in public health, healthcare settings, community programmes, arts therapies, and arts in humanities and healthcare. It aimed to raise the profile of the arts in health, support the development of initiatives, encourage strategic partnerships to enhance health and wellbeing, and provide a foundation for future development of the field in Wales.

In April 2014, Arts Council of Wales produced a publication in partnership with Wellbeing Wales, an organization that is challenging inequality in Wales by using wellbeing as a means to focus action and measure progress. *Wellbeing Assessment of Arts Council of Wales funded events, presenters, and venues* explored the impact of arts events organized by Arts Council of Wales on the wellbeing of people who attended.(18) It drew on UK wellbeing policy, identifying ways that the arts had supported economic and material wellbeing, community and society wellbeing, environmental wellbeing, and physical and psychological wellbeing. It was accompanied by *Wellbeing case studies of Arts Council of Wales venues and exhibitions* to give practical demonstrations of the work: www.arts.wales/c_research/wellbeing-case-studies.

In July 2016, the *Draft Strategic Equality Action Plan 2016-2021* was produced as a way of engaging and informing the arts sector on diversity and equalities. One of the specific targets was to ensure that participatory arts programmes and events are consistently accessible and relevant to all. One of the key objectives from 2016 onwards is to develop a major strategy for arts in health in Wales, with a particular focus on arts and mental health. More information about the consultation is available at www.arts.wales.

USA

Americans for the Arts is the leading not-for-profit organization committed to advancing the arts in America. It looks to develop local environments for the arts to thrive, advocate for increased resources for the arts and arts education across America, and foster individual understanding and appreciation for the arts. Some of the many papers on arts in health to emerge from this organization include fact pages on *Why healthcare institutions invest in the arts* (2008), summaries from conferences such as the Mini-Conference on Creativity and Aging in America held in May 2005, and monographs featuring in-depth issue papers on aspects of arts in health such as arts in hospitals (produced 1993-2010). These are available on the website www.americansforthearts.org.

In 2013, a policy roundtable in Utah led to the report *Arts and Healing: Body, Mind and Community*. This report proposed that the arts could play an important role in rehabilitation for people who had experienced mental and physical traumas.(19) It covered topics such as how the arts can aid pre-deployment of military personnel, arts for preventative care in parallel with the National Prevention Strategy of 2011, and arts for collective community identities. It made recommendations to the Department of Veterans Affairs, proposed partnerships with the Global Healthcare Alliance, and discussed opportunities for working with digital arts leaders such as Google and Yahoo.

In the same year, the 2013 white paper *Arts, Health and Wellbeing across the Military Continuum* framed a national plan for action, summarizing research into the arts and the military, overviewing practice in the USA and current policy initiatives, before making specific recommendations for future policy. (20) These recommendations emerged from the Arts and Health in the Military National Roundtable in November 2012 and the National Summit: Arts, Health and Wellbeing Across the Military Continuum.

Americans for the Arts has also established the *New Community Visions Initiative*; part of a 3-year suite launched in 2015 of large-scale initiatives called *Transforming America's Communities Through the Arts* which aims to general dialogue at a state and national level around the creation of healthy communities as well as encouraging arts programming and partnerships, all under the banner of improving healthy living over time. The programme brings together arts councils, arts boards, and city offices across the USA, and the emerging publications cover topics such as artists and communities and arts, health, and wellness.

Americans for the Arts is also being supported by other bodies working at a state level. For example, the South Dakota Arts Council along with Sanford Health and the University of South Dakota are working to develop arts in health programmes for rural settings in South Dakota. The State of Florida Division of Cultural Affairs is working with partners in the Kresge Foundation, the Florida Office of Rural Health, and the University of Florida's Arts in Medicine Programme to develop the Arts in HealthCare in Rural Communities project.

Further information and downloadable publications are available from the website www.americansforthearts.org.

Health policy papers

UK

Early health policy papers referencing the arts come from the late 1990s. One of the key drivers in setting the precedent for the consideration of the arts within health policy was the UK Nuffield Trust for Research and Policy Studies in Health Services. In 1998, the Trust organized a conference entitled *The Role of Humanities in Medicine: Beyond the Millennium*. The conference reviewed the use of humanities and the arts in medicine and health in the UK and the USA. The conference led to a 12-point action plan to support the arts in health, focusing on professional education, arts in therapy and healthcare environments, and the arts in community development. A year later, the conference was repeated and the Nuffield Trust published the report *Arts, Health & Wellbeing: from the Windsor I conference to a Nuffield forum for the medical humanities*.(21)

In the same year, the UK Department of Health published *Saving Lives: Our Healthier Nation* (1999), an action plan to tackle poor health, which mentioned the role of the arts in promoting social cohesion by building strong social networks, contributing to healthy neighbourhoods.(22) And in 2000, the Health Development Agency published a landmark piece entitled *Art for Health: a review of good practice in community-based arts projects and initiatives which impact on health and wellbeing*.(23) The paper discussed the complexity in tackling health inequalities, and suggested that social approaches to the organization and delivery of public health could have significant potential for health improvement. This built on ideas from the mid-1990s that social capital (including civic engagement, social relationships, and social support) could impact on health outcomes. The arts were identified as one of the ways of supporting social capital and broader health, with the report self-identifying as 'a very welcome first step in documenting the evidence on best practice in "arts for health" in England'.

Following on from this surge in activity, in 2004, the Nuffield Trust published another paper strategic for the arts sector, health sector, and policymakers: *Creative arts and humanities in healthcare*.(24) The paper highlighted the importance of the arts to healthcare, but noted that they do not always fit easily within the UK's target-driven national healthcare system. So the paper demonstrated how the arts could bring new opportunities to deliver on healthcare priorities. It looked at what patients, artists and healthcare staff want from arts in health programmes and made some strategic action recommendations.

On 25 November 2010, a new opportunity for the arts was outlined in a speech by the then-UK Prime Minister David Cameron in which he committed to 'start measuring our progress as a country, not just by how our economy is growing, but by how our lives are improving; not just by our standard of living, but by our quality of life'. This led to an increasing emphasis within the UK on measuring national wellbeing. In the 2010 paper *Confident communities, brighter futures. A framework for developing wellbeing*, the arts were explicitly discussed in two separate sections for their wellbeing benefits: 'participation in the arts and creativity can enhance engagement in both individuals and communities, increase positive emotions and a sense of purpose' and 'actively being involved in creativity and the arts helps people to connect with a wider sense of meaning and fulfilment, which can increase wellbeing'.(25) In fact, visiting museums and galleries and engaging in the arts were both listed as national indicators relevant to promoting purpose and participation. In response to this there were a number of acts produced that aimed to support wellbeing. For example, the *Well-being of Future Generations (Wales) Act* of 2015 was produced by the Welsh Government.(26) It is a new law that makes public bodies including local authorities, local health boards, Arts Council of Wales, National Library of Wales, National Museum of Wales, Public Health Wales NHS Trust, and Welsh Ministers think long term and work in a sustainable way, collaborating and taking a more joined-up approach to prevent problems. As an example, the act made it a duty for public bodies, including public arts bodies, to set wellbeing objectives. In this act, wellbeing was defined as having seven goals, one of which was to create a Wales of vibrant culture that encouraged people to participate in the arts. In October 2015, Arts Council of Wales published a response to this, demonstrating how the arts could and do fulfil each of the seven wellbeing goals.(27) Government wellbeing publications have continued to discuss the arts as integral to wellbeing, such as in the June 2013 *Wellbeing Policy and Analysis* update.(28)

Alongside the focus on wellbeing, there has also been an increasing emphasis within the UK and more widely on mental health (for more on the distinction between the two, see Chapter 2). The UK government's *No health without mental health* is a cross-government mental health outcomes strategy for people of all ages. Published in 2011, it set out plans to mainstream mental health. It included the following statement on the role of arts in mental health: 'There are many things individuals can do to improve their own mental health; for example, drinking within safe limits, taking regular exercise and participating in meaningful activities, such as arts and sports activities and experiencing the natural environment'.(29) Also in 2011, the British Medical Association published a report entitled *The psychological and social needs of patients*, which discussed the positive effect of arts and humanities programmes on in-patients. (30) The report included three pages on how different art forms could enhance patient experience as well as further information on the design of hospitals. Local NHS trusts have also produced their own reports discussing what the arts can bring to hospitals and community health centres, such as the 2011-2013 strategy published for the East Midlands by Derbyshire Community Health Services, Leicester City Primary Care NHS Trust, and Lincolnshire Partnership NHS Foundation Trust: *Reflecting upon the value of arts and health.*(31)

In addition to specific policy papers, the UK's National Institute for Health and Care Excellence (NICE) has also included the arts in a range of guideline papers over the past few years. For example, *Community Engagement to Improve Health* published in February 2008 suggests the running of community arts in health workshops as health promotion activities. Similarly, the *Looked-after children and young people* public health guideline from October 2010 created in partnership with the Social Care Institute for Excellence (SCIE) encourages directors of children's services, commissioners, social care teams, schools, and public health bodies to ensure access to creative arts 'to support and encourage overall wellbeing and self-esteem' in young people under the age of 25 who are in care. This was reiterated in the April 2013 quality standard paper. Similarly, the NICE Pathways document 'Mental wellbeing and independence in older people overview' encourages the integration of the arts directly into the care pathway for older people. The guidance from 2015 suggests establishing group activities including 'singing programmes, in particular, those involving a professionally-led community choir; [and] arts and crafts and other creative activities' as well as other 'activities related to hobbies and interests'. Again, this was also mentioned in the quality statement for older people in care homes in December 2013. In 2013, the clinical guidelines for *Psychosis and schizophrenia in young people: prevention and management* and in 2014 the clinical guidelines for *Psychosis and schizophrenia in adults: prevention and management* each made eight references to the arts, including 'Consider offering arts therapies to all people with psychosis or schizophrenia, particularly for the alleviation of negative symptoms'. Arts therapies are recommended to help people develop new ways of relating to others, express themselves and accept and understanding their feelings. The arts are even labelled as 'more efficacious psychological treatments' than counselling or supportive psychotherapy for people with psychosis or schizophrenia. There is also a brief mention of arts therapy in the *National Dementia Strategy* from the Department of Health from 2009. All of these documents are available via www.nice.org.uk.

This growing acceptance of the importance of arts in health has led to the development of several new commissioning models for the arts within the

UK's National Health Service. 'Arts on prescription' (sometimes known as 'arts on referral') is a type of social prescribing. In general, this does not aim to replace conventional therapies but is added alongside to support people in their recovery such as increasing social support networks, self-esteem, confidence, and transferrable skills. Nevertheless, reduced reliance on medication has been reported from some evaluations, although research into the effectiveness and potential cost-savings of the scheme is still very much under way. Funding has come broadly from arts budgets as well as charitable funding, while 'prescriptions' for patients to access the arts have come from local authorities, clinical commissioning groups, hospital trusts, and doctors' practices. Although the model has been running for a while, Health Education England produced a new resource in 2016 entitled *Social prescribing at a glance*.(32) An alternative model is cultural commissioning, by which the arts and culture are directly commissioned through the health budget (sometimes with additional external funding too). NCVO (an organization that champions the voluntary sector) provides comprehensive resources on cultural commissioning including a report on a large-scale pilot that took place across 2015-2016: www.ncvo.org.uk. Further information on commissioning models is available in Chapter 7.

Tying all of this together, the Royal Society for Public Health produced a statement paper in 2013 entitled *Arts, Health and Wellbeing Beyond the Millennium: How far have we come and where do we want to go?*(33) This led to the launch of a Special Interest Group in Arts, Health and Wellbeing which is helping to support research, practice, and policy development in the UK (see Chapter 4). And in January 2014, an All Party Parliamentary Group (APPG) in the UK was launched with the aim of informing a vision for political leadership in the field of arts, health, and wellbeing to support practitioners and stimulate progress. Since its conception, the APPG has held a series of roundtables bringing together cross-party politicians alongside leading arts organizations and health organizations. The group has made policy recommendations for government departments including the Department for Culture, Media and Sport, and ran a major national enquiry into the arts in health, the results of which were published in 2017. Minutes from the meetings, annual reports from the APPG and the recommendations for policy are available through the National Alliance for Arts Health and Wellbeing website: www.artshealthandwellbeing.org.uk/APPG.

Australia

The Australian government, like the UK government, has also discussed the arts in Department of Health publications. For example, in the *Fourth National*

Mental Health Plan: an agenda for collaborative government action in mental health 2009-2014, arts-based services were recommended as services to support mental health.(34) Art and music were also mentioned in the 2006 report for the National Mental Health Promotion and Prevention Working Party *Pathways of recovery: preventing further episodes of mental illness.*(35) Furthermore, the arts, including drama, drawing, pottery, creative writing, and painting classes, are part of the Support for Day to Day Living in the Community (D2DL) programme which transitioned to the National Disability Insurance Scheme (NDIS) in 2016 and is being rolled out across 2016-2019. Details are available on the government website www.health.gov.au.

Alongside this activity, the Australian National Rural Health Alliance, which is committed to improving the health and wellbeing of the 7 million people in rural and remote Australia, has published a series of reports on the value of the arts to healthcare. For example, the 2011 *Submission on the National Cultural Policy Discussion Paper* advocated the place of the arts in healthy lives, citing previous work by the alliance developing arts in health projects in Australia and their impact.(36) It called for Australia's cultural policy to recognize arts in health as a legitimate and established area of cultural practice, recommended the development of a national arts in health policy and strategy, and asked the Minister for the Arts to convene an ongoing network of arts and public health practitioners to address barriers to understanding and practice. In 2014, the alliance also published a supplementary submission to the National Mental Health Commission's *Review of Mental Health Services and Programmes.*(37) The submission discussed ways of supporting Aboriginal and Torres Strait Islander people, including the value of the arts for health, explaining 'Being involved in art and cultural activities has real potential to help address some of the social determinants of health'. As one of the recommendations from the submission, the alliance suggested that 'Agencies with responsibility for devising and implementing policies in mental health, should take account of the demonstrated significant social, therapeutic and economic benefits of arts in health projects'. Further submissions advocating for the arts have included the 2016 submission to the Standing Committee on Communications and the Arts, *Inquiry into Broadcasting, Online Content and Live Production to Rural and Regional Australia* subtitled *The Common Wealth of Arts and Health* available through the website www.ruralhealth.org.au.

Australia's *National Arts and Health Framework* was produced in 2015 by Australia's Health Ministers and Cultural Minsters to enhance the profile of arts in health in Australia. It grew out of work from the Institute for Creative Health in Australia which convened a forum at Parliament House Canberra in 2012 with key stakeholders. This led to the establishment of a Ministerial Working Group tasked with developing the framework. As part of the development of this framework, the Australian Health and Hospitals Association also reviewed international evidence for arts in health. The resulting framework was endorsed by Ministers of Health and Ministers of the Arts in every Australian state and territory, marking a pivotal step forwards for the field in Australia. The framework is aimed at government agencies, departments, and organizations (including arts agencies) with a role in promoting health and wellbeing and in delivering healthcare and services. It acknowledges the value and benefits of arts in health practice, endorses collaborative relationships between arts and health sectors nationally as well as across the spheres of government, and recommends continuing research in the field. Importantly, the framework considers questions such as how arts in health activity relates to arts and disability programmes and provides an in-depth list of resources for people working in Australia. The framework is available at www.instituteforcreativehealth.org.au.

Nordic countries

In 2000, the Swedish Governmental Commission on Public Health published a report on its future public health plans in Sweden.(38) For the first time, the report contained a chapter on the importance of cultural activities as a vehicle for public health work. This publication led to greater cultural interest as a part of public health in many counties and municipalities in Sweden. In 2009, this was followed up with the Cultural Politics Commission, which continued to stress the importance of culture in health promotion, and the Ministry of Health and Social Affairs and the Ministry of Culture allocated money to support pilot projects on arts and culture as rehabilitation.(39) Since then, there have been several regional evaluations launched and increased coordination between the ministries for health and social security and culture. For example, Skåne county is coordinating research on the associations between cultural participation and rates of sick leave, following government interest in reducing the rate of sick leave. The Swedish Parliament also started a Society for Culture and Health in 2007. This has tried to exert political pressure to encourage a dialogue among politicians, researchers, and cultural organizations. In collaboration with the Centre for Research on Culture and Health at the University of Gothenburg, the society has also organized several panel discussions.

Activity is not just occurring in Sweden. In Norway, the Norwegian Government instigated a number of projects bringing together culture and health totalling 15 million Norwegian crowns from 1997 to 1999. As in Sweden, one of the factors that encouraged this was high rates of sick leave. Another factor was the UNESCO project during the World Decade for Cultural Development 1988-1998, which raised awareness around the importance of culture from a public health perspective, including through an International Conference on Culture and Health in Oslo in 1995. Over the 3 years of Norwegian Government funding, 20 counties and municipalities took part, coordinated through the Centre for Culture, Health and Care in Levanger. Since the funding finished, counties and municipalities have been encouraged to continue the work at a local level.(40) However, there is still high-level support. For example, Arts Council Norway's EEA Grants focus on areas where there are demonstrable needs, including children and health as one of their areas of priority. In 2014, Norway established the Norwegian National Institute for Culture, Health and Care and some of the Norwegian Healthy Life Centres are experimenting with Arts on Prescription. Norway also has a public health law and a cultural law that emphasizes the importance of arts in health promotion and care.(40)

Meanwhile, in Finland, the Arts Promotion Centre Finland appoints regional artists for set terms of 3 years, including representatives for arts and wellbeing in each region. There are also state subsidies to support embedding art and culture services within social welfare and healthcare activities. In 2007, the Finnish Government adopted a Policy Programme for Health Promotion and launched a programme to enhance the contribution of art and culture to health and wellbeing. In 2008, the Minister for Culture and Sport commissioned an expert review in preparation for the programme. The review, entitled *Art and Culture for Well-being—proposal for an action programme 2010-2014* was published in 2010 and proposed three priority areas: culture for promotion social inclusion, culture for health promotion, and culture for supporting wellbeing at work.

In addition to country-specific activity, there have also been collaborative initiatives between countries. In 2013, the Nordic Ministers for Culture commissioned a report entitled *Turning Point*.(41) It mapped ongoing initiatives in culture and health in Nordic countries and internationally and existing research in Nordic countries, calling for a Nordic knowledge resource for culture and health and a research project exploring the socioeconomic gains afforded by the link between culture and health. Part of the reason for this investment in Nordic countries is that some of the countries have gathered extensive statistical data on cultural activities over the past few decades. For example, Statistics Sweden, the national agency for population statistics, has been producing statistics on cultural activities every 8 years since the 1970s, while the HUNT Databank in Nord Tröndelag in Norway has gathered data on cultural engagement as part of its wider studies in 125,000 citizens.

Summary

As this chapter has demonstrated, there has been a rich body of political activity underpinning the field of arts in health, in particular over the past decade. Some of this activity has been driven by national arts bodies, championing the value of the arts in health and wellbeing and advocating for their inclusion within core arts funding and practice. Other activity has been led by health bodies, including health departments within governments and health services themselves. While key case studies of countries where there has been a particularly large volume of activity have been provided, this is by no means the full extent of involvement. Arts in health is gradually being incorporated into policy developments across the world. As a few illustrative examples, UNICEF and the Uganda Ministry for Health have commissioned arts in public health projects jointly. The Indian Council for Mental Health recognizes and endorses arts in health. And the US Department of Health and Human Services (USDHHS) has set goals for its Healthy People 2020 initiative, which include AH-2 'Increase the proportion of adolescents who participate in extracurricular and/or out-of-school activities' and DH-13 'Increase the proportion of adults with disabilities aged 18 years and older who participate in leisure, social, religious or community activities', which could pave the way for more cultural engagement.

It should also be noted that the lack of political endorsement in some countries does not mean that arts in health has not flourished nor been supported; far from it. Indeed, alongside political work, there has also been a mass of activity in countries globally, including large-scale project delivery, international conferences, long-term collaborations between arts organizations and health organizations, and the formation of national bodies and boards for arts in health. In the next chapter, we will consider what 'arts in health' actually encompasses, mapping the development of some of the different strands of activity within the field over the past few decades and charting how, both with and without political endorsement, they have moved from local to national and even international scales.

References

1. **World Health Organization**. WHOQOL-BREF: introduction, administration, scoring and generic version of the assessment: field trial version [Internet]. 1996 Dec [cited 2016 Nov 14]. Available from: http://www.who.int/substance_abuse/research_tools/whoqolbref/en/.

2. **Eastern Regional Arts Committee**. The Picture of Health: a framework for the practice of arts in health settings. 2004 Dec.

3. **O Cuiv R**, Leargas Consulting. Mapping the Arts in Healthcare Contexts in the Republic of Ireland. Arts Council of Ireland; 2001.

4. **Arts Council of Ireland.** Partnership for the arts in practice 2006-2008 = Comhpháirtíocht ar son na n-ealaíon cleachtais 2006-2008. Dublin: Arts Council; 2005.

5. **Arts Council of Ireland.** Arts and Health Policy and Strategy. Arts Council of Ireland; 2010.

6. **Arts Council of Ireland.** Making Great Art Work: Leading the development of the arts in Ireland [Internet]. Dublin: Arts Council of Ireland; 2015 [cited 2016 Nov 4]. Available from: http://www.artscouncil.ie/arts-council-strategy/.

7. **Staricoff RL.** Arts in Health: A Review of the Medical Literature [Internet]. London: Arts Council England; 2004 [cited 2016 Nov 4]. Available from: https://www.researchgate.net/publication/237332598_Arts_in_Health_A_Review_of_the_Medical_Literature.

8. **Staricoff RL, Clift S.** Arts and Music in Healthcare: An overview of the medical literature 2004-2011 [Internet]. London: Chelsea and Westminster Health Charity; 2011 Jul [cited 2016 Nov 4]. Available from: http://www.lahf.org.uk/sites/default/files/Chelsea%20and%20Westminster%20Literature%20Review%20Staricoff%20and%20Clift%20FINAL.pdf.

9. **Staricoff RL, Duncan J, Wright M, Loppert S, Scott J.** A study of the effects of visual and performing arts in health care. London: Chelsea and Westminster Hospital; 2002.

10. **Cayton H.** Report of the Review of Arts and Health Working Group [Internet]. Leeds: Department of Health; 2007 Apr [cited 2016 Nov 4]. Available from: http://www.artsandhealth.ie/wp-content/uploads/2011/09/Report-of-the-review-on-the-arts-and-health-working-group-DeptofHealth.pdf.

11. **Cayton H, Hewitt P.** A prospectus for arts and health [Internet]. London: Arts Council England; 2007 [cited 2016 Nov 4]. Available from: http://www.artsandhealth.ie/wp-content/uploads/2011/09/A-prospectus-for-Arts-Health-Arts-Council-England.pdf.

12. **Royal Society of Arts and Arts Council England.** Towards Plan A: A new political economy for Arts and Culture [Internet]. Manchester: Royal Society of Arts and Arts Council England; 2013 [cited 2016 Nov 4]. Available from: https://www.thersa.org/about-us/media/2013/03/a-new-political-economy-for-arts-and-culture.

13. **Centre for Economics and Business Research Ltd.** The contribution of the arts and culture to the national economy [Internet]. London: Arts Council England and the National Museums Directors' Council; 2013 [cited 2016 Nov 4]. Available from: http://www.artscouncil.org.uk/sites/default/files/download-file/The_contribution_of_the_arts_and_culture_to_the_national_economy.pdf.

14. **Fujiwara D, MacKerron G.** Cultural Activities, Artforms and Wellbeing | Arts Council England [Internet]. London: Arts Council England; 2015 [cited 2016 Nov 4]. Available from: http://www.artscouncil.org.uk/cultural-activities-artforms-and%C2%A0wellbeing.

15. The Culture White Paper [Internet]. London: Department for Culture, Media and Sport; 2016 [cited 2016 Nov 4]. Available from: https://www.gov.uk/government/publications/culture-white-paper.

16. **Arts Council of Wales.** Review of Arts and Health Activities in Wales [Internet]. Arts Council of Wales; 2006 [cited 2016 Nov 3]. Available from: http://www.arts.wales/c_research/review-of-arts-and-health-activities-in-wales.

17. **Arts Council of Wales.** Arts in Health and Well-being—An Action Plan for Wales [Internet]. Cardiff: Arts Council of Wales; 2009 [cited 2016 Nov 4].

Available from: http://www.artshealthandwellbeing.org.uk/resources/policy/arts-in-health-and-well-being-action-plan-wales.

18. **Lles Cymru Wellbeing Wales**. Wellbeing Assessment of Arts Council of Wales funded events, presenters, and venues [Internet]. Cardiff: Arts Council of Wales; 2014 [cited 2016 Nov 4]. Available from: http://www.arts.wales/c_research/wellbeing-assessment-events-presenters-venues.

19. **National Arts Policy Roundtable**. Arts and Healing: Body, Mind and Community [Internet]. Utah: Americans for the Arts; 2013 [cited 2016 Nov 4]. Available from: http://www.americansforthearts.org/sites/default/files/pdf/2014/by_program/reports_and_data/legislation_and_policy/national_arts_policy_roundtable/2013-NAPR-Report-Arts-and-Healing.pdf.

20. **Americans for the Arts**. Arts, Health, and Well-Being Across the Military Continuum [Internet]. Washington, DC: Americans for the Arts; 2013 [cited 2016 Nov 4]. Available from: http://www.americansforthearts.org/by-program/reports-and-data/legislation-policy/naappd/arts-health-and-well-being-across-the-military-continuum-white-paper-and-framing-a-national-plan-for.

21. **Philipp R**. Arts, Health and Wellbeing. From the Windsor I conference to a Nuffield forum for the medical humanities [Internet]. London: The Nuffield Trust; 2002 [cited 2016 Nov 4]. Available from: http://www.nuffieldtrust.org.uk/sites/files/nuffield/publication/arts-health-and-well-being-nov02.pdf.

22. **Department of Health**. Saving Lives: Our Healthier Nation [Internet]. London: Department of Health; 1999 [cited 2016 Nov 4]. Available from: https://www.gov.uk/government/publications/saving-lives-our-healthier-nation.

23. **Health Development Agency**. Art for health. A review of good practice in community-based arts projects and initiatives which impact on health and wellbeing [Internet]. London: Health Development Agency; 2000 [cited 2016 Nov 4]. Available from: http://www.pdsw.org.uk/assets/Uploads/Breathe-Art-for-Health-good-practice-document-NHS-Health-Development-Agency-2000.pdf.

24. **Stephens G**, **Titchen A**, **McCormack B**, **Odell-Miller H**, **Sarginson A**, **Hoffman C**, et al. Creative arts and humanities in healthcare: swallows to other continents [Internet]. The Nuffield Trust; 2004 [cited 2016 Nov 4]. Available from: http://www.nuffieldtrust.org.uk/publications/creative-arts-and-humanities-healthcare-swallows-other-continents.

25. **Department of Health**. Confident communities, brighter futures: a framework for developing well-being [Internet]. London: New Horizons; 2010 [cited 2016 Nov 4] p. 98. Available from: http://webarchive.nationalarchives.gov.uk/+/www.dh.gov.uk/en/Publicationsandstatistics/Publications/PublicationsPolicyAndGuidance/DH_114774.

26. **Welsh Government**. Well-being of Future Generations (Wales) Act 2015 [Internet]. 2015 [cited 2016 Nov 4]. Available from: http://gov.wales/topics/people-and-communities/people/future-generations-act/?lang=en.

27. **Arts Council of Wales**. Consultation on the Statutory Guidance. Response from the Arts Council of Wales. Arts Council of Wales; 2015.

28. **Cabinet Office**. Wellbeing: policy and analysis: an update of wellbeing work across Whitehall [Internet]. Cabinet office; 2013 [cited 2016 Nov 4]. Available from: https://www.gov.uk/government/publications/wellbeing-policy-and-analysis.

29. **Department of Health**. No health without mental health. A cross-government mental health outcomes strategy for people of all ages [Internet]. London: Department of

Health; 2011 [cited 2016 Nov 4]. Available from: https://www.gov.uk/government/uploads/system/uploads/attachment_data/file/213761/dh_124058.pdf.

30. **British Medical Association.** The psychological and social needs of patients [Internet]. BMA Science & Education; 2011 [cited 2016 Nov 4]. Available from: http://www.ahsw.org.uk/userfiles/Other_Resources/Health__Social_Care_Wellbeing/psychologicalsocialneedsofpatients_tcm41-202964_copy.pdf.

31. **Derbyshire Community Health Services, Leicester City Primary Care NHS Trust, Lincolnshire Partnership NHS Foundation Trust.** Reflecting upon the value of Arts & Health & a new approach for the East Midlands 2011-2013. 2013.

32. **Health Education England.** Social prescribing at a glance. Manchester; 2016.

33. **RSPH.** Arts, Health and Wellbeing Beyond the Millennium: How far have we come and where do we want to go? London: Royal Society for Public Health; 2013, pp. 1–119.

34. **Australian Government Department of Health and Ageing.** Fourth National Mental Health Plan: an agenda for collaborative government action in mental health 2009-2014 [Internet]. Australian Government Department of Health and Ageing; 2009 [cited 2016 Nov 4]. Available from: http://www.health.gov.au/internet/main/publishing.nsf/content/mental-pubs-f-plan09.

35. **Rickwood D.** Pathways of recovery: preventing further episodes of mental illness (monograph) [Internet]. Australian Government Department of Health and Ageing; [cited 2016 Nov 4]. Available from: http://www.health.gov.au/internet/main/publishing.nsf/content/mental-pubs-p-mono.

36. **ABC National Cultural Policy Submission.** National Cultural Policy discussion paper [Internet]. ABC National Cultural Policy Submission; 2011 [cited 2016 Nov 4]. Available from: http://about.abc.net.au/reports-publications/national-cultural-policy-discussion-paper-october-2011/.

37. **National Mental Health Commission.** Contributing Lives, Thriving Communities—Review of Mental Health Programmes and Services [Internet]. 2014 [cited 2016 Nov 4]. Available from: http://www.mentalhealthcommission.gov.au/our-reports/contributing-lives,-thriving-communities-review-of-mental-health-programmes-and-services.aspx.

38. **SOU.** Hälsa på lika villkor [Health on equal terms]. Stockholm: Commission of the Swedish Government; 2000.

39. **SOU.** 16 Kulturutredningen [Commission on culture]. Stockholm: Commission of the Swedish Government; 2009.

40. **Theorell T, Knudtsen MS, Horwitz EB, Wikström B-M.** Culture and public health activities in Sweden and Norway—Oxford Medicine. In: Clift S, Camic PM, editors. Oxford Textbook of Creative Arts, Health, and Wellbeing: International perspectives on practice, policy and research [Internet]. Oxford: Oxford University Press; 2015 [cited 2016 Nov 14]. Available from: http://oxfordmedicine.com/view/10.1093/med/9780199688074.001.0001/med-9780199688074-chapter-21.

41. Kultur kan stärka välfärden i Norden—Kulturradet [Internet]. 2014 [cited 2016 Dec 8]. Available from: http://www.kulturradet.se/Kultur-och-halsa/Nyheter/Nyheter-2014/Norden/.

Chapter 4

Defining arts in health

What is arts in health?

Despite ancient historical roots and global activity, a standardized definition of arts in health still does not exist. Influential proposals of definitions include 'creative activities that aim to improve individual or community health using arts-based approaches, and that seek to enhance healthcare delivery through provision of artworks or performances'(1) and 'a range of arts practices occurring primarily in healthcare settings, which brings together the skills and priorities of both arts and health professionals'.(2) However, no single definition has become standard. Indeed, the exact name of the field is itself unclear. Some refer to 'arts and health', intended to signify the bringing together of two worlds, giving equal weighting to both. Others prefer 'arts in health', seeing it not as the complete alignment of two fields, but rather the use of the arts as a way of supporting individual health or healthcare systems. Others still refer to 'arts for health', implying more of an advocacy role. Whichever term is used, the core ingredients of the combining of arts and health remain the same. Nevertheless, arriving at a more specific definition than this can be rather challenging, in part because one of the defining features of the field of arts in health is its variety.

Arts in health activity encompasses a broad range of art forms, from visual arts such as paintings and photography, to crafts and sculpture, to performance art and theatre, to all genres of dance and music, whether watched or performed, to design elements including architecture, to film, new media, and technology. In addition, every major health condition has at one point or another been brought into the mix, whether physical health conditions or mental health conditions; acute or chronic; inherited or acquired. Even the target participants of arts in health activity vary enormously, from people at risk, to those with the condition and those who have recovered; encompassing not only patients but also relatives, friends, and healthcare staff; focusing both on individuals and on entire communities and nations; taking place across both high and low income countries; and cutting through different populations within society. Given this diversity, a number of people have tried to categorize arts in health into different subfields.

Continua models

One model, called the 'Arts and Health Diamond' proposed by Macnaughton, White, and Stacy (2005) in an article in *Health Education* has suggested that activity within arts in health exists on two axes: the first moving from the extremes of focusing on the individual effects to focusing on the social effects, with the other moving from focusing on the health services to focusing on the art itself (see Figure 4.1).(3) According to this model, projects can situate themselves somewhere within the four points of the grid or diamond, moving from art to health and from social to individual. However, the model implies that for a project to be more embedded within health services it has to move towards the 'health' end of the spectrum, and thus has to have less of the arts involved, moving away from the 'arts' end of spectrum. This could be seen to imply that rather than sitting alongside one another, the arts and health sit as polar opposites.

Another continua categorization by Gary Ansdell splits activity also onto social and individual but has a second axis that moves from mind to body (see Figure 4.2). Ansdell's model specifically was developed for music therapy, but its principles are very interesting, and indeed it provides an alternative framework to Macnaughton, White, and Stacey's if extrapolated to the larger field of arts in health.

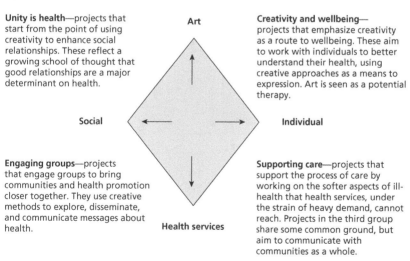

Key dimensions of arts/health

Unity is health—projects that start from the point of using creativity to enhance social relationships. These reflect a growing school of thought that good relationships are a major determinant on health.

Art

Creativity and wellbeing—projects that emphasize creativity as a route to wellbeing. These aim to work with individuals to better understand their health, using creative approaches as a means to expression. Art is seen as a potential therapy.

Social ← → **Individual**

Engaging groups—projects that engage groups to bring communities and health promotion closer together. They use creative methods to explore, disseminate, and communicate messages about health.

Health services

Supporting care—projects that support the process of care by working on the softer aspects of ill-health that health services, under the strain of heavy demand, cannot reach. Projects in the third group share some common ground, but aim to communicate with communities as a whole.

Figure 4.1 Arts and Health Diamond. Reproduced from Jane Macnaughton, Mike White, and Rosie Stacy, *Health Education*, 105 (5), pp. 332–339, http://dx.doi.org/10.1108/09654280510617169, © Emerald Group Publishing Limited all rights reserved.

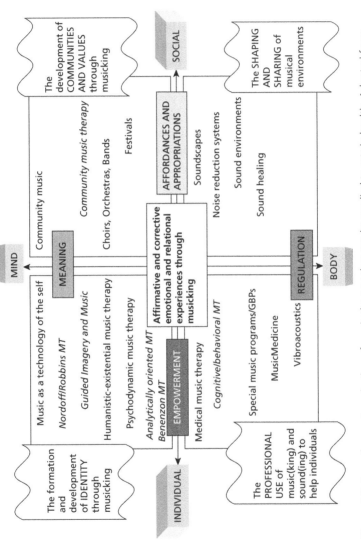

Figure 4.2 A continua categorisation of music therapy that can be applied to arts in health. Adapted from Ansdell, G. Musicology: Misunderstood guest at the music therapy feast? In: D. Aldridge, G. Di Franco, E. Ruud, and T. Wigram (eds.) *Music Therapy in Europe*. The 5th European Music Therapy Congress (Napoli, April 2001), pp. 1-33 © ISMEZ, 2001.

Ansdell's model looks at the aims of the activity, and proposes that different projects can be situated along two continua: the first moving from the extremes of focusing on the individual effects to focusing on the social effects (similar to the Arts and Health Diamond), with the other moving from focusing on the mind to focusing on the body. According to this model, projects that are more focused on the mind and individual can lead to the formation and development of identity, whereas those that focus on the mind and are more social can help with the development of communities and values. Similarly, projects that focus more on the mind generate meaning, whereas those that focus more on the body help with regulation. This is certainly a useful way of categorizing activities to differentiate between different strands of work. However, there is a challenge to continua models in general: many projects have multi-layered effects. As discussed in Chapter 2 when looking at psychosomatic medicine and psychoneuroimmunology, projects that intend to affect the mind may well also have regulatory effects on the body. Similarly, projects that are delivered to social groups can also have deep personal resonance and empowering effects for individuals. Consequently, although continua models can help to contextualize the core techniques and aims involved in a project, the complexities and diversity of the field of arts in health arguably go beyond just two continua.

Venn diagram model

An alternative to the continua models is a Venn diagram model. For example, Raymond MacDonald proposed a Venn diagram approach for categorizing work in music, health, and wellbeing (see Figure 4.3). While this is a subset of the field already, the principles of the Venn diagram approach could be extended to arts and health more broadly. This approach differentiates between the settings in which people receive music (or the arts more generally), specifically subdividing into community, educational, everyday, and therapeutic settings.

This model is attractive in that the circles overlap, such that projects can be classified in more than one way. However, it is arguable that there are more than just these four domains, even for music alone. Indeed, a later article by MacDonald added MusicMedicine as an additional circle; an off-shoot of music therapy.(4) The differences between these two areas of work will be discussed later, but this highlights that activity cannot necessarily be split into just these four domains. Yet if we increase the number of domains, we also increase the complexity of any potential model, with the risk of providing more confusion than clarification.

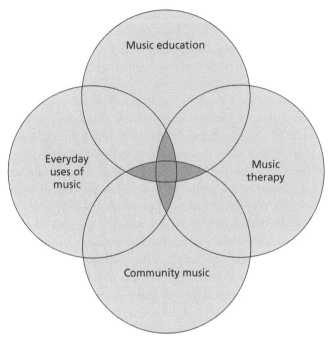

Figure 4.3 A conceptual framework for music, health and wellbeing. This material was originally published in Raymond MacDonald, Gunter Kreutz, and Laura Mitchell, 'What is Music, Health, and Wellbeing and Why is it Important?', in *Music, Health, and Wellbeing* edited by Raymond MacDonald, Gunter Kreutz, and Laura Mitchell, p. 8, Figure 1.1 © Oxford University Press, 2012 and has been reproduced by permission of Oxford University Press http://www.oxfordscholarship.com/view/ 10.1093/oso/9780199586974.001.0001/acprof-9780199586974?rskey=Ta1RzS& result=1. For permission to reuse this material, please visit http://www.oup.co.uk/ academic/rights/permissions.

Does a model exist?

Given these challenges with fitting arts in health activity into a model, a key question is does such a model exist? Changes over the last decade of practice have arguably signalled a change in the way that we now see arts in health, albeit a change that has happened so gradually as to be almost imperceptible. As opposed to having a toolbox of arts in health projects and selecting the one that appears to best suit the participant group and health needs at hand, arts in health projects are generally bespoke for each situation; specially designed to fit the specific needs of those involved. This approach arguably renders any model impossible and at the same time removes some of the boundaries around the field of arts in health to offer seemingly limitless possibilities for types of activity. On the one hand this can be seen as a positive in that it affords so many options to the field; however, some form of categorization is still necessary to describe succinctly what arts in health involves.

Consequently, for the purpose of describing some of the key areas of activity for this book, arts in health activity has been split into seven categories[1]:

1. Arts in the healthcare environment

2. Participatory arts programmes for specific patient groups

3. General arts activities in everyday life

4. Arts in psychotherapy

5. Arts in healthcare technology

6. Arts-based training for staff

7. Arts in health education

These categories are by no means exhaustive, partly because new types of activities are emerging so quickly. Furthermore, there is significant overlap between some of them. For example, the increasingly ubiquitous nature of healthcare technology means that arts in healthcare technology projects can also overlap with general arts activities in everyday life. However, these categories can be of help in mapping activity within the field. The rest of this chapter considers each of these categories in turn, looking at what the category encompasses, case studies of practice, and sources of further reading. It also gives an overview of how these areas of activity have developed over the past century from wider arts in health activity described in Chapter 1. In general, each of these areas has had a rich and unique history in each country in which it has developed. But such full histories move beyond the confines of this book. So, instead, examples have been selected from different countries to illustrate how each area of activity developed and give a flavour of how different organizations took root and spread, with further reading recommended for those who wish to know more.

Types of arts in health

Arts in the healthcare environment

Overview

Arts in the healthcare environment refers to the use of the arts in the design or enhancement of spaces within healthcare institutions such as hospitals, doctors' surgeries, hospices, care homes, and community clinics. It ranges from the architectural planning of buildings, to their enrichment through a variety of art forms. Examples of arts in the healthcare environment could include:

- ◆ Colour schemes and design to create relaxing environments for in-patients
- ◆ Personalized bed areas to re-humanize clinical wards
- ◆ Ambient sounds or background music in critical care spaces to support calmness
- ◆ Artistic wayfinding such as signage and maps to reduce disorientation
- ◆ Artwork and films to provide distraction in waiting areas
- ◆ Gardens to enhance wellbeing
- ◆ Exhibitions and public concerts in healthcare settings to uplift patients, staff, and visitors

History

The use of arts in the healthcare environment, as we saw from Chapter 1, has a long history. However, since the mid-twentieth century, there has been a heightened awareness of its importance, mainly because of a series of pivotal moments and key individuals and organizations that have helped to drive forwards the field and shape the way that the arts are conceptualized within modern hospitals.

One of the defining moves was from the commissioning of individual artworks for hospitals, such as works celebrating the donor whose generosity had enabled the hospital to be built, to the acquisition of high volumes of artwork for each hospital, so that art was not just found in key areas of the hospital but was available across networks of corridors and wards. An organization that played a role in this move is Paintings in Hospitals, which was founded as an arts lending organization in 1959, providing artwork across the UK to hospitals on rotation. It was founded by Sheridan Russell, formerly the head almoner at the National Hospital for Nervous Diseases in London. He started borrowing paintings from friends and galleries and hanging them in his department. The positive response he got for this work led to him establishing Paintings in Hospitals in partnership with the Nuffield Foundation, with each artwork chosen to ensure it would support comfort and relaxation in patients and relatives. The organization has since developed to operate satellite schemes for its collection of nearly 4,000 artworks and it also leads arts workshops and creative projects.(5)

However, the mid-twentieth century also saw the appetite for artwork in hospitals expand into a desire for a more embedded approach to arts in hospitals that not only placed paintings onto walls but also redesigned the walls themselves. For example, in the 1930s in Mexico, there was a flourishing of mural painting that resulted in awe-inspiring artworks in hospitals. Interestingly, the style ranged from serene images of nature and health, as displayed in the Hospital de la Raza in Mexico City painted by Diego Rivera, to dramatic and tragic images of mourning, as produced in the Hospicio Cabanas in Guadalajara by José Clemente Orozco.(6) As with hanging artworks on walls, there were larger-scale moves to roll out murals in certain countries. In 1979, the King's Fund, an independent charity that aims to improve health and care in England, established a scheme called 'Murals for Hospital Decoration', which was later renamed the 'Art in Hospital Scheme.' It commissioned young artists to paint murals for NHS hospitals in Greater London, aiming to transform the feel of the hospital spaces. The success of this scheme led to a larger-scale project being rolled out over the following decade which funded over 40 commissions totalling around £20,000 of investment per year.(7)

This early work led to the launch of a larger programme by the King's Fund that looked even broader than the walls and reassessed the environment itself: 'Enhancing the Healing Environment'. Its main areas of focus were end-of-life environments, including those in hospitals, mental health trusts, and hospices, and dementia environments. Specifically, the programme expanded the 'arts' in hospitals into a more comprehensive examination of the environment as a whole, including its layout, natural light, sound, ease of access, and usage by patients. The programme also combined research and evaluation to identify which sorts of environments could help targeted patient groups, such as dementia patients, and developed toolkits to measure the suitability of different environments for patient groups. This more scientific approach to the use of arts in hospitals has had a global impact in terms of how healthcare environments are imagined and designed, pushing not just for aesthetic beauty but for the arts to help improve the functioning of hospitals. In total over the lifetime of the Enhancing the Healing Environment programme, more than £2.25 million was invested in projects in the UK alone and over 250 teams from hospitals, hospices, mental health trusts, and prisons were involved.

Case study

Title: De Hogeweyk Dementia Village

Aims and objectives: Hogeweyk was established in the Netherlands with the aim of radically changing how people visualized care for those with severe dementia. Drawing on evidence showing that traditional nursing homes can provide greater confusion for dementia patients by removing them from environments with which they are familiar, leading to altered behaviour and depression, Hogeweyk aimed to de-institutionalize residential care, transform sterile environments into supportive ones, and provide 'life as normal'.

The project: As opposed to a nursing home, Hogeweyk is a nursing village, complete with restaurants, gardens, a grocery store, pub, theatre, and hair salon. Residents can walk around freely as the site is entirely enclosed and secure. Staff dress in street clothes and are specifically trained to work with individuals with dementia. Around 150 residents live in 23 small houses, each with six to seven bedrooms, two bathrooms, and a kitchen. Residents are housed with like-minded people, with lifestyle groups identified from a Dutch national database. These groups include 'homey', for people who focus on housekeeping and family and want a simple life; 'craftsman', for people who are traditional, hardworking, and early to rise; 'aristocracy', for people who prefer a more formal and classic living design and are accustomed to having household staff; and 'arts and culture', for international travellers who are more adventurous. These groups guide the design of the living spaces, background music, and meal choices.

Research: The programme draws heavily on research into how environments can be transformed to support dementia patients, including data suggesting the importance of exercise, fresh air and daylight, views of nature, social contacts, and small group activities. Dementia-friendly design is used in the architecture, public spaces, and interior design of the buildings. Evaluation of the programme has shown decreases in challenging behaviours, the use of incontinence materials, the need for sedatives, and the need for ground food. The programme has received high satisfaction ratings from residents, families, and staff. Importantly, the programme costs around the same per month as other nursing homes, making it a viable financial option for families. Similar villages are now being built in other countries.

Further information: For more information about the programme including photographs of the site and evaluation findings, visit http://hogeweyk.dementiavillage.com/

Q *The Arts in HealthCare: Learning from Experience* edited by Duncan Haldane and Susan Loppert gives a rich insight into the history and use of art in hospitals across the world, with a particular focus on the UK, US, Australia, Austria, and Japan.(8) *Art in Hospitals: A Guide* by Lesley Greene was produced in 1989 to provide guidelines on how to commission artworks for hospitals.(9) The King's Fund has published a range of resources, including its guide to *Developing supportive design for people with dementia*, its guide to *Environments for care at end of life*, specific tools for assessing whether a care home, house, health centre, or hospital is dementia-friendly, and a range of guidelines and audit tools for hospices. These are all available through its website www.kingsfund. org.uk. There is also a database of completed projects available to browse. Finally, *Healing Spaces: The Science of Place and Wellbeing* by Esther M. Sternberg explores every angle of healthcare environments from the visual attraction to the acoustic balance, the logic of wayfinding, the incorporation of gardens, and how these principles translate into the world outside hospitals too.(10)

Participatory arts programmes for specific patient groups

Overview

Participatory arts programmes aim to get people taking part. They are normally targeted at a specific audience such as a patient group or people supporting a patient such as carers, and are designed to meet an identified health or wellbeing need. They can take place in healthcare institutions such as hospitals but can also take place in broader settings such as in the local community, including public spaces or participants' homes. Examples of participatory arts programmes include:

+ Dance-physio classes for amputees
+ Dementia reminiscence sessions
+ Singing workshops for people with chronic lung disease
+ Drumming workshops for people with depression
+ Museum object handling for people with Alzheimer's disease
+ Magic tricks to improve motor skills for movement impairments
+ Hip-hop groups to improve support networks and reduce isolation in vulnerable teenagers

History

As with arts in the healthcare environment, participatory arts programmes for specific patient groups have developed organically from activity across history. However, there has been growing interest and activity over the last century across a range of countries. In particular, a common pattern within these countries has been the move from individuals developing their own projects to larger, even nationwide, programmes being delivered at scale. This has been supported by the formation of national alliances acting as umbrella organizations, linking together projects and providing support for larger-scale funding and activity.

For example, in the UK during World War II, a highly successful venture was the Entertainments National Services Association (ENSA), which brought live music to wounded servicemen in military hospitals. After the war, Sheila McCreery, an employee at the newly established Arts Council, had the idea of continuing this scheme in the new National Health Service hospitals. In 1947, 22 pilot concerts were given by famous artists and the success of this led to the development of the Council for Music in Hospitals (CMH). In 1999, CMH was rebranded as Music in Hospitals and still delivers over 4,000 concerts per year in hospitals around the UK.(11) Similarly, the USA has large-scale national programmes that have developed over the past few decades, such as Musicians on Call; an organization that provides music to patients in hospital, reaching over 500,000 patients since it was started in 1999.

Alongside the expanding work of these charities, national networks also have been established. Some of these have struggled with issues such as funding and been forced to close, such as the National Network for the Arts in Health (NNAH) founded in the UK in 2000 and disbanded in 2006; the Society for Arts in Healthcare founded in 1991 in the USA and later rebranded as the American Arts & Health Alliance before it too was forced to close; and the Australian Network for Arts and Health established in 1997 but closed in 2004. Nevertheless, over the past decade, new organizations have been founded. For example, in the UK, the National Alliance for Arts, Health and Wellbeing was formed in 2012. Comprising nine regional organizations across England, it advocates on behalf of work in the field and acts as a hub of information as well as encouraging the use of the arts by health and social care providers and working in partnership with the Special Interest Group in Arts, Health and Wellbeing run by the Royal Society for Public Health. In the USA, one example of national work is the Society and the National Endowment for the Arts (NEA), which has undertaken programmes of work mapping the field of arts in healthcare institutions to try and integrate the arts within healthcare on a national level. And in Australia, the Australian Centre for Arts and Health (ACAH) leads an annual conference while the Institute for Creative Health (ICH) sponsors national awards and has worked with Creative Partnerships Australia, a government organization established to increase private sector support for the arts.

Case study

Title: Breathe Magic Intensive Therapy Programme

Aims and objectives: Approximately 1 in 1,300 young people has hemiplegia: a paralysis affecting one side of the body. Of the young people affected, 65% could benefit from intensive motor therapy, and of those, 60% also suffer from psychosocial comorbidities. However, there are limited intensive motor therapies available, with few that concurrently integrate psychosocial therapies and even fewer that are fun for children.

The project: Breathe Magic Intensive Therapy is a service designed by occupational therapists, academics in the field of neuroscience, and Magic Circle magicians, which incorporates traditional therapy exercises into magic tricks so children have a clear incentive and goal to carry out their rehabilitation. As part of a 12-day summer Magic Camp and follow-up workshops, young people with hemiplegia aged 7–19 undertake 78 hours of one-to-one intensive therapy in a group setting, learning not just how to do the magic tricks but also how to be a magician, speaking confidently, making eye contact, and holding the audience's attention.

Research: Breathe Magic is built on a medical model called the Hand Arm Bimanual Intensive Therapy programme (HABIT), which has been researched in its own right. In addition, further research around the programme has shown and replicated clinically significant improvements in bimanual motor skills and independence following the programme, reported improvements in psychological wellbeing, communication skills, self-esteem, and parent-child relationships, and shown reduction in the hours of care and support needed by each child. The programme has been shown to be comparable cost-wise to other treatments such as Botulinum toxin injections and, through its combined psychosocial and physiological approach supporting mental health and encouraging independence among young people, it also helps people with hemiplegia to engage more and contribute to society, with wider potential economic gains. To date, camps have been run in Wales, Australia, and England, where it has been commissioned across the National Health Service. A new programme is under way to try and scale the project to further locations.

Further information: For more information and to see research papers associated with the programme, visit www.breatheahr.org.

Q Many of the national associations for arts in health have bespoke websites with links to regional organizations, conferences, frameworks, and minutes from meetings. In the UK, these include the National Alliance for Arts, Health and Wellbeing: www. artshealthandwellbeing.org.uk, and the Royal Society for Public Health Special Interest Group in Arts, Health and Wellbeing: www.rsph.org.uk/resources/special-interest-groups/arts-health-wellbeing.html. In Australia, these include the Institute for Creative Health: www.instituteforcreativehealth.org.au, and the Centre for Arts and Health: www. artsandhealth.org.au. In the USA these include the National Endowment for the Arts: www.arts.gov. For more information on other countries, *The Oxford Textbook of Creative Arts, Health and Wellbeing* (2015) provides a summary of global activity.(12)

General arts activities in everyday life

Overview

In addition to bespoke arts activities for people with diagnosed conditions, general arts and cultural engagement can also offer a variety of benefits for health and wellbeing. These can include visiting cultural sites, physically taking part in arts activities, and more receptively engaging with the arts such as through television or reading. Sometimes arts organizations market activities specifically to enhance health or wellbeing, but other times benefits can be felt from taking part without specific health-related aims. Examples of general arts activities in everyday life could include:

- Learning an instrument to support cognition
- Attending a concert to de-stress
- Visiting a gallery to feel inspired
- Leading a book club to develop social support networks
- Taking up ballet for bone strength
- Joining a pottery class to improve self-esteem
- Listening to the radio to improve mood

History

Much of the history of general arts activities has involved the same organizations and activity as participatory programmes in healthcare settings with specific patient groups. This is perhaps surprising given that the two have very different designs: participatory projects in healthcare settings focus on specific target participant groups and often have deliberate aims, whereas general arts activities in the community are often not designed with any specific intention of supporting health but rather for public enjoyment. However, there is a blurred line between the two: an arts organization may develop a strand of community work with a focus on health and wellbeing. Or individuals may decide to attend a concert, for example, deliberately to help them relax and feel less stressed. Indeed, more and more arts organizations are developing wellbeing and engagement strands to support people engaging as part of a healthy lifestyle. Consequently, although the two activities have different starting points, they can be very much aligned.

This alignment has particularly been encouraged by four developments in the last century. First, as described in Chapter 2, the way that healthcare is delivered has changed significantly over the last 100 years. With the rise of public health, there has been a gradual widening of arts in health activity beyond the confines of hospital walls to include community health centres, public spaces, and, more generally, people's individual daily lives. Second, there has been an increasing pressure on arts organizations to measure impact. Measuring impact in charities has been under way since at least the late nineteenth century. However, data suggest that this has been driven forwards in particular over the past decade by changes in funders' requirements as a result of tougher financial climates and a desire to show that investments are worthwhile.(13) As a result, arts organizations (alongside other charities and not-for-profit organizations) have had to identify myriad ways their work has an effect on different people who interact with them. For example, in the UK in 2014, Arts Council England identified four major areas in which the arts could have an impact: culture, education, society, and economy. In 2015 this was adjusted to society, the economy, education, and health and wellbeing.(14) This identification of health and wellbeing as one of the ways that the arts have an impact has, in turn, led to development of more programmes specifically targeting that impact, both from charities and also from commercial organizations. For example, global music streaming service Spotify has developed a service called 'Genres and Moods', which encourages people to listen to playlists targeted at improving how they feel. Third, community arts movements that emerged in the 1960s brought together arts, public health, and education leading to more socially engaged arts.(1) Finally, a broader awareness of the health and wellbeing benefits of the arts in healthcare settings has helped to raise the profile of the arts in general life. This follows on from the developing wellbeing agendas globally which were discussed in Chapter 2, which have made a space for the arts through their encouragement of staying active, connecting, continuing to learn, taking notice, and giving.

Case study

Title: The Whitworth Art Gallery

Aims and objectives: The Whitworth is a public art gallery and part of the University of Manchester. It aims to make fine art, textiles, and wallpapers accessible to a wide range of visitors, bringing together its rich history with contemporary culture in Manchester. The Whitworth's aspirations include developing internationally significant exhibition programmes, diversifying audiences to reflect the city and region, using the collections for teaching and learning, and developing dialogues and engagement with its visitors.

The project: The Whitworth runs a vibrant programme aimed at attracting a broad range of people, from Tuesday talks from leading artists and thinkers, to Thursday Lates which provide sociable and eclectic late-night openings, to Saturday Supplements workshops that help people to engage with the key themes of current exhibitions, and family half-term events to get children engaged with the arts. They also run programmes specifically for pregnant women, new mothers, toddlers, young people in pupil referral units, and older adults with dementia. The Whitworth has also held exhibitions and events in parks, shopping centres, pubs, care homes, hospitals, and skate parks. Their +Culture Shots programme also specifically takes events into hospital settings to show how culture can enhance the health and wellbeing of healthcare professionals, their patients, and families.

Research: The Whitworth is part of a 3-year Arts Council England Research Grants Programme entitled 'Not So Grim Up North' in collaboration with University College London (UCL) (2015–2018). The project aims to identify how museum activities can support health and wellbeing in different demographic groups and support recovery and rehabilitation. It focuses specifically on the effects for people living with dementia, stroke rehabilitation patients, mental health service users, and addiction recovery service users.

Further information: For more information about the various programmes, visit www.whitworth.manchester.ac.uk and www.healthandculture.org.uk. For more information about the research programme, visit www.healthandculture.org.uk/not-so-grim-up-north.

Q For further information about national public arts funders and an insight into arts activities, national arts council websites have a wealth of information. For example:

- *Americans for the Arts:* www.americansforthearts.org
- *Arts Council England:* www.artscouncil.org.uk
- *Arts Council of Northern Ireland:* www.artscouncil-ni.org
- *Arts Council of Wales:* www.arts.wales
- *Creative New Zealand—Arts Council of New Zealand:* www.creativenz.govt.nz
- *Creative Scotland:* www.creativescotland.com
- *Australia Council for the Arts:* www.australiacouncil.gov.au
- *Canada Council for the Arts:* www.canadacouncil.ca

Arts in psychotherapy

Overview

As well as activities led by arts organizations, the arts can also be used in health as established psychological therapies. Arts therapies are delivered by trained professional therapists to support people's psychological, emotional, cognitive, physical, communicative, or social needs. They can be delivered in individual or group settings. In these settings, the arts are often used as a bridge to strengthen and support patients and help them develop skills and strategies that can be transferred to other areas of their lives. Examples of the arts in psychotherapy could include:

+ Drama therapy to reduce antisocial behaviour in teenagers
+ Art therapy to express difficult feelings in people who have been bereaved
+ Music therapy to communicate without words for children with autistic spectrum disorders
+ Dance therapy to reconnect with the body for people coping with chronic illnesses
+ Poetry therapy to reduce symptoms of post-traumatic stress in military veterans
+ Play therapy to distract children having painful procedures
+ Sand tray therapy to regain control over anger

A common confusion lies around how arts therapies are different from participatory arts programmes for specific patient groups. Interventions delivered as part of music therapy, for example involving group drumming, could be very similar to community-led group drumming projects. Indeed, historically there was some overlap in the 1950s and 1960s between the British Society for Music Therapy and the charity Music in Hospitals. However, they soon moved away from one another with their key difference being that arts therapies must be delivered by trained professional therapists and have specific psychotherapeutic aims, whereas arts in healthcare settings or in everyday life are delivered normally by musicians or professional workshop leaders who do not have training as a therapist. Although there remains debate around the similarities and differences in approach between the two areas of work, the involvement of a trained therapist is still, in many countries, a defining distinction between arts therapy and other arts interventions.

History

Each individual form of arts therapy has had its own unique history, tracing back through history as discussed in Chapter 1. Although some arts therapies existed in the early twentieth century (the National Society for Musical Therapeutics in America, for example, was founded in 1903), it was in the mid-twentieth century that the arts therapies really began to emerge into their own areas of practice. Many of the early ideas within arts therapies came from psychoanalysis, drawing on theories of Sigmund

Freud and Carl Jung, among others. For example, American psychologist Margaret Naumberg, who became known as the 'Mother of Art Therapy', drew on similar methods to psychoanalytic practices of the day, developing a dynamically oriented art therapy that used art as a symbolic communication of unconscious thoughts.(15) Dancer and choreographer Marian Chace, drew on Jung's writings on the use of the arts to alleviate trauma to develop dance classes to help patients in Washington express their emotions, which became one of the early examples of dance therapy.(16) And psychiatrist and psychosociologist Jacob L. Moreno drew on the work of psychoanalysts such as Freud and Wilhelm Reich to develop 'psychodrama'; a form of spontaneous dramatization and role-play that helped clients explore their own lives.(17)

However, arts therapies did not just rely on psychiatry and psychoanalysis. They also drew on more general arts engagement. For example, in Australia, the Red Cross played an important role in the development of music therapy. In 1950, the Victoria branch of the Red Cross, which had been organizing concerts, formed a Music Therapy Committee. This was followed in 1954 by a Red Cross music library, which was established in Melbourne and started sending recordings to hospitals throughout Victoria to stimulate discussion groups led by occupational therapists. By 1984, the Red Cross Music Therapy committee had employed four music therapists and was working in 14 hospitals.(18) As another example, in the UK the British artist Adrian Hill, known for his depictions of the Western Front in World War I, used his own experiences of recovering from tuberculosis while in a sanatorium to draw aspects of his ward. Finding the process therapeutic, he went on to set up further arts projects in sanatoriums. Hill disliked the use of psychiatric terms in conjunction with art. However, he began using the term 'art therapy' to describe his work as he felt it would appeal to those working in the medical profession.(15)

The professionalization of arts therapies quickly followed. Among other examples, in the UK, the Society for Music Therapy and Remedial Music was formed in 1950 which became the British Society for Music Therapy in 1967, with the Guildhall School of Music and Drama leading the first training courses a year later. In 1966, the American Dance Therapy Association was formed. In 1975, both the Australian Music Therapy Association and Canadian Association for Music Therapy were founded. And in 1979 the North American Drama Therapy Association (NADTA) was incorporated for both Canada and the USA.

The precise forms of arts therapies in practice today vary enormously between country and even between different schools of thought. For example, within music therapy alone, there are a broad range of different models, including guided imagery and music (known as the Bonny method), a receptive music therapy method involving active music listening; analytically oriented music therapy (known as the Priestley model), a method based largely on improvization; creative music therapy (known as the Nordoff-Robbins model), originally developed for children with learning disabilities and hearing-impairments; free improvization therapy (known as the Alvin Model) also based around improvization including through unconventional ways of making sounds; and behavioural music therapy, which focuses on using music to modify adaptive behaviours and extinguish maladaptive behaviours.(18) Furthermore, arts therapies are now used across a range of settings, including hospitals, schools, hospices, care homes, prisons, community spaces, and bespoke therapy centres, as well as clients' own homes.

Case study

Title: MusicWorks

Aims and objectives: The Cape Flats is an expansive, low-lying area to the southeast of Cape Town. The area is known as 'apartheid's dumping ground' as during the apartheid many people were forcibly removed from inner city suburbs of Cape Town to the Flats. Over the past decade, young people in the Flats have been left vulnerable by the ravages of drug and alcohol abuse, violence, and high incidences of HIV/AIDS infection. As a result, many children are exposed to trauma and suffer from the debilitating effects of rage, distrust, grief, anxiety, and depression.

The project: MusicWorks provides one-on-one and group-based music therapy delivered by qualified music therapists for young children in the Flats. Music therapy is used to give a voice to children and young people who are normally unheard and support their development. Young people create songs to tell their individual stories and play instruments to help deal with strong emotions such as anger and grief.

Research: MusicWorks has captured a plethora of case studies from their work illustrating how the music therapy programme supports children who take part. They have identified the sessions as encouraging playfulness, expression, resilience, and hope in children, as well as supporting healing, strength, and empowerment.

Further information: For more information, including case studies of the project featured in the annual reports, visit www.musicworks.org.za.

Q For a broader overview of the history of art therapy, Susan Hogan's *Healing Arts: The History of Art Therapy* provides a rich overview.(15) For more information on art therapy practice, Judith A. Rubin's *Introduction to Art Therapy: sources and resources* is comprehensive and is accompanied by a DVD of over 400 images and 250 video clips to give the reader a real insight into the field.(19) For music therapy, *A comprehensive guide to music therapy* provides a comprehensive exploration of the theoretical foundations of music therapy and its application with various clients in clinical practice.(18) For dramatherapy, the

Routledge International Handbook of Dramatherapy provides a thorough overview of activity around the world, alongside comparisons of different theoretical approaches and case studies of practice,(20) while *Current Approaches in Drama Therapy* considers much more the history and psychoanalytic aspects of different models and methods.(21) For more information on dance therapy, Sharon W. Goodill's *An Introduction to Medical Dance/ Movement Therapy* gives a concise overview.(22) For more detail, *Dance Movement Therapy: Theory, Research and Practice* brings together chapters on a variety of topics from dance for post-traumatic stress disorder to dance for holistic birth preparation alongside considerations of social and cultural issues in practice.(23)

Arts in healthcare technology

Overview

Technological developments are also now broadening the ways the arts can be incorporated into healthcare, especially allowing the arts to be brought into areas where issues such as infection control can prevent artists themselves entertaining patients. Examples of the arts in healthcare technology could include:

- Guided music and imagery for chronic pain
- Live streaming of nature for patients in isolation
- Relaxation films to reduce anxiety in waiting areas
- Games apps for distracting children having anaesthetics
- Recorded lullabies to calm premature babies

History

One of the more recent developments in arts in health has been the integration of technology into arts in health projects. Some forms of this have existed for a while, such as 'musicmedicine'. Most commonly implemented in the USA, musicmedicine (also written as 'musicmedicine' or 'music-medicine') usually involves the use of recorded music to support patients. Unlike music therapies, musicmedicine does not need a trained therapist to be present and so lacks the interpersonal relationship that is key within music therapy. Instead, the music is initially selected by either a musician or a therapist, or patients are simply invited to bring in their own music when visiting hospital, and then this music is played at the allotted time when it is felt it could be of benefit. The use of recorded music in hospitals could arguably be traced back to the Guild of St Cecilia (discussed in Chapter 1) in the 1890s, who wanted to provide music on demand for patients, so tried to set up a system of transmitting live music via telephone to London hospitals so it could be heard by many patients at once, providing an effect similar to listening to a recording. Recorded music is now used widely in waiting areas, pre-surgical settings, and neo-natal intensive care units, where research has explored the impact on psychological and physiological measures of distress and anxiety.

A development of the use of recorded music has been the use of guided music and imagery. This builds on music therapy techniques and was developed by music and psychotherapist Helen L. Bonny in the USA in the 1970s. Through music the client is encouraged to relax and then embark on a journey exploring the mental imagery created by the music. Bonny created specific music programmes herself that drew on famous pieces of music by composers such as Beethoven, Mozart, and Debussy, arguing that the music took on the form of co-therapist during the sessions.(18)

More recently, other technologies have been brought into arts in health practice, including the development of arts-based apps and films and some early work with augmented reality and gadgets. These developments have yet to spin into mini movements of their own. However, work within arts, health, and technology has been inspired by two main fields to date. First, the burgeoning world of healthcare technology is providing new opportunities in terms of hardware and software capabilities that are beginning to be used within arts in health. For example, the use of 'gamification' in healthcare (by which routine activities such as taking medication are turned into challenges with the aim of leading to sustainable modifications in people's behaviour and improved health outcomes) is opening opportunities for the arts to be used as incentives or rewards for healthy behaviours. And wearable technologies incorporating biofeedback are providing opportunities for using the arts, such as music, to modulate arousal states and mood. Second, there is an increasing emphasis within the arts world for technology to be used to enhance the artistic experience, generate data, and support the reach of arts organizations. This is epitomized in the work of NESTA, an innovation charity that has published reports on how arts and technology are interacting and highlighted potential growth and opportunity areas.

Although one of the least developed areas within arts in health at the moment, arts in healthcare technology has the potential to expand over the coming years. Not only would this help to ensure that the work within arts in health continues to keep track with developments within the field of healthcare and the way that healthcare is delivered, but it would also enable arts in health to reach harder-to-access groups of people, including those who are geographically or socially isolated, and could be taken to scale internationally with much greater ease than physical programmes.

Case study

Title: Open Window

Aims and objectives: This project was undertaken in response to the expressed needs of patients in the National Bone Marrow Transplant Unit at St. James Hospital, Dublin in Ireland. Patients who are in protective isolation for the treatment of leukaemia have to endure stays of up to 4 weeks with restricted access to their families and the outside world. Consequently, the project aimed to reduce this perceived isolation and enhance wellbeing and patient experience.

The project: A 'digital window' was projected onto the wall opposite the bed of each patient in an isolation ward within the hospital, which they could control personally. This 'window' opened onto a number of 'virtual places' that were either specific locations in the outside world where patients requested that an internet-enabled camera was placed, or pre-recorded films made by an artist looking through windows onto different views of nature. The digital window was delivered by artist Denis Roche working in partnership with the Human Connectedness group in the Massachusetts Institute of Technology MediaLab.

Research: A randomized trial of the effect of Open Window on patients experiencing stem cell transplantation was undertaken between 2006 and 2009. Participants who had access to Open Window had significantly reduced levels of anxiety and depression the day before their transplant, as well as reduced anxiety at day 7 and at day 60 post transplant. They also reported better experiences of undergoing stem cell transplantation, including feeling less isolated and more connected with the outside world.(24)

Further information: A video clip about the project is available at www.vimeo.com/6301289 and more information about the public is available through searching 'Open Window' at www.publicart.ie.

 The NESTA reports on Innovation Technology and Imagining Technology, as well as their Digital Culture report, are available via the NESTA website www.nesta.org.uk.

Arts-based training for staff

Overview

As well as arts programmes aimed at supporting patients and the general public, arts in health also includes programmes specifically developed to support staff. In some cases, this includes the arts being embedded into the initial training of doctors or other healthcare professionals. In other cases, it involves the arts being integrated into the day-to-day practice of staff or being offered as an additional opportunity to support their health and wellbeing. Examples of arts programmes for staff could include:

◆ Creative relaxation workshops to reduce burnout

◆ Photography to improve diagnostic skills

◆ Music in theatre to help surgeons concentrate

- Role play sessions to improve patient communication
- Expressive poetry to improve job satisfaction
- Staff choirs to enhance teamwork

History

Arts-based training within healthcare has arisen as part of a larger global movement of applying arts-based methods in business. The aim of this work is to use the arts, especially participatory arts, as an instrument for team-building, leadership development, problem-solving, and communications training. The field began to grow in particular in the late twentieth century, primarily in the UK and USA, and has since spread all over the world. One of the most famous examples of this is the 'Serious Play' concept developed by the LEGO company, by which teams are encouraged to strategize, communicate, and problem-solve through the use of 3D LEGO modelling.

Within healthcare, arts-based training arose through a growing awareness of the needs for development of the interpersonal skills of healthcare professionals to enable respectful and understanding care. In 1927, a history of medicine programme was established at the University of Zagreb in Croatia as part of a move to integrate the humanities into the medical programme to broaden the perspectives of students and support the demands of life as a practising doctor. This was followed by others, such as the National University of La Plata in Argentina, which launched a medical humanities programme in 1976, and Dalhousi University and the University of Manitoba in Canada. In the 1990s, the number of medical schools offering similar programmes suddenly burgeoned, with programmes in the USA flourishing, including at Stony Brook University, the University of California, and the University of Missouri-Kansas City.

In 1996, the University of Oslo developed a course entitled 'Medicine and the Arts', which covered visual arts, architecture, literature, and music, and explored their role as sources of personal and professional development and sources of insight into patients' experiences.(25) Following suit in 1997, in response to a publication from the General Medical Council in the UK entitled *Tomorrow's Doctors: recommendations on undergraduate medical education* (1993), three Scottish medical schools proposed a special study module in medicine and literature, which they explained was adaptable to other art forms too. They cited the importance of the module in broadening 'the intellectual armamentarium of tomorrow's doctors', as well as promoting the ability to tackle challenges, adapt to changes, develop a critical and questioning attitude, and stimulate interest and education.(26) The module included creative writing workshops, reading groups, performances of short plays, magazine designs, field visits to theatres, and poetry readings. The sample bibliography focused on books that were related to health and medicine, such as scientific experiments in Mary Shelley's *Frankenstein* and Virginia Woolf's study of mental illness in *Mrs Dalloway*.

Since then, a whole range of modules and training programmes have developed in an attempt to support the training of doctors and, more broadly, the continuing professional development of healthcare professionals. Many of these programmes are focused on the development of interpersonal skills, including supporting empathy and communication, but many also tackle issues such as coping with the physical and emotional demands of healthcare work with aims to improve wellbeing and reduce burnout, and others have specific aims to enhance clinical skills such as critical thinking in diagnostics and visual awareness in imaging.

Case study

Title: Performing Medicine

Aims and objectives: A major concern for medical students in the UK is their performance in their Objective Structured Clinical Exams (OSCEs). These exams are designed to test competency in skills such as clinical examinations, medical procedures, and communication. The exams are hands-on either with real or simulated patients (either actors or electronic patient simulators), with candidates rotating through 'stations' assessed by different examiners. The Guys', King's and St Thomas' School of Medical Education in London (GKT) identified that many students who failed a year and had to retake attributed failing to their performance in these exams. Consequently, GKT wanted to identify a way of supporting these students.

The project: An Academic Support Programme was designed by theatre company Clod Ensemble and delivered to students in their third, fourth, or fifth years at GKT. It ran for a day a week and included 10 taught, practical study days, delivered by Performing Medicine Associate Artists. The programme used exercises and methods drawn from dance, theatre, and live art practices, which addressed areas such as non-verbal communication, voice, teamwork, reflective practice, power and status, ways of seeing, care and compassion, and difference, with sessions run by Clinical Faculty focusing on learning styles, effective patient history-taking, and application of clinical knowledge.

Research: An impact study from King's Learning Institute of the pilot (2013-2015) found that 87% of the Year 4 students felt the programme had directly improved their OSCE skills. In addition, 90% felt it had improved their communication skills and learning techniques and 94% felt they could manage stress better. The variety of the artistic forms involved and the multi-disciplinary perspective on medicine were found to be strengths of the programme.

Further information: A video of student responses to the programme is available via the Performing Medicine website along with further information on the programme: www.performingmedicine.com. Further information on Clod Ensemble is available at www.clodensemble.com.

Q For further information on the use of arts-based methods in business, Steven S Taylor and Donna Ladkin explore four processes by which arts-based methods can contribute to the development of managers and leaders.(27) 'The effectiveness of arts-based interventions in medical education: a literature review' in the journal *Medical Education* summarizes the evidence base to date.(28) *Artful Creation: Learning-Tales of Arts-in-Business* by Lotto Darsø maps international involvement in arts-based training, replete with case studies and interviews with visionary business people alongside methods and guidelines for arts organizations and businesses planning on working together.(29) For more information about medical humanities in medical programmes, the journal *Academic Medicine* hosted an open-access special edition in October 2003 (volume 78 issue 10), which gave overviews of some of the leading programmes around the world.

Arts in health promotion

Overview

Health promotion is defined by the World Health Organization as the process of enabling people to increase control over, and to improve, their health. As well as arts interventions themselves being linked with improved health, the arts also can be used as engaging tools for delivering healthcare messages to different populations. This could include:

+ Visual arts publicity campaigns to raise understanding about oral health

+ Concerts to raise awareness and money to combat poverty

+ Songs for teaching children about sexual health and HIV

+ Touring theatre performances that dramatize issues around mental health

+ Pop-up dance performances in public spaces to highlight new exercise guidelines

History

Although the phrase 'health promotion' only came into national and international policy in the 1980s, what it describes is an old concept. One of the earliest public health texts we have was written by Hippocrates around 400 BC and is entitled *On Airs, Waters and Places*, intended as a guide to prevent travellers from getting ill in new places. Chapter 2 discussed the modern rise of public health, in particular the emphases on sanitarian reforms and social hygiene. Following on from this, and in particular since the 1970s, there has been a growing focus on health promotion and primary healthcare, not just combating disease but promoting good health.(30)

In support of this, the Ottawa Charter for Health Promotion was signed at the First International Conference on Health Promotion organized by the World Health Organization in 1986. The charter had five areas of focus: building health public policy, creating supportive environments, strengthening community action, developing personal skills, and reorienting healthcare services towards the prevention of illness and promotion of health.(31) To achieve this, the charter called for advocacy as to the importance of health and the factors that affect it; the empowering of individuals to take responsibility for their health to help them have a higher quality of life; and mediation between governments and independent organizations to foster good health. This governmental lead has been followed at more local levels, such as in the 1987 Healthy Cities Initiative, which aimed to tackle health inequalities.

Much of the use of the arts within public health has occurred organically rather than through the development of specific organizations (as has happened in other areas of arts in health), often driven by public health agencies themselves. For example, following the signing of the Ottawa Charter, in Australia between 1987 and 1995, state government health promotion organizations were established in Victoria, South Australia, Western Australia, and the Australian Capital Territory. All four agencies used arts sponsorship to support the promotion of health messages. Interestingly, the success of this activity led to a greater receptiveness for other arts in health work, including the development of more community arts programmes.

However, one of the challenges to health promotion is the continued presence of health inequalities globally. Sanitarian reforms and developments in infrastructure including social and housing reforms that would ensure a basic level of public health have yet to take place in many countries, and rapid urbanization, migration, and conflicts contribute to social instability with detrimental effects on health. The 1948 WHO Constitution called 'the enjoyment of the highest attainable standard of health' one of the 'fundamental rights of every human being'.(32) But this is a right that has yet to be universally available. Consequently, health promotion across the world takes place on many different levels depending on the baseline conditions that exist in each country. Importantly, given the continuing presence of these health inequalities, the arts have not just been employed to support health promotion in countries that already enjoy a good level of basic health. They have been mobilized also as part of attempts to challenge these health inequalities. For example, the 1985 Live Aid concert organized by Sir Bob Geldof and Midge Ure raised funds for famine in Ethiopia. Watched by an estimated global audience of 1.9 billion across 150 nations, the event used the arts, including music, dance, and film, to bring attention to the health challenges being faced in certain countries and to demonstrate the enormous divide between social and economic standing in different parts of the world.

In the context of global poverty and mortality, it is possible to see the arts in health as the icing on a cake: a wonderful element when the core ingredients of food, water, shelter, and basic health are there, but meaning-less, perhaps even flippant, without them. However, the involvement of the arts in health promotion messages such as Live Aid actually highlights that it is the opposite. The inclusion of the arts within health, here in the context of health pro-motion, turned a critical health message that could otherwise have been ignored as part of a longer list of global issues into something accessible and emotive with which people actively wanted to engage. The arts enabled fundraising for the Ethiopian famine to have a far greater reach than would have been possible in their absence. For this reason, the inclusion of the arts continues to be a mainstream in major public health initiatives, at local, national, and international levels.

Case study

Title: Arts in Ebola Response

Aims and objectives: Across 2013-2016, the arts were mobilized throughout West Africa with the aim of raising awareness about Ebola, dispelling myths, and encouraging protective behaviours. In particular, projects aimed to reach communities with low literacy levels and local dialects, and also challenge some of the perceived resistance to government messaging by empowering local communities to take action themselves.

The project: A number of arts projects were developed to try and stop the spread of Ebola. As just three examples:

- 'Spread Knowledge to Stop Ebola' programme was developed by WeOwnTV; a San Francisco-based non-profit organization. It involved Sierra Leoneans themselves being trained in film-making and creating short films in their own words to raise public under-standing about Ebola. The films built on local oral traditions and storytelling and combated misinformation

- 'Stop Ebola Now: Through Creative Storytelling' was a programme with UNICEF Liberia that involved the development of a five-episode radio serial drama that addressed the reality of the Ebola epidemic. The programmes were sensitive to local cultural values and perceptions of Liberian audiences. The programmes contained songs and jingles alongside drama to help fight myths, including those surrounding survivors to help them reintegrate into communities. User kits were also made available online to support other local radio shows in local dialects

- Songs such as *Ebola in Town* by Rapper Shadow were released that warned about how Ebola could be caught. With the most crucial messages looped over an electro-dance beat, the rap song became popular in Liberia along with a 'no-touching' dance

Research: An evaluation of the artistic response to the Ebola outbreak has been published in BMJ Outcomes and is available in their article collection online: outcomes.bmj.com/imple-mentation-reports/. Reviews and opinions about the various programmes have been collated by the University of Florida: www.arts.ufl.edu/academics/center-for-arts-in-medicine/artist-repository/, and the university is currently developing a framework for the use of the arts in public health messaging.

Further information: WeOwnTV's programme is available here: www.sierraleone.weowntv.org. The kits produced by Stop Ebola Now are available here: www.mediaimpact.org/

ebola/guide.html. *Ebola in Town* can be heard here: www.soundcloud.com/shadowmrgn/ebola-in-town-d-12-shadow-kuzzy-of-2kings.

Q For more information on global health promotion movements, the original WHO discussion document on health promotion from 1974 entitled 'Health Promotion: a discussion document on the concept and principles' is available via the WHO website, as is more information on the Healthy Cities initiative: www.euro.who.int. Further details on the arts in health promotion are included in the *Oxford Textbook of Creative Arts, Health and Wellbeing* (2015).(12)

Related fields

This chapter has outlined seven key areas of arts in health. However, it is by no means an exhaustive list. As discussed at the start of the chapter, there is a constant development of new ways in which the arts can be integrated with healthcare and programmes are becoming more and more bespoke to the health challenge they address. A further difficulty in cataloguing arts in health activity is that the field does not exist in isolation but also intersects with related fields, including, but not limited to, cultural studies, sociology, psychology of the arts, and medical humanities.

To explore one example, medical humanities encompasses a broad range of academic disciplines that are applied to understand more about the social, historical, and cultural dimensions of medicine, including the arts (such as the visual arts, and performing arts), humanities (such as literature, philosophy, religion, history, and ethics) and social science (such as cultural studies, sociology, and anthropology).(33) Medical humanities can include:

♦ Narrative accounts of the experience of doctors and patients

♦ Artistic representations of health conditions, the body, and the mind

♦ Philosophical considerations of medicine as an art or a science

♦ Literary explorations of sensitive topics such as death and bereavement

♦ Cultural and historical analyses of ethical challenges in medicine

♦ Linguistic considerations of the terms used within medicine.

Related to medical humanities is the more recent field of health humanities, which takes a similar approach but focusing on wider health, wellbeing, and social care, aiming to create healthier and more compassionate societies.(34)

As is immediately evident, medical and health humanities occupy a similar space to arts in health. A prime example of overlap is in arts-based training for healthcare professionals, which draws on medical humanities approaches as a way of improving understanding and practice. However, the fields of arts in health and medical/health humanities currently still operate relatively independently, as evidenced by separate journals, conferences, and societies, even though researchers and practitioners can cross between the two. Unsurprisingly, there has been a great deal of debate as to how medical/health humanities and arts in health differ. An article in the journal *Medical Humanities* in 2002 suggested 'an attractively neat way of distinguishing them might have been to case medical humanities in a reflective and theoretical role, as it were considering and commentating upon the essentially practical and therapeutic role intended for the arts in health'.(35) If we consider arts-based training through this lens, a clinician's involvement with the arts and humanities remains under the auspices of medical humanities until the involvement starts to have specific therapeutic aims. However, as Evans and Greaves acknowledge, this can be an artificial divide. It is reductive to suggest that medical humanities cannot have therapeutic implications without this crossing the divide into a separate field, as even if there are not specific therapeutic aims, involvement with medical humanities can indirectly lead to therapeutic outcomes. For example, the medical humanities can naturally contribute to senses of identity and community. And arts in health interventions can be reflective too, not just having therapeutic outcomes but also helping to alter public perceptions of conditions and enhance cultural sensitivity.

Consequently, Evans and Greaves question whether there is a sharp divide between medical humanities and arts in health, asking 'Does an individual therapeutic effect stemming directly from the clinical encounter stand wholly distinct from a more general therapeutic effect stemming from interventions in policy or in the education of practitioners? Alternatively, could both be seen on a continuum?'. Certainly, although medical humanities and arts in health continue to exist as two distinct fields, they are in fact very much related, and care should be taken not to force an artificial separation between them because, as the breadth and depth of the use of arts within health and medicine continues to grow, the opportunities for intersect between the two are blossoming.

Another related field is that of museums, health, and wellbeing. While museums and galleries are considered by some to be part of the arts in health movement (and for the purposes of this book they are considered together), in the UK in particular museums and health has begun to emerge out of the wider field of arts in health as its own entity with its own National Alliance. The seminal book on the topic *Museums, Health and Well-being* (2013) described how the more passive role of museums and galleries in reflecting on our heritage, acting as custodians of objects of cultural importance, can place them apart from current active arts practice.(36) Indeed, research suggests that symbolic significance of these objects is a factor in their therapeutic effects as they can help individuals to convey and uncover emotions.(37) However, museums and galleries are increasingly developing active programmes, such as object handling projects, multi-art performances (where other art forms, such as music, are used to reinterpret previous works of art), and also hosting participatory arts in health interventions too such as fine art, crafts, and creative writing. These programmes bring the activity of museums and galleries more in-line with arts in health programmes. Furthermore, the role of museums and galleries as sites for social interaction is undisputed. Growing research in arts in health and museums, health and wellbeing is highlighting the social benefits of both (as discussed in Chapter 2), creating further links between the two. However, the separation of museums and health into its own strand is certainly helping its visibility, funding, and programme development. Whether the development of this strand remains relatively practical, or whether museums and health does indeed separate into either its own strand within arts in health or its own movement altogether, or whether 'museums and health' and 'arts in health' become united under a broader umbrella of 'culture in health' remains to be seen.

 For more information on Museums and Health, the journal *Arts & Health* hosted a special issue focusing on culture, museums, and wellbeing: volume 7, issue 3 (2015).

Summary

This chapter has provided an overview of the breadth and rich diversity of arts in health, and importantly shown how it can work in tandem with other disciplines. As we have seen, this is a field that depends on its flexibility and creativity. As a result of this, the construction of more rigid models or definitions of what arts in health is might not provide further clarification but could in fact be detrimental. Consequently, even the broad sub-areas that have been outlined in this chapter should be referenced with caution. As will be shown in the next chapter, far more important than what aspect of any potential model an arts in health project fits into, is what that project aims to accomplish, how well targeted it is, and with how much sensitivity it is integrated into a person's care. The next part of this book will move from a contextual to a more practical focus and explore how such projects can be conceptualized, planned, delivered, and evaluated.

Note

1. I submitted an earlier version of this categorization as infographics as part of consultancy work with Breathe Arts Health Research to King's Cultural Institute in December 2015 and they were published online in January 2016.

References

1. **White M, Hillary E.** Arts Development in Community Health: A Social Tonic. Radcliffe Publishing; 2009. 262 pp.

2. **Arts Council of Ireland.** Arts and Health Policy and Strategy. Arts Council of Ireland; 2010.

3. **Macnaughton J, White M, Stacy R.** Researching the benefits of arts in health. Health Educ. 2005 Oct 1;105(5):332–9.

4. **Macdonald R.** Music, health and wellbeing: a review. Int J Qual Stud Health Well-Being. 2013 Aug;8:1–13.

5. **Walshaw T.** The Picture of Health: An introduction to Paintings in Hospitals [Internet]. [cited 2016 Nov 3]. Available from: http://www.wallacecollection.org/blog/2016/07/the-picture-of-health-an-introduction-to-paintings-in-hospitals/.

6. **Cork R.** The Healing Presence of Art: A History of Western Art in Hospitals. 1 edition. New Haven Conn.; London: Yale University Press; 2012. 496 pp.

7. **Nitkiewicz R.** Art in hospitals [Internet]. The King's Fund. [cited 2016 Nov 3]. Available from: https://www.kingsfund.org.uk/library/blog/art-hospitals.

8. Haldane D, Loppert S, eds. The Arts in Health Care: Learning from Experience. London: King's Fund; 1999.

9. **Greene L.** Art in Hospitals: A Guide. London: King Edwards Hospital Fund for London, Greater London Arts; 1989.

10. **Sternberg EM.** Healing Spaces: The Science of Place and Well-Being. Harvard University Press; 2010. 352 pp.

11. Music in Hospitals [Internet]. Music In Hospitals. [cited 2016 Nov 3]. Available from: http://www.musicinhospitals.org.uk/about/.

12. Clift S, Camic PM, editors. Oxford Textbook of Creative Arts, Health, and Wellbeing: International perspectives on practice, policy and research. OUP Oxford; 2015. 368 pp.

13. **Ní Ógáin E, Lumley T, Pritchard D.** Making an impact: impact measurement among charities and social enterprises in the UK. London: New Philanthropy Capital; 2012 Oct.

14. **Mowlah A, Niblett V, Blackburn J, Harris M.** The value of arts and culture to people and society [Internet]. Manchester: Arts Council England; 2014 [cited 2016 Jun 27]. Available from: http://www.artscouncil.org.uk/exploring-value-arts-and-culture/value-arts-and-culture-people-and-society.

15. **Hogan S.** Healing Arts: The History of Art Therapy. London: Jessica Kingsley Publishers; 2001. 338 pp.

16. **Sandel SL, Chaiklin S.** Foundations of Dance/Movement Therapy: The Life and Work of Marian Chace. Columba, Maryland: Marian Chace Memorial Fund of the American Dance Therapy Association; 1993. 472 pp.

17. Fox J (ed.). The Essential Moreno: Writings on Psychodrama, Group Method, and Spontaneity. New York: Springer Publishing Company; 1987. 263 pp.

18. **Wigram T, Pedersen IN, Bonde LO.** A comprehensive guide to music therapy: theory, clinical practice, research, and training. London; Philadelphia: Jessica Kingsley Publishers; 2002.

19. **Rubin JA.** Introduction to Art Therapy: Sources & Resources. New York and Hove: Taylor & Francis; 2009. 357 pp.

20. **Jennings S, Holmwood C.** Routledge International Handbook of Dramatherapy. London and New York: Routledge; 2016. 662 pp.

21. **Johnson DR, Emunah R.** Current Approaches in Drama Therapy. Charles C Thomas Publisher; 2009. 541 pp.

22. **Goodill SW.** An Introduction to Medical Dance/Movement Therapy: Health Care in Motion. London and Philadelphia: Jessica Kingsley Publishers; 2005. 242 pp.

23. **Payne H.** Dance Movement Therapy: Theory, Research and Practice. Hove: Routledge; 2013. 286 pp.

24. **McCabe C, Roche D, Hegarty F, McCann S.** 'Open Window': a randomized trial of the effect of new media art using a virtual window on quality of life in patients' experiencing stem cell transplantation. Psychooncology. 2013 Feb 1;**22**(2):330–7.

25. **Frich JC, Fugelli P.** Medicine and the arts in the undergraduate medical curriculum at the University of Oslo Faculty of Medicine, Oslo, Norway. Acad Med J Assoc Am Med Coll. 2003 Oct;**78**(10):1036–8.

26. **Downie RS, Hendry RA, Macnaughton RJ, Smith BH.** Humanizing medicine: a special study module. Med Educ. 1997 Jul;**31**(4):276–80.

27. **Taylor SS, Ladkin D.** Understanding Arts-Based Methods in Managerial Development. Acad Manag Learn Educ. 2009;**8**(1):55–69.

28. **Perry M, Maffulli N, Willson S, Morrissey D.** The effectiveness of arts-based interventions in medical education: a literature review: Effectiveness of the arts in medical education. Med Educ. 2011 Feb;**45**(2):141–8.

29. **Darsø L.** Artful Creation: Learning-Tales of Arts-in-Business. Frederiksberg: Samfundslitteratur; 2004. 213 pp.

30. **Mold A, Berridge V.** The history of health promotion. In: Cragg L, editor. Health Promotion Theory. McGraw-Hill Education (UK); 2013.

31. **WHO.** The Ottawa Charter for Health Promotion [Internet]. Ottawa: WHO; 1986 Nov [cited 2016 Nov 3]. Available from: http://www.who.int/healthpromotion/conferences/previous/ottawa/en/.

32. **World Health Organization.** Constitution [Internet]. Geneva; 1948 [cited 2015 Dec 7]. Available from: http://www.who.int/about/mission/en/.

33. **Cole TR, Carlin NS, Carson RA.** Medical Humanities: An Introduction. Cambridge University Press; 2014. 463 pp.

34. **Crawford P, Brown B, Baker C, Tischler V, Abrams B.** Health Humanities. Palgrave Macmillan UK; 2015. 194 pp.

35. **Evans HM, Greaves D.** Medical humanities among the healing arts? Med Humanit. 2002 Dec 1;**28**(2):57–60.

36. **Chatterjee H, Noble G.** Museums, Health and Well-Being. Farnham, Surrey, England ; Burlington, VT, USA: Routledge; 2013. 158 pp.

37. **Lanceley A, Noble G, Johnson M, Balogun N, Chatterjee H, Menon U.** Investigating the therapeutic potential of a heritage-object focused intervention: a qualitative study. J Health Psychol. 2012 Sep;**17**(6):809–20.

Part II

Designing and delivering arts in health interventions

Chapter 5

Conceptualizing and planning interventions

In 1854 in the midst of the Crimean war, British nurse Florence Nightingale was sent by the British government, along with a team of other nurses and nuns, to care for wounded soldiers in Turkey. On arrival, Nightingale began a series of improvement measures within the hospital, including reducing overcrowding by spacing beds apart, providing ventilation, removing animals from the hospital basement, and flushing out sewers.(1) Within 6 months, the rate of mortality from disease dropped from 42.7% to 2.2%. Nightingale, later recognized with a fellowship from the Statistical Society (1860) among other awards, had set up one of the first hospital quality improvement systems involving the identification of a problem, the development of a potential solution, the establishment of a measurement system to track progress, and the monitoring of this progress over time, as well as generating buy-in from her peers to support the ongoing use of her improvement.(2) Since then, programmes within healthcare systems across the world that aim to improve or innovate have flourished, aided by new research findings, educational and training programmes for healthcare professionals, developments in technology, and the discovery of a range of drugs and treatments.

In particular, following World War II, there was a burgeoning of interest in industrial models of improvement and innovation and how they could be applied to healthcare settings. Models developed by industry giants such as Ford and Toyota, along with management concepts from disciplines such as services marketing, human resources management, organization studies, psychology, and organizational behaviour have gradually been incorporated into healthcare systems around the world, dramatically improving the ability of countries to deliver streamlined, mass-volume yet person-centred care.

Improvement and innovation models are not and should not be confined just to core healthcare activity, but have a fundamental value to play in the development and running of all activity within health. Indeed, some of the longest-running and most successful arts in health interventions are those that, consciously or unconsciously, followed such models during their design, implementation,

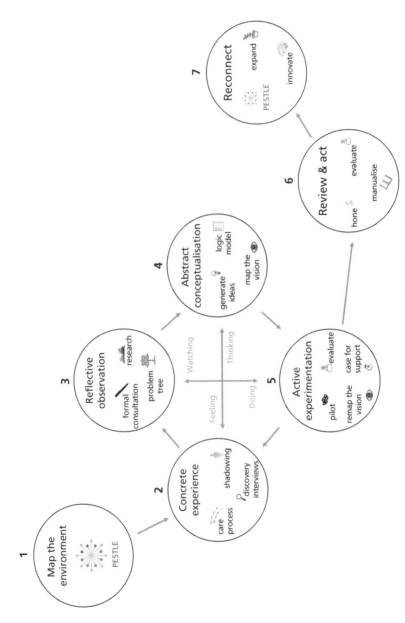

Figure 5.1 The seven steps of designing and delivering an arts in health intervention.

and ongoing evaluation. The next two chapters will explore how a range of models drawn from psychology, business, industry, healthcare, and sales when organized into seven logical 'steps' can help to conceptualize, design, implement, and evaluate arts in health interventions. These steps are represented graphically in Figure 5.1. In particular, these chapters propose a 'problem-based solution' model, where the key is identifying a specific problem, weakness, or challenge that can then be overcome with an arts-based solution. This is not to suggest an instrumentalist approach whereby the arts only have a value in solving healthcare problems. However, when seeking to bring the arts into healthcare, finding a particular problem or challenge can be an effective way of defining the niche for a new intervention and encouraging financial, institutional, and individual support.

In particular, these next two chapters will demonstrate how following this problem-based solution approach and especially these seven steps is not, as it might appear on the surface, a more cumbersome way of integrating the arts within healthcare, but is actually an effective and sustainable way of approaching new interventions likely to reflect the needs of patients, public, and staff, engage the highest artistic quality, and encourage buy-in from key stakeholders.

Step 1: Map the environment

The first step in the development of an arts in health intervention is to understand the environment within which it is going to be implemented. Different environments provide different opportunities and barriers for interventions, so identifying what these are can help with early decisions as to whether an idea has the potential to be developed or whether conditions are such that it is a case of either wrong time or wrong place. The size of the 'environment' is an important consideration. On a 'macro' level, the national or even international environment could have an influence on whether there will be an appetite for an intervention; whether it is timely, fits into available funding streams, and draws on available resources. But equally strategies and resources at the more local organizational level (or 'micro' level) will play a key role in whether an intervention succeeds. Consequently, mapping different scales of environment can provide crucial information to help assess the viability of launching a new intervention.

PESTLE analysis, thought to be first outlined in an earlier form by Harvard professor Francis Aguilar in a 1967 book *Scanning the Business Environment*, was initially a marketing principle to help companies track the environment in which they were planning on launching a new product or service.(3) However, its principles can be of real value when initially planning an arts in health intervention. PESTLE analyses can be carried out on both macro and micro environments, scaled according to the size and ambition of the intervention.

🔍 *Practising Public health: A Guide to Examinations and Workplace Application* (2015) edited by Adam DM Briggs, Paul A Fished, and Rob F Cooper is just one example of a discussion of the value of PESTLE within healthcare.

PESTLE is an acronym for six aspects of an environment that should be considered to gain a full picture of whether conditions are supportive of an intervention:

1. Political—when conceptualizing an arts in health intervention, political activity has the potential to support or hinder its realization, even if it is operating on a small scale. For example, cuts in the numbers of nurses in a hospital, whether as part of a national change or at an individual organizational level, could put pressure on remaining staff, reducing their time capacity and subsequent availability to be involved in a new project for a period of time after the change. However, the same cuts could provide an opportunity for conceptualization of a new project once this period of resettling is over if the project can alleviate some of the pressures on those remaining staff, such as engaging patient attention during busy handover periods or increasing patient experience and perceptions of the quality of care. Consequently, keeping abreast of relevant political developments at national, local, and also healthcare institution levels is important in tailoring the aims of a project and timing its delivery.

2. Economic—the announcement of new funding streams that might be relevant to an arts in health intervention could be an important steer in design and implementation plans. Similarly, more general funding such as either a government increase in spending on a particular health area or even an announcement of financial cuts could provide rationales for new interventions, whether to complement new health schemes or provide support where there is likely to be an even greater need. The continual monitoring of funding activity could be important at each stage of a project, whether supporting the initial pilot or helping a successful small-scale project to expand. If an intervention is seeking core healthcare funding, understanding the application process for such funding will be crucial, at which point being aware of forthcoming economic changes on a larger level will also be important.

3. Social—the social and demographic characteristics of an environment can also influence initial plans for an intervention. National pressures such as an ageing population or awareness campaigns around health conditions

such as diabetes or mental health could provide fertile ground for developing a related arts in health intervention. But aside from specific changes, simply being aware of the social make-up of an environment is important. For example, data on the number of patients coming through a hospital with a specific condition or the number of people living in a particular nursing home could give an indication of how many potential participants there are for a new activity. Or understanding the cultural or ethnic diversity of a particular geographical area could guide the artistic design of an activity.

4. Technological—the use of technology within healthcare is rapidly expanding. Developments in security systems have enabled the electronic storing and transfer of patients records. The internet has radically altered the way the public engage with information on health conditions. Hardware such as tablets and smartphones have transformed the way patients provide data and receive updates, not to mention the extraordinary speed in developments of medical technologies from diagnostic tests to surgical apparatus to wearable monitors. Some of the most innovative uses of technology have come from transferring ideas from other sectors, such as the use of 'gamification' as a way of encouraging medication adherence.(4) Tracking technological developments both inside and outside healthcare can help to develop truly innovative projects. Even for projects involving active participation at a set location and time, technology can be used to extend the impact through follow-up resources, or disseminate educational tools or project data to other patients or stakeholders.

5. Legal—there may also be important laws that should be explored before a project is developed. Entertainment licensing may affect the delivery of live arts performances or the use of recorded music, or the replication of artwork or screening of films may incur a cost. It may be necessary to adhere to healthcare regulations such as staffing levels in healthcare institutions, health and safety rules, or patient safeguarding protocols. Even at a local level, organizational policies may affect the ease with which a project can be implemented. Understanding these challenges up front can ease the process of finding solutions, rather than being presented with obstacles further down the line.

6. Environmental—being aware of environmental changes is also important to new interventions. For example, if a participatory project proposes to involve older adults, timing a pilot to start in winter could affect attendance. Similarly, a project aiming to help people with respiratory conditions might have different uptake in polluted cities compared with more rural areas. Or high tourist seasons could change the demographic of patients in an area. So an awareness of environmental factors could guide planning for a new intervention.

Q More information about PESTLE analysis can be found on the website www. pestleanalysis.com.

Overall, PESTLE analysis has three core purposes. Understanding this overall environment through PESTLE analysis can highlight the opportunities for innovation, increase buy-in, and even support funding, or conversely flag the barriers that must be overcome to achieve success. Furthermore, what PESTLE analysis should reveal is a promising target group for an intervention, be that people with a specific health condition, people working in a particular department or institution, or people who reside within a chosen area. This group will become the focus of Step 2 of this seven-step process. Finally, while PESTLE analysis is a strategic first step in any intervention conceptualization, it can also be of value as an ongoing process; an exercise returned to at strategic points in the development of an intervention to monitor potential forthcoming challenges or highlight opportunities for growth.

Following this first 'scoping' step, the next four steps in the seven-step process move from learning more about an environment or situation to practically improving it. A helpful way to understand these next steps is to use the 'Reflective Cycle': a four-step process developed in the 1980s by David Kolb, an educational theorist who trained at Harvard University.(5) Shown in Figure 5.2, the 'Reflective Cycle' explores the poles of two key continua (marked in the centre of the diagram): processing (from passive watching to active doing) and perception (from thinking to feeling). These continua are particularly pertinent for arts in health interventions as they actively promote a balance between observing a system to identify what could be improved and directly engaging in changing that system, and between the science of planning a successful intervention and the creativity of designing something innovative. Importantly, the flexibility of the 'Reflective Cycle' means that it can be applied to a range of situations, whether working in a hospital, care home, primary school, or community setting. Each of the next four steps outlined in this chapter and in Chapter 6 provides further details on how the four stages can be carried out to make it a productive tool for arts in health interventions. Each of the four steps have been split into substeps with specific purposes.

Q David Kolb has written extensively about experiential learning and its role in the 'Reflective Cycle' in his book *Experiential Learning: Experience as the source of learning and development* (1983).(5)

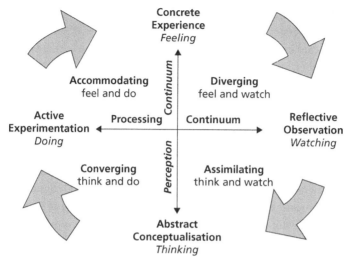

Figure 5.2 Kolb's Learning Cycle. Reproduced from Kolb, David A., *Experiential learning: experience as the source of learning and development*, 2nd Ed., p. 41, Figure 4.1 ©2015. Reprinted by permission of Pearson Education, Inc., New York, New York.

Step 2: Gain concrete experience

Once a target group of interest has been selected, the key is to identify the needs of the target group and understand the experience they face, for example in coping with their health condition. As this forms the first phase of Kolb's cycle, the 'divergent' phase, emphasis is on having as broad an experience as possible to avoid any options being shut down too soon. Below are three suggestions for how concrete experience can be undertaken. These methods are highly complementary so could be undertaken alongside one another to provide a solid foundation for the development of a project:

Map the care process

Every health condition carries with it a necessary 'process' that people with the health condition follow. A process map is a visual representation of the multidisciplinary system of events that occur for a person through the process of their care. These processes can range from formal stages in a treatment model that get followed closely by people with specific diagnoses, to broader and looser types of activity that somebody with a health condition engages in, such as appointments with their local doctor, routine medications, and visits to hospital for scans or treatments such as surgery. These processes also differ between countries and regions and even within specific health conditions depending on the age of the person, the severity of their condition, and other factors such as their healthcare insurance policies. Even if an intervention is being planned for staff or members of the 'healthy' general public, it will be important to understand their routines and the people and places with which they might engage. Although each person may follow a slightly different process, there will often be certain similarities in the activities they undertake.

Understanding these broad routes is important as it allows the identification of timepoints at which problems or challenges might exist. For example, it might show if treatment is particularly complicated or painful at any particular point, if patient experience is known to fall short of expected standards during part of the process, or if there are aspects of people's physical or psychological recovery that are not fully supported. Some arts interventions may be appropriate for very specific parts of a person's care, whereas others may be the sort of activity that people can engage with on a regular basis throughout their treatment. It is also useful to gather data on the numbers of patients involved in care processes to assess the extent of a potential target group.

Information on care processes can be gathered from a range of sources including healthcare professionals who are involved with the target participant group, from patient-facing literature on health conditions such as leaflets or websites, from national documents mapping patient care, from institution-specific protocols on intranets or with divisional managers, or from patients themselves. Even if the proposed intervention has already been conceptualized for a specific section of a care process for a particular patient group, it can still be important to go back and undertake a care process analysis to confirm that the proposed project is being timed for the most appropriate moment in that process or to ascertain whether it could have value if it is offered at additional points of care as well.

Shadow the target group

Once the care process is understood, it is important to ascertain how this process is perceived by the patients themselves. A process may be experienced quite differently by patients in reality compared with how it appears on paper. Experiencing care processes is most easily undertaken through shadowing a patient or staff journey (depending on the target participant group). For example, sitting in a hospital waiting area can reveal what factors lead to it being a relaxing or daunting experience; or seeing people attend weekly clinics can show whether patients are likely to find a further weekly arts activity an enhancement or an exhaustion. Although it may not be appropriate to shadow an entire care process, as it may take several months for a patient to follow a full process, shadowing sections of the care process that have been flagged as potentials for an intervention from the care process analysis can be a valuable task.

As Kolb's Reflective Cycle demonstrates, the key aspect of this step of the process is in 'feeling'. A useful tool that may help with shadowing is 'thick description'. Developed in the mid-twentieth century as an ethnographic tool, thick description involves observing and recording in fine detail what is noticed, including factual details as well as contextual details about the environment in which the observations are made and sometimes even interpretations of how details make the observer feel.(6) The more details that can be provided, whether they seem relevant at the time of writing or not, the richer the body of data there will be. Essentially, this enables an experience to be recorded, but it also means that small details that might not seem important at the time of shadowing can later be revisited and better appreciated. For example, through thick description, it might be that the person shadowing a waiting area in a hospital writes down three times over the course of a day that they were startled by an unexpected noise, or they overheard another patient's conversation with a doctor. These small details might be easily forgotten over the course of the day, but if they are recorded along with other information about the waiting area, when they are returned to, it may become clear that some sort of arts intervention that directs patients' attention away from background noise and towards a more pleasant stimulus may reduce waiting anxiety, provide extra privacy for staff and patient conversations, and ultimately improve the experience.

Undertake discovery interviews

In addition to trying to experience the practical steps in a patient's care process, gathering the views of patients as well as staff and relatives is crucial to get to the heart of the physical and emotional experience of a section of a care process. Even through shadowing, it is not possible to experience something as a patient or staff member will. Furthermore, it is also often a mandatory step in funding applications to involve patients and the public (patient public involvement, also known as 'PPI'). A simple way of gathering such information is via discovery interviews; a technique becoming increasingly popular within healthcare systems. Although they can be undertaken over the phone, it is often best to interview people in the location in which the intervention is being planned, such as a hospital waiting area, community centre, or nursing home.

Discovery interviews typically involve small numbers of people either spoken to individually or in small groups, aiming to get an overview of broad issues that can then be tested with much larger numbers of people in a formal paper consultation process (see Step 3 later in this chapter). With this in mind, it is best in discovery interviews not to use questions that are too guided as they may skew patients' responses. Even if there is already a potential project idea, it is best to ask open questions to see whether the need for the project you have in mind is as evident among patients and staff as you might initially think.

As they are intended to be exploratory, the discovery interviews should not ask any personal details or sensitive information. To avoid issues around data protection, it is simplest not to audio record them at this early stage in project planning, although with appropriate consent from participants it may be possible to do so if this is felt to be important (see Chapter 8 for more information on audio recording and consent). In line with the 'problem-based solutions' model being proposed here, it can be helpful to start with open questions, such as what 'challenges' to working practice or experience patients, staff, and relatives face. In response to the problems, interviewees can then be asked what 'solutions' they might propose. Although the solutions that are discussed may not be feasible or effective, they may provide helpful steers for a new intervention. Simply gathering this information alone can be a valuable starting point, and the short nature of the questions means that several patients and staff can be interviewed, avoiding bias that might arise from asking just a few people; discovery interviews work best when they involve a range of patients and relatives of different ages and backgrounds, and staff in different roles and across different levels. If there are already ideas for a potential project, following on from these initial questions, it may be relevant to pose some additional questions that might provide more information for the project design. However, interviewers should avoid pushing one particular idea too much as this is still an early stage in the consultation process and is more focused on 'feeling' and 'experience' rather than actively finding solutions. The interviewer should also ensure that no promises are made about changes or innovations in these early stages.

Q For more information on how to run discovery interviews in healthcare settings, South East Wales Cardiac Network have put together a comprehensive toolkit entitled ' "How to" kit: undertaking discovery interviews', available through www. wales.nhs.uk.

Overall, discovery interviews can provide some valuable early detail about where the space for a new intervention lies and help identify some of the barriers that might be in place. This process can also ensure patient and public involvement in the early stages of designing an intervention, and can identify project 'champions' who may be able to act as ambassadors for a project and help with its running or evaluation later on. These immersive activities of Step 2 should provide an understanding of the experiences of patients, staff, and relatives in the target group, which can then be explored more critically and objectively in Step 3.

Step 3: Conduct reflective observation

Following on from the 'feeling'-based observational work of Step 2, Step 3 involves a more structured observation process that can be broken down into three stages.

Carry out a formal consultation

The care process analysis, shadowing, and discovery interviews should have yielded a substantial amount of information from various sources. To make sense of this information, grouping findings into common themes can be valuable, identifying which patterns emerge from multiple sources and looking for how the views of the different groups (e.g. staff, patients, relatives, or members of the public) both converge and differ. Although Step 2 was inherently exploratory and not intended to be deeply analysed, there is still a general rule that if a problem seems to occur multiple times from multiple sources, it is less likely that it is a rogue view and more likely to be a common opinion affecting at least a proportion of the target group.

The ideas that begin to surface from Step 2 can be more thoroughly tested through a formal consultation. The aim of the formal consultation is threefold:

1. To gather more comprehensive data about the section of the care process and the target group that have been selected to have a 'benchmark' of what the current situation is like

2. To test whether problems identified in Step 2 are commonly felt by a wider sample of the target group and are indeed commonly perceived problems (rather than individual views)

3. To gather additional open feedback that could have a bearing on how an intervention is designed

Unlike discovery interviews, the formal consultation should aim to involve larger numbers of participants. The exact number will depend on the care process and the target group involved. For a busy hospital waiting area that sees 200 people a day, for example, it may be advisable to collect at least 100 consultation forms across a range of days (e.g. weekdays and weekends) and times of day (e.g. morning, evening or night). However, for a nursing home that has only 20 residents and 10 staff, it might be that collecting responses from two-thirds of these provides enough information to get a good overview of opinion. If a low volume of forms is needed, it may be possible for somebody to hand these to respondents individually. For a high volume, or for forms that need distributing on both day and night shifts, it may be possible to add them to a routine already in place. For example, if all visitors to a waiting area are given a registration form on arrival, the receptionist may be able to hand over a consultation form at the same time. When visitors return their registration form, they can return the consultation form too, meaning that forms are distributed without additional staff time being involved. Alternatively, if there is a bank of email addresses of people who attend a particular community centre, say, it could be that the form can be emailed to them as an online survey for people to complete in their own time.

To gather information on the three themes, a formal consultation questionnaire could contain the following types of questions:

1. Demographic questions—It is important to ascertain when and by whom consultation forms are completed. Asking the date and time of day is advised, as well as asking for people's age and gender along with other demographic factors that are likely to stratify responses. However, to preserve anonymity, the form should allow questions to be optional and not ask too many personal questions that could lead to a participant being identified. It may also be helpful to know how many times a person has experienced the section of the care process under focus, such as how many times they have visited the waiting area or how long they have had a particular condition and been visiting a clinic for a particular treatment as this may affect their responses. As a guide, demographic questions often take up around 10% of a consultation form

2. Baseline data—Another important element of a consultation is gathering information on the current situation. This is helpful for a number of reasons, including (i) illuminating more about the initial problem to help understand it, (ii) providing additional evidence that the current situation is inadequate to support buy-in or funding for the planned intervention, (iii) providing a baseline against which the impact of an arts intervention can be measured. Depending on the area of interest, this might be identifying people's overall view on a hospital waiting room environment, or assessing how supported people feel during a treatment programme. It might also involve constructing a set of 'standards': targets that the part of the patient's care process should aim for, such as 'create a waiting environment that 90% of people feel is calming' or 'have every patient undergoing a particular treatment feeling moderately or very well supported in their care'. Some organizations such as hospitals may already have their own set of standards that can be used here. Alternatively, standards could be established in consultation with

patients and staff during discovery interviews. Testing whether standards are met in this consultation can demonstrate if there is a shortfall in the current situation and show to people involved what the arts intervention is aiming to achieve. Consultation questions can be numeric or text-based. For baseline data, numeric answers will provide the easiest benchmarking information but text-based answers will illuminate more about a problem, so both are advisable. As a guide, baseline data could take up around 30% of a consultation form

Q Brace's *Questionnaire Design: How to Plan, Structure and Write Survey Material for Effective Market Research* (2008) provides a good introduction to designing questionnaires for market research such as this.(7)

3. Test the validity of identified themes—The core part of the consultation form should be testing whether the themes that emerged from the small sample involved in the discovery interviews are representative of the larger population and also to tease out more about these themes or clarify issues surrounding them. This should involve around 50% of the consultation form. The themes tested should include the initial problems, to see whether other people agree that they are problems, and some of the proposed solutions that may have been suggested in the discovery interviews, or that may already be being considered for an arts intervention. Results can then be analysed to give the average value or most common response. A common problem in testing themes is inadvertently biasing responses, such as pushing agreement with a particular 'solution'. There are a number of ways to avoid this, including phrasing questions in a neutral way, providing a range of answers so people highlight the ones they think are best, or providing sliding scales of agreement (such as 'Likert' scales).

Q Matell and Jacoby discuss Likert scales in more detail in an article from 1971 entitled 'Is there an optimal number of alternatives for Likert scale items?'.(8).

4. Invite open responses—The consultation form can end with an invitation for more opinions on an issue. This can extend the work of the discovery interviews. However, unlike discovery interviews, it is not possible to ask people more questions based on their answers, and people are also less likely to spend time explaining their thoughts properly. So to provide useful data, as well as providing truly open-ended responses such as 'do you have any comments', open-ended questions can be more targeted, such as

asking people if there are any other problems with the part of the care process being explored, or if they have specific solutions to help with one of the identified problems

Consultations may need to be slightly different for staff, patients, and relatives, but as much as possible the questions should be kept similar so that results can be compared between groups. And as with discovery interviews, it is important to canvas the views of a wide range of people, including patients of different ages and staff in different roles and levels of seniority.

In analysing consultation forms, descriptive statistics should be calculated, such as the current levels of 'standards' and the percentage of people agreeing with the identified themes. Graphics such as bar charts are helpful for quickly understanding the data. It is also useful to examine a diagram of the demographics of participants who were involved, to check whether they were representative of the people being targeted with the intervention (such as the right age range). If responses have been gathered from lots of people, it may also be worth exploring whether there were differences in response between certain groups, such as men and women or older and younger people. For open-ended responses, it can help to group feedback into themes. Although this is just a planning stage, care should be taken over the interpretation of the consultation data as this could make the difference between a pleasant arts activity and a really well-targeted and high-impact intervention.

Research related projects

At this stage, it is also useful to carry out two other types of research:

1. Research studies that have been carried out exploring previous arts (or similar) interventions with the target group should be identified. The evidence base available may point to certain solutions being particularly effective, or highlight which are the key factors in an intervention that contribute to its efficacy. Conversely, research studies may show which interventions did not work and discuss why. Both of these angles will help to build a strong case for support to discuss with stakeholders or funders. Understanding how successful interventions were designed will also guide the planning stage for the intervention being developed. Studies can be found through entering keywords into search engines and databases including Google Scholar, PubMed, and PsychINFO, and there are also a wealth of research studies in the fact file in Part IV

2. It can also be revealing to identify which arts in health interventions already exist in different organizations. There may be other successful projects already running for the target group that can be learnt from, or there may

equally be projects that have not been successful in their aims because of unforeseen problems. Starting to consider the range of arts options available at the same time as determining the needs of the target group may help solidify thoughts prior to the main generation of ideas on appropriate interventions, as discussed later in Step 4. Examples of practice and details of where to find out more about existing projects is also given in the fact file in Part IV.

Develop a problem tree

Another exercise that can support the reflective observation process of Step 3 is mapping out a problem tree. The care process analysis should have revealed particular challenges that were then elucidated further through the shadowing, discovery interviews, and consultation. A problem tree is a way of narrowing down which problem is going to be addressed and clarifying both how this problem fits within a wider framework and what its components are. If a suite of problems have been identified, a diagram of how these problems relate can be drawn up.

Within problem trees, the core problems form the 'roots' of the tree, and the consequences become the 'branches'. Some of the problems may be similar to one another and can be grouped together, with roots linking into one another. Others may be subcomponents of larger problems, forming sub-sections of individual roots. Some of the consequence branches may come directly from specific roots, whereas others may be broader and the effect of the sum total of the roots. By highlighting the relationships between problems, problem trees help to break down the larger challenge into manageable and definable chunks and show how tackling one or two of the problems could have a wider impact. They can also help establish which are the key problems that most need to be addressed.

Of course, the arts may not be able to solve all problems. It may be that the most effective way of using the arts is not to tackle the largest problem but rather to remove a series of smaller problems at specific levels, presenting a complete solution to some clearly defined and manageable problems. Alternatively, it may be that an arts intervention is best placed trying to improve the situation relating to one or more larger problems, even if solving them entirely is not feasible. Both possibilities have their own respective merits. However, it is generally easier to engage stakeholders and funders with interventions that solve a very targeted problem. That said, if the problem selected is too specific it may not translate into much of a change overall (not changing much of the external structure of the tree), thus not leaving much room for an arts intervention to achieve meaningful effects. So a balance between these extremes is important.

Q The Australian website 'Evaluation Toolbox', which aims to support community sustainability engagement programmes, contains a section on Problem Trees under its 'tools': www.evaluationtoolbox.net.au.

Overall, Step 3 should have built on the contextualizing work of Step 1 and the observational work of Step 2, meaning that there is a clear target group, stage of the care process, and problem that an intervention is going to tackle, and the environment within which this work is going to be undertaken is understood. This should form a firm foundation for Step 4, which involves developing an effective and targeted intervention.

Step 4: Undertake abstract conceptualization

Based on the work undertaken in the three previous steps, Step 4 involves putting the learning that has been accumulated into practice, involving, as the heading implies, the actual conceptualization of an arts in health intervention. For some projects, it may be that ideas for an intervention have not been formally discussed until this step. For other projects, it may be that an intervention has been in mind right from the start, and the first three steps have involved consolidating what was already felt intuitively, refining ideas, and honing the aim of the intervention. Either way, Step 4 is important. For projects where an intervention has yet to be designed, it will highlight the range of potential ideas for an intervention. For interventions that may already have been mapped out, it can help to expand horizons, ensuring that what is proposed is as rich and effective as possible. There are three activities that can be undertaken as part of this conceptualization process.

Generate ideas

Generating ideas for an intervention can appear a daunting task. Either there may not be a clear intervention for the specific circumstances, or there may be a plethora of options that make it hard to pick just one. To guide the process of ideas generation, there are several different types of 'thinking' that have been proposed from different fields of practice.

Design thinking was originally developed in design engineering for use when developing new product ideas and is discussed in the book *The Sciences of the Artificial* by Herbert A Simon in 1969.(9) Design thinking is a useful foil for the development of arts interventions in healthcare when following the guidelines of this book as it encourages focus not just on the problem that is going to be solved (and how an intervention can tackle that specific problem), but also on imagining what a utopian future situation might be like. Indeed, this is where the true potential of the arts within health can be harnessed: the arts can be more than a 'fix-it' solution but can be rich, varied, and creative. For example, if the problem identified is that patients post surgery are not doing their rehabilitation exercises, the solution might well involve setting up specific classes that post-surgical patients can attend to do their exercises together to ensure they get done. This would be a problem-based solution. If we are looking at incorporating the arts, the equivalent problem-based solution could be a dance-based exercise class with the aim of making the exercise more engaging. However, design thinking would encourage the identification of a more utopian goal. This is where the arts can be of real value. The utopian vision might be that people are not just exercising more but experience a growth in self-confidence and feel proud of their achievements, leading them to encourage more exercise among their friends and family. A way of achieving this through the arts could involve getting participants to choreograph some of their own routines, put on a performance for family and friends, or make their own film raising awareness about dance for health. It might involve the use of CDs for participants to dance to music at home or trips to watch professional dance performances to inspire participants further. This more creative and varied activity, developed as part of design thinking through the aim of achieving more than just exercise, could lead to combined longer-term physical and psychosocial benefits. When undertaking design thinking, it can be valuable to hold a session for open ideas generation in which participants are encouraged to suggest as many ideas as they can, building on what other people say, even if they do not seem immediately feasible. Later, the full range of creative opportunities can then be honed down to an ambitious yet realistic intervention.

In addition, it may be useful to employ *open innovation*. This term was promoted in relation to technology by Henry Chesbrough, the faculty director of the Centre for Open Innovation at the Haas School of Business at the University of California.(10) It involves bringing in outside ideas and opinions as well as relying on internal ideas. In relation to arts in health, open innovation need not be confined just to technology. It might involve setting up a patient-public involvement (PPI) group involving patients or staff engaged in the area to discuss ideas, or partnering with an external organization to jointly develop a brief, or running an ideas competition in which people can propose projects that meet the brief. As with *design thinking*, open innovation can be an iterative phase, involving initial ideas, further project development, and even the piloting of suggestions. For example, if a project is being considered that involves the creation of a website page with short artistic educational films to encourage people to manage their diabetes, design thinking may lead to the development of more ambitious ideas about the content of the films, their target audience, and their aims. Open innovation may lead to working up ideas with an app company instead who propose developing an app rather than a website. At this point, it may be worth discussing the idea with a PPI group or even showing some proof-of-concept graphics ideas to some patients to see if they like the concept; maybe even putting out a competition call for artists to design their own logos for the project, with the winner going on to design the graphics for the films.

As the project develops through design thinking and open innovation, it is also worth applying *systems thinking*,(11) which is another concept developed in engineering, as well as in ecosystems research. Systems thinking involves considering an arts intervention not as a single individual entity but as a dynamic and complex system comprising different inter-related parts and nested within wider systems such as the healthcare organization involved. Consequently, an arts intervention does not act in isolation but can have wide-ranging knock-on implications (partly shown through developing a problem tree and the care process analysis undertaken in Steps 2 and 3). This may be a positive activity with respect to an arts intervention as it may demonstrate a larger reach of an intervention than initially anticipated. For example, a dance intervention in a hospital specifically designed to improve mental wellbeing among cancer patients could also improve body strength, social support networks, and self-esteem. However, systems thinking also involves considering other inputs that might jeopardize these potential benefits. For example, cancer treatments may lead to reduced energy levels and weaker bones, meaning that participants actually lose confidence as they see their strength diminishing. So the intervention may not be able to achieve its initial aims unless it is designed carefully. Furthermore, systems thinking also involves isolating potential implications for the project. For example, if some patients are quite frail, it may be necessary to have a nurse or a physiotherapist in the room while the intervention is taking place, which could have budget implications or place extra strain on staff. Early identification of the potential and the possible problems of an intervention allows planning to take place to make necessary adjustments, thus making the intervention run more smoothly.

Interventions should also be assessed to see if they have potential longevity: *futures thinking*. Investing in DVD players to show films in waiting areas does not make economic sense if these DVD players are going to be out of date within a couple of years. And murals painted onto a corridor wall may have to be removed if the area is scheduled to be repainted in a few months. As well as identifying hurdles such as these, cleaning, repairs, and general upkeep also should be factored into the design of projects so that there is budget set aside. Otherwise the project will not be sustainable in the long term. Sometimes it may be possible to plan in 'redevelopments' of the project, such as through periodic 'improvement' meetings, perhaps involving the PPI group. Or it may be possible to budget for upgrades of equipment where necessary. Even if it is not known whether an intervention will continue after its initial pilot phase, planning for this eventuality in the early stages will increase the likelihood of it being continued and demonstrate a more thought-through intervention, which may help with funding applications.

Plan a logic model

Based on the ideas that have been generated, it should be possible to construct a logic model. Logic models (also known as logical frameworks or programme matrices) are tools that allow graphical depiction of the logical relationship between components including inputs, interventions, and impacts. Working backwards, it should now be clear what the desired impacts are for the intervention, including short-, medium-, and long-term effects. The ideas generation process should have identified what the intervention will consist of to achieve these impacts, including the actual arts activities (whether performative, visual, aural, technological, or other) and how people will engage with them (whether actively taking part, a more receptive engagement, or a subconscious involvement). In mapping out the logic model, it should become clear whether the intervention is entirely matching the planned impacts, or whether adjustments must be made to align them more effectively.

The final category to plan for is the inputs: what is invested to allow the intervention to happen. Depending on the nature of the intervention, inputs involve several categories. Below is a checklist of some of the key logistical features that may be involved. These may not be necessary for each intervention and there may be others added to the list for specific projects. Nevertheless, this list offers an important starting point in mapping the requirements of a project and ascertaining what financial and physical resources are necessary:

- Personnel
  - Staff required to project manage an intervention
  - Staff required to run the intervention sessions
  - Key stakeholders within the organizations involved
  - Project champions (to encourage buy-in or recruitment)
  - A patient-public involvement group
  - The participants themselves

- ◆ Funding
  - Pilot funding
  - In-kind support
- ◆ Infrastructure
  - Location or venue
  - Technologies required
  - Instruments, equipment, or resources
  - Transport
  - Staff training
- ◆ Marketing
  - A project website
  - Advertisement leaflets and other collateral
  - Social media channels
- ◆ Safeguarding
  - Organizational permissions
  - Ethical approval or permissions
  - Criminal record checks
  - Occupational health checks
  - Contracts for staff involved
  - Appropriate insurance and indemnity
  - Risk assessments
  - Vulnerable working policies

These processes and physical items are discussed in detail later in the book, in particular in Chapters 7 and 8. Mapping out these requirements in detail is an important part of logic modelling as it shows what the intervention will actually require. At this stage, it may become clear that a project is overly ambitious as the requirements are beyond the capabilities of staff and resources available. Alternatively, the logic model may lead to further elements of a project being added into the plan. Project planning tools, such as Gantt charts (which illustrate a project schedule), help map out the activities to take place and show where multiple streams of work may need to coincide. This can help in distributing staff appropriately and planning for project budgets. Appropriate lead time is needed to manage each of these elements, as well as a contingency plan if these deadlines are not met. In particular, sufficient time should be mapped out for participant recruitment.

Q For more information on logic models, Lisa Wyatt Knowlton and Cynthia C. Phillips's *The Logic Model Guidebook: Better Strategies for Great Results* (2012) provides a comprehensive guide to planning and using logic models.(12)

Map the vision

As well as confirming the fine-tuned details of an intervention, it can also help to step back and maintain sight of the overall big picture of the project. 'Balanced scorecards' can be used to tie together the work of Steps 1, 2, 3, and 4, mapping the vision and strategy for an intervention. Balanced scorecards were originally developed in business to keep track of the execution of activities and monitor consequences. They have been applied within healthcare systems, for example to monitor performance at an organizational level and report to healthcare funders. However, they are also important later in the project development process as a way of planning a measurement and management system. They will be discussed again in this second capacity in Step 5 (Chapter 6).

A balanced scorecard typically looks at several different areas of performance. Exactly what these are will vary according to the type of project and its setting. Nevertheless, there are generally four key areas as well as an overarching vision and aim for the project: the target group, finance, internal process, and learning and growth.(13) Once the intervention has been devised, it is advisable to map what the vision and strategy will be for each of these for areas, and in particular to ascertain how this could be achieved in an initial pilot of the proposed intervention. The balanced scorecard exercise can be particularly helpful in ascertaining whether a project is feasible and preparing for running a pilot in Step 5 (discussed in Chapter 6).

Target group

Following the previous work of Steps 1-3, it should be clear what the project hopes to achieve. In this section of the balanced scorecard, the aims and vision for this target group should be set out. Although it may still be too early to tell exactly what a project can achieve in measurable terms (something that will become much clearer with a pilot), understanding the broad headings of this planned impact is important. This could include both physical and psychological health-related outcomes or enhanced patient experience. However, the vision should be broader than this and also consider the values of the project that will mean it appeals to participants and a wider vision for the project. For example, a clay modelling group may have the aim of supporting people who have been bereaved in coming to terms with their loss. But the vision would also go beyond this and perhaps include the development of a safe space and social support network for participants, and also aim to build resilience and self-esteem through the acquisition of a new skill and a medium through which the participants can express their experiences.

Finance

The intervention should also have an initial plan for how it will succeed financially and be sustained in the long term. The vision may be for the project to receive core healthcare funding, or for it to receive a multi-year charitable grant, or for it to be financially self-sustaining. Different funding models are discussed in Chapter 7 and selecting an appropriate one is an important part of the balanced scorecard exercise. It is anticipated that at this early stage, the precise funders may not be known, but the strategic plans and financial vision of how to make the intervention financially viable should be outlined. Importantly, the plans for how a *pilot* will be funded must be outlined clearly at this stage to show how the project can be tested in practice.

In addition to planning where the money is going to come from, it may be possible to map out the target 'cost-per-head' for involvement, or to plan rough budgets for the intervention. There may be economies of scale, meaning that if a certain number of people are involved the overall cost will be reduced. However, any anticipated costs for maintenance, such as technology updates, training of new staff to be involved, or refreshing of resources, should be planned too. These costs may change following a pilot, but knowing what they are anticipated to be is one way of ascertaining whether a project ends up above or below its initial projected costs once it is piloted.

Internal processes

There should also be consideration of how the project will fit in with existing internal processes. It may be that the intervention is contingent on a particular programme of care continuing in an organization, or certain staff members being involved. The complexity of the processes should also be mapped out so it is clear how the project will be managed. If there is a vision for the project becoming part of routine care and therefore assimilated within part of a care process, this should be outlined too.

Learning and growth

For the project to achieves its aims, especially the impact on the target audience, plans should be put in place for how it will be improved to sustain the initial vision. This may involve decisions to propose annual meetings of a steering group to monitor progress, or relevant conferences could be planned for a project team member to attend. Learning and growth should be outlined at this early stage to ensure that the required resources are built into the project's design. Attempting to set up steering groups from scratch later in a project can be more challenging, so securing the involvement of key stakeholders early on and planning for their roles in the future can provide a firm foundation for the project.

As previously mentioned, there may be other headings within the balanced scorecard that are particularly pertinent to an individual project, so this is by no means the limit of its use. The exercise can be an important step in ascertaining whether there is indeed the potential for the project to be carried out, or whether there are further obstacles that could become a hindrance. We will return to this balanced scorecard in the Chapter 6.

> Q BMcD Consulting have produced a report entitled *A Review of the Use of the Balanced Scorecard in Healthcare* (2011). The review explores how it has been used, the main factors associated with its successful implementation, and provides learning from case studies.(13) The review is available on their website www.bmcdconsulting.com.

Summary

The overall aim is that by the end of Step 4 there is a well-designed and thoroughly planned arts intervention that meets a clear need and has targets ready for testing. It is not necessarily expected that this will be the final version of the intervention. Indeed, interventions often work differently in reality compared with theory. Nevertheless, interventions that have involved a careful planning process are more likely to have a smoother piloting and implementation phase, so time invested in these early stages can reap rewards later down the line. In Chapter 6, we move from considering how to plan an intervention to how to implement and evaluate it. It is here that the ideas developed in this chapter can really come to fruition.

References

1. **Nightingale F.** Notes on Hospitals [Internet]. Longman, Green, Longman, Roberts, and Green; 1863 [cited 2016 Feb 7]. 240 pp. Available from: http://archive.org/details/notesonhospital01nighgoog.
2. **Sheingold BH, Hahn JA.** The history of healthcare quality: The first 100 years 1860–1960. Int J Afr Nurs Sci. 2014;1:18–22.
3. **Aguilar FJ.** Scanning the Business Environment. 1st THUS edition. New York: Macmillan; 1967.
4. **King D, Greaves F, Exeter C, Darzi A.** 'Gamification': Influencing health behaviours with games. J R Soc Med. 2013 Mar 1;**106**(3):76–8.
5. **Kolb DA.** Experiential Learning: Experience as the Source of Learning and Development. 1 edition. Englewood Cliffs, N.J.: Financial Times/ Prentice Hall; 1983. 288 p.

6. **Geertz C.** Thick description: toward an interpretive theory of culture. Interpret Cult. 1973;3–30.

7. **Brace I.** Questionnaire Design: How to Plan, Structure and Write Survey Material for Effective Market Research. 2 edition. London ; Philadelphia: Kogan Page; 2008. 320 pp.

8. **Matell MS**, **Jacoby J.** Is there an optimal number of alternatives for Likert scale items? I. Reliability and validity. Educ Psychol Meas. 1971;**31**(3):657–74.

9. **Simon HA.** The Sciences of the Artificial. Cambridge, Massachusetts: MIT Press; 1996. 252 pp.

10. **Chesbrough HW.** Open Innovation: The New Imperative for Creating And Profiting from Technology. First Trade Paper Edition. Boston, Mass.: Harvard Business Review Press; 2006. 272 pp.

11. **Weinberg GM** . An introduction to general systems thinking. Dorset House Publishing, US; 2011.

12. **Knowlton LW**, **Phillips CC.** The Logic Model Guidebook: Better Strategies for Great Results. Los Angeles, London, New Delhi: SAGE Publications; 2012. 193 pp.

13. **McDonald B.** A Review of the Use of the Balanced Scorecard in Healthcare [Internet]. BMcD Consulting; 2012 Apr [cited 2016 Oct 31]. Available from: http://www.bmcdconsulting.com/index_htm_files/Review%20of%20the%20Use%20of%20the%20Balanced%20Scorecard%20in%20Healthcare%20BMcD.pdf.

Chapter 6

Implementing and evaluating interventions

In Chapter 5, we explored how to conceptualize and plan an arts in health intervention, moving from broad considerations of the national or even international environment to the specific problems of a select participant group at a select point in their health journey. We then expanded out again, considering how an intervention could solve not just the immediate challenge identified but lead to a wider improvement for the target group and their network, and planning how this intervention could be put into action and developed in a way that had the possibility of turning into a long-term project. Whereas Chapter 5 focused on 'thinking', this chapter explores how to turn thinking into action and how to implement, evaluate, and maximize the potential of the intervention.

Step 5: Carry out active experimentation

Step 5 follows on from Step 4 and involves the final stage in David Kolb's Reflective Cycle, as discussed in Chapter 5: active experimentation. This step is very much a test of the detail and insight gathered through the previous four steps, with the most successful interventions being those that are built on firm foundations. Active experimentation can be split itself into four stages, the first of which involves piloting the intervention.

Pilot the intervention

Piloting can be valuable for three reasons. First, it gives an opportunity for an intervention to be road-tested. Although the previous steps may have revealed rich information about the health challenge identified and how it could potentially be solved, in reality things may work differently. Aims and expectations may need to be altered, or methods of working changed to maximize impact. Road-testing can be of enormous value for artists and healthcare professionals involved. The arts have not developed exclusively to support health; not by any means. However, in being applied in health, similar to being applied in educational settings for example, there are certain restrictions that may be imposed by practicalities such as the participant group, the location or the institutions involved. These can be idiosyncratic and change for each intervention. Consequently, in designing arts in health interventions there may be a necessary shift in working practice for artists, or a process of acclimatization to the new environment. In a well-designed intervention, this should not mean a compromise of any of the artistic components or aims. However, it may take some time for the boundaries to be understood and the opportunities for flourishing identified. Similarly, the process of acclimatization also applies to health professionals. As discussed in Chapter 5, arts interventions offer enormous creative potential, meaning that an initial challenge identified need not just be 'met', but can be met in a way that goes beyond a simple solution and offers something more engaging and effective with other potential gains. It may take time for the effects of this creativity to be realized and understood. For example, if a project aims to allow nurses opportunities to express their worries and stresses, an arts activity involving creative poetry workshops for nurses may require a few pilot sessions before the artists leading the workshops can identify which language and methods encourage the nurses to engage in poetry; something very different and, on the surface, quite far removed from their day-to-day work. Equally, it may take time for the nurses to feel comfortable enough to engage in the process and express themselves through poetry when some might feel that a feedback form about what they find good and bad about the job would have been more efficient. However, over the course of a pilot it may be that poetry writing not only encourages those who might have been nervous about speaking up to express themselves, but also provides greater solidarity among staff and a greater awareness in the hospital as a whole about the challenges faced by nurses. Therefore, piloting offers an opportunity to assess which elements of an intervention work in meeting the challenge as well as which may need to be altered, improved, or streamlined to maximize the artistic and health outcomes.

Building on this first point, another important reason for piloting an intervention is that it allows staff and stakeholders to see what a project involves so they are properly bought-in. Some projects may be led by healthcare staff or have involved staff engagement right from the start, including the identification of the initial challenge, through the consultation process, and through the design of the activity. This can be a real strength for a project as these staff can help to engage other staff, facilitating smooth implementation. However, if healthcare staff have not been as involved in the development of an intervention, they may be more cautious, for example because of concerns that the project will not be suitable for their patients, will distract them from doing their work, or will even create more work for them. Some may, understandably, be sceptical as to the value of the intervention. This may lead to a general reserve around agreeing to entire projects straight away. However, a single or short series of pilot sessions can allow staff to see a project in action before they have to make a decision about it becoming a long-term feature. This can prevent the appearance that an arts intervention is being 'thrust' on a hospital ward, nursing home, or community centre and instead help to give staff more ownership of the project as they can then feed into its evaluation and future plans, ensuring it is as well suited as possible to its environment.

Finally, piloting can also help in sourcing funding for a longer project. Many larger funders require evidence that an intervention is feasible, can be carried out, and has the potential to achieve its aims. Even for small funding sources, demonstrating that an idea can be realized is one of the most important parts of an application. To help to leverage this funding for a longer project, a short pilot (for which the costs may be relatively low) can be used as a proof of concept as well as giving an opportunity for evaluation data to be gathered. In Chapter 7, we explore some of these funding models in greater depth.

When undertaking a pilot, there are a few guidelines that should be followed. First, for a pilot to be effective, it should be run as closely as possible to how it is proposed that the actual intervention will run. This will give an opportunity to test as many of the key features as is feasible, limiting the amount of risk with the full intervention later on. However, to make it a smaller undertaking, the overall length of the intervention may be reduced, or the numbers involved may be decreased. Nevertheless, the temptation to involve only those participants who have already had significant involvement in the planning of the intervention should be avoided as they are likely already to be advocates of the project, and this could lead to skewed evaluation data.

Evaluate the pilot

As part of the experimentation stage and the undertaking of a pilot, it is also critical to gather evaluation data. There are many different types of evaluation and ways of carrying them out. However, there is no single optimum way of designing or undertaking an evaluation: the most effective evaluations are those that identify what information is most needed to test the potential of the intervention and support its future development and involve a bespoke evaluation design. This can be split into three core questions:

1. Is the intervention well designed and suitable for its participants?

2. Does the intervention run smoothly and fit in with the care process?

3. Does the intervention show signs that it will, in its full form, be able to achieve its aims?

To answer these three questions, there are three types of evaluation that can be carried out:

1. Formative evaluations—Formative evaluations have the aim of improving a project's design and performance. A formative evaluation may assess whether the project is suitable for the target participants, ascertain whether it has integrity as an intervention, and identify what changes are needed to improve its design

2. Process evaluations—Process evaluations explore the successes and challenges related to how an intervention runs. This may include identifying not just what worked well but also what the potential obstacles were and how these could be overcome; assessing how well the intervention fits in with other processes involving participants, staff, or institutions; and confirming whether the logic model from Step 4 appears to hold in practice as well as in theory and whether the inputs-intervention-impacts flow holds strong

3. Outcome evaluations—Outcome evaluations ascertain whether an intervention had the desired effect on participants. This may include confirming whether the main outcomes show signs of being achieved, exploring whether there are other subsidiary effects, and identifying how the intervention could be adapted to improve its impact

Evaluating a pilot is, of course, not going to give a complete picture of how the actual intervention will run, as the pilot is, by nature, a simplified or smaller-scale version. However, a project that does not produce strong results for the three types of evaluation is unlikely to find success on a larger scale. A key issue is how to go about running these evaluations, as different qualitative and quantitative methods can be involved in an evaluation.

Quantitative evaluations

These involve numerical data and often take the form of questionnaires distributed to participants, families, or staff. Quantitative evaluations may directly ask participants if an intervention achieved its aims, such as asking older adults in a dance for falls prevention programme if they think they fell fewer times during the programme than before. This direct approach can yield useful responses, but it can also lead to bias as participants feel they are expected to respond positively. Techniques to avoid this include using evaluation forms both before and after the pilot, for example asking people at the start how many times on average they fall a month and asking the same question again at the end; or providing multiple choice responses, such as listing a number of possible outcomes participants may have experienced, both likely and unlikely, positive and negative, including 'falling less frequently' and see if participants select that as an option.

Alternatively, quantitative evaluations may use measures that have been validated (a procedure that demonstrates that they accurately measure what they claim to measure) to ask participants about their experience. For example, validated depression measures typically will not ask participants directly if they 'feel depressed', but rather ask them about symptoms that are associated with depression to build up a picture of whether participants show signs of depression. Such validated measures have the benefit of often having national or local average data against which responses can be benchmarked. However, for pilot evaluations, this level of detail may not always be necessary. Quantitative evaluations may also assess more objective data, such as records in a nursing home about how many falls there have been on a ward since the participants engaged in the dancing programme.

A helpful thing to include in quantitative evaluations is a section of the original consultation form used in Step 3 (see Chapter 5). The baseline data gathered before the intervention will provide a benchmark against which data from the pilot evaluation can be compared. If recorded music is being integrated into a waiting area to improve the patient experience, the question on patient experience used in the consultation form can be replicated in the evaluation form to see whether the recorded music did indeed have an impact. Quantitative evaluations need not only cover outcome data, but also can ask participants and staff about their experience of the intervention to provide information for the process evaluation, and ascertain their views on the intervention experience for the formative evaluation. For pilot evaluations in particular, it is good to invite participants to be honest and give plenty of opportunity for negative responses as this will help the intervention to improve. In light of this, although quantitative data can provide clear and powerful statistics, these are best informed by qualitative approaches too, to understand the results better.

Qualitative evaluations

These can include focus groups, interviews, observations, and free-response questions. Focus groups involve a selection of participants being invited to join a group discussion. Questions asked may cover the core themes of the formative, process, and outcome evaluations. Group discussions may provide a range of views on problems or successes. However, sometimes participants may feel concerned about being a dissenting voice, so individual interviews also can be helpful. Interviews and focus groups are often most effective when they have a planned outline structure to ensure that the important questions are asked, but also allow flexibility for participants to provide information that may not have been planned for; a semi-structured style.

As well as face-to-face feedback, free-responses boxes in evaluation forms can also provide a completely anonymous way of participants feeding back, which can provide very honest information. However, with free-response boxes, there is not the opportunity to ask for clarification or enquire more about a problem. So this method of evaluating is often best used in tandem with a face-to-face approach.

In some instances, observation of activities may also provide helpful information. This could involve informal observation of sessions to ascertain whether participants appear engaged, facilitators feel at ease, and activities are manageable and enjoyable. Having a list of questions or lines of enquiry during an informal observation can help to order what is observed. Facilitators also can be asked for their own observations of how sessions have run. For more objective observation, there are some specific observation tools available, such as the Arts Observation Scale, which is a mixed-methods observation tool for pilots that can be used to assess changes in mood, relaxation, and distraction across an intervention.(1) This can be particularly helpful for interventions in which it may not be possible to collect questionnaire feedback, such as when working with people with severe dementia.

Related to qualitative methods are creative and arts-based methods. These include more artistic ways of gathering evaluation data. On a simple level, this could include taking photographs or recordings of the activities, or maybe creating a short film. This can often support the development of the project by showing stakeholders and possible funders exactly what the intervention involves. Alternative methods include showcasing any outputs from the intervention, such as pictures or sculptures made or recordings of performances. Arts-based methods can also involve capturing experience through the arts, such as asking participants to create graphical representations of their experiences in the intervention or analysing the outputs from an intervention as evaluation materials in their own right. This may be suitable for certain participant demographics, such as younger children for whom feedback forms may not be suitable. More details on qualitative and quantitative techniques are provided in Chapter 10.

Evaluations can either be approached in a 'top-down' way, with evaluation forms designed by staff or external organizations and provided to those involved, or the evaluation can be undertaken in a more collaborative way, such as through participatory action research methods, in which participants themselves sit at the centre of the process and play a key role in guiding the form it takes.(2) They can also either focus on groups of people involved, or just zone in on the experience of one or more individual participants as case studies. Case studies can sometimes be confused with anecdotal evidence, but they should, if conducted well, provide more in-depth information. Case studies may choose to focus on a 'typical' participant as a way of giving insight into how the intervention may be received by a wider pool of participants. Or they may focus on an outlier who for some reason had a different experience, either as a way of highlighting the flexibility of an intervention or giving an example of how the intervention might need to be adapted in the future. Case studies often involve information gathered from multiple sources, including perhaps interviews with the case participant or group, reports from observations of that individual, staff, or family member, and arts-based methods. It must be noted that case studies give only a snap-shot view. As such, they often work well alongside other quantitative and qualitative data as a way of illustrating more tangibly the effects noted from a larger group.

For all evaluation activities, ethical considerations are important. In general permission should be obtained from participants before any photographs or filming are undertaken, feedback forms should be anonymous, and any data presented should not be easily linked back to the original participants so, where appropriate, names and other identifying features should be removed. Ethical considerations are discussed further in Chapter 12.

As this is simply an evaluation of a pilot, the evaluation should be proportional to the size of the pilot. For small pilots, the evaluation need not take up too much time or resource either for participants or staff involved in gathering and analysing the data; evaluation will be returned to more thoroughly once the intervention is properly up and running. Consequently, it may not be possible to capture every potential project impact. However, the results of the pilot evaluation should be carefully considered. On the one hand, they may provide important information about how an intervention needs to be modified: it is common that interventions that appear to have strong logic models and to be suitable for the participant group do not always work as well in practice. Alternatively, evaluations that produce strong results can become a powerful source of support for the larger intervention, including helping to improve staff buy-in and convince external partners of the value of being involved with the project. However, care should always be taken that evaluations do not merely become advocacy, recommending the project rather than exploring how it went, but rather are designed in a balanced way and the results dealt with accordingly.

Q Public Health England has produced an evaluation framework for 'Arts for health and wellbeing', which includes more information on undertaking evaluations and a proposed tool for reporting the outcomes of evaluations.(3)

Remap the vision

Once an intervention has been piloted and the evaluation data gathered, it is important to weigh up the different aspects of the project as a whole by returning to the balanced scorecard. This gives a chance to ascertain whether the original vision and strategy for the intervention has been maintained. If a project has moved off initial target, this may signal that adjustments are needed. However, it may also be that the intervention has merely settled into a more appropriate niche. In this case, it may be that the initial vision and strategy needs to be updated.

As well as updating the balanced scorecard, an important development following the pilot is to turn the visions and goals of the project into clear and concise objectives. These objectives will set out more specifically what the intervention has the potential to achieve. Objectives should, if possible, be 'SMART' to maximize their clarity to readers. SMART objectives were set out by George T Doran in 1981 in the journal *Management Review*.(4) Doran proposed that if people focused their attention onto five criteria when setting objectives, then they would have a higher chance of succeeding. The criteria areas that objectives should aim to contain are:

◆ Specific: clearly defined and well targeted to the participant group

◆ Measurable: it should be possible to track whether the objective has been achieved

◆ Assignable: stakeholders involved in the project should confirm that the objectives are suitable and specific people should be assigned to make them happen

◆ Realistic: it should be possible to achieve them through the intervention

◆ Time-related: there should be enough time to achieve the objectives, yet not so much that they lose their value

So, for example, an objective should not be 'the dancing class will improve mobility', but rather 'a 6-week programme of weekly hour-long dance classes will lead to 90% of participants self-rating that they feel more generally mobile than before they started the programme'. Often interventions will have more than one objective. However, more than five or six objectives for each of the four headings in the balanced scorecard could lead to a diffuse project rather than one that is clearly defined. These objectives will become what is tested as part of the full evaluation and, if relevant, the framework for what is taken forwards as a research idea. Consequently, they are an important output from the pilot evaluation.

> Q Project Smart is an online resource that contains further information on establishing SMART objectives as well as containing a wealth of other information for establishing effective projects. www.projectsmart.co.uk.

Draw up a case for support

Equally important following the pilot evaluation is the development of a case for support. The case for support should draw together all the learning and evidence from the steps so far. Cases for support are most commonly used for funding applications and they explain exactly what a project is, what it aims to do, and what is involved in running it. Cases for support may not be formally necessary for projects, such as where funds are already committed. However, in addition to their role in funding applications, cases for support can also provide important overviews of a project to convince people of its need and value or engage project partners and form the template document for website pages, presentations to stakeholders, or award applications, giving it a life beyond the initial set-up of the project. So it is advisable to develop one for each intervention even if one is not directly requested. These different aims mean that cases for support will differ depending on the audience, and, depending on which funding sources are being considered for a project, there may be specific formats that they need to take. Nevertheless, there are certain core sections within a case for support that will be similar across all uses, and having a draft version at hand can help to ensure that the project is well mapped out and will save time when people ask for further information about the intervention or when there is a need to present information on the project at short notice.

A case for support should be concise with a clear argument as to the need for an intervention and how the proposed intervention meets that need as well as what the project requires to run. If there is no formal requirement for a case for support that sets the structure or format, a good length to aim for is one to two pages. The key parts of a case for support include:

1. Executive summary—This should outline the project in a few sentences, including who it aims to reach, what it aims to do, how it will do it, and what the implications of this are. The executive summary often summarizes what the rest of the document says, although care should be taken to ensure that there is not obvious repetition within the document

2. Aims and objectives—The initial vision and the measurable objectives that were set up as part of the balanced scorecard should be translated into the case for support too. If a project is designed in such a way that it is possible to achieve a high number of objectives, these could be summarized

3. Evidence—Part of the job of the case for support is to convince people that an intervention can achieve the aims it has set out to achieve. In Step 3, research was undertaken into existing interventions or research projects relevant to the intervention. Summarizing these can help to demonstrate the potential of the intervention. Data collected from the pilot study will also be of value.

Often the addition of photographs or quotations from participants can help to make an intervention more tangible

4. Logistics—The case for support should detail who is involved in the intervention, what processes are required to make it run, and where and when it takes place. This should include references to any partners or project leaders. This section should include enough information that a reader can understand how the project will run, but it need not include every ingredient; the case for support is not intended to be a full manual for the project, but rather a summary overview

5. Support—If funding or other support is still required, this should be outlined clearly in the case for support. For funding, providing a short summary of the budget and the amount sought could be an introduction to a larger document with a full budget once a potential funder shows interest. If other support is sought, such as arts partners, healthcare staff, or more practical support such as institutional buy-in or a location for the intervention, this can all be detailed too. If there are any benefits that supporters may receive, such as their logo on publicity material, involvement in an advisory group, or an invitation to see the outputs of the project, these can be mapped out too. The case for support should also list a key contact who can provide further information

By the end of Step 4, the project should be ready for proper implementation. Chapters 7 and 8 look at the practicalities of implementing a project in more detail. If all the previous steps have been followed well, there should be a high chance of the intervention providing value to its participants. Chapter 10 explores how to go about developing a research project to ascertain much more information about this potential value. However, the rest of this chapter focuses on the future of the intervention itself.

Step 6: Review and act

Following the implementation of an intervention, the sixth step in the process is to review critically its running and its impact and take steps to ensure its longevity. There are three stages that can be particularly helpful in this review process to ensure that it is running as efficiently and effectively as possible.

Hone the intervention

As a project settles into a rhythm, it will become apparent which parts of the process required to run the intervention are essential to its continuation and which parts could perhaps be simplified to maximize its efficiency. One simple way of assessing this is to apply 'lean thinking'. Initially developed by Toyota in the 1950s, lean thinking helped to turn a Japanese car company on the edge of bankruptcy into one of the largest motor companies in the world.(5) Toyota invested time and training in understanding and reasoning with processes involved in car manufacturing. This included ways of eliminating waste and improving flow. Lean thinking values include:

1. Spending time with the intervention to see how it works first hand, rather than relying on reports from others

2. Valuing every element of a process, stopping at any part that appears doubtful and correcting defects

3. Planning the time required for each stage in the intervention so that capacity can be properly understood

4. Mapping what the real demand is and adjusting to that, rather than trying to force numbers higher or lower to suit the intervention

5. Identifying parts of tension in the process and spreading the workload to accommodate these better

6. Commitment to making small changes one step at a time with the aim of improving a process overall

To implement these values within healthcare, lean thinking is often discussed through the '5 Ss'; five processes to organize, standardize, and eliminate non-valuable steps.(6) The exact terms used for each of the Ss vary depending on different sources. However, the steps are broadly the same across different models:

- **Sort**—The intervention should be organized so that things that are not essential can be identified and separated out from things that are integral to the intervention. Resources and staff time also should be sorted, with only the necessary amount of equipment/technology/consumables ordered for each intervention and just the necessary staff members or number of staff hours involved. There might be features that were initially thought to be important, such as musical instruments in a session or additional art supplies, which have been found to be superfluous or underused

- **Set in order**—All parts of the process surrounding the intervention should be scrutinized, including how participants are engaged, how they are managed through the intervention, and how they are followed-up as well as the processes required in actually running the intervention. Where processes can be cut back or simplified, this should be undertaken. Similarly, physical items required in an intervention should be ordered and stored as simply as possible

- **Shine**—Clutter should be removed from the intervention and the elements that remain should be cleaned. This might involve redesigning publicity to make it more targeted to the participant group or including more details about the intervention once it has settled into a regular mode. Or it might involve refreshing social media awareness or website pages

- **Standardize**—The elements and processes that remain should be turned into standard operating procedures so it is clear the value and importance they hold for the future running of the intervention. This process will be supported by 'manualizing', which is discussed in 'Manualize the intervention' later in this chapter

- **Sustain**—Finally, plans should be put in place for how the intervention can continue to run effectively including preparing budgets and sourcing funding, mapping staff support, and setting up more rolling recruitment campaigns

> For more information about lean thinking, Robert Chalice turns the 5 Ss into 46 separate steps to support streamlined interventions within healthcare in his book *Improving Healthcare Using Toyota Lean Production Methods* (2007).(7)

Evaluate the intervention

Once an intervention is up and running properly, it is important to return to evaluation. As with the pilot evaluation, the full intervention evaluation should consider the three types of evaluation described before: formative, process, and outcome. Much of the same methods from the pilot evaluation may be employed, including questions to check whether previous problems have been successfully overcome. However, the evaluation now has two further goals. First of all, a full evaluation will be able to explore the effects of an intervention in much greater detail. Sometimes intervention evaluations are used as a precursor to research projects. Second, a full evaluation can be used to set benchmarks for future monitoring and audits. Audits in healthcare are intended to be more resource-efficient evaluations once an initial evaluation has taken place and they ascertain whether interventions are continuing in line with the standards they aspire to. Chapter 9 considers the relationship among evaluation, research, and audits in more detail.

Consequently, the evaluation project for the full intervention may repeat methods from the pilot evaluation in greater detail, but crucially it should also draw on the SMART outcomes from the balanced scorecard, using these as a set of measuring standards and ascertaining whether they have been achieved.

If they have, it is a sign that the intervention is running well and a simplified version of the process can be repeated periodically (as an audit) to ensure these standards are maintained. If the standards have not been met, this demonstrates that aspects of the intervention need to be altered, for which the rest of the evaluation (especially the formative and process evaluations) will help to provide more information. For some projects, it may be that the initial targets are simply not met, perhaps because of circumstances beyond the control of those involved. In this instance, it may be that initial ambitions were too high and that they must be readjusted, followed by checking whether all stakeholders and partners are still interested in pursuing the intervention. Or it may be that an intervention has to be withdrawn and rethought before being implemented again. It is possible that interventions that do not meet their targets can still continue. However, it is rare that interventions that are not providing measurable outcomes are able to secure long-term funding, so even if the outcomes have changed, identifying what they are and finding a way of measuring them is important.

Project evaluations are often made public, and this should be encouraged. Positive results may encourage similar projects to be developed elsewhere, while honesty over obstacles and challenges will prevent other teams from repeating the same mistakes. Project evaluations with good results may be further developed into research projects. This will be explored in Chapter 10.

Manualize the intervention

Another important part of Step 6 is 'manualizing' the intervention: comprehensively documenting what the intervention involves so that it can be maintained properly and with appropriate quality, or even developed in more locations. Manualizing an intervention combines several stages from the process just described, so can grow organically out of previous work. A helpful tool in manualizing is the TIDieR checklist, a template for intervention description and replication.(8) TIDieR suggests that there are 12 essential pieces of information that must be logged for an intervention to be well understood by people who have not been involved and replicated in other locations.

1. Brief name

Although the precise name of an intervention may change depending on when and where it is taking place, if the intervention claims to be associated with the initial project, it will need in some way to be identified back with this project, so a brief name or phrase describing the intervention is necessary. Precision in the name is also a way of being able to link back any future research reports or outputs from projects with the initial intervention.

2. Why

A rationale, theory, or goal of the elements essential to the intervention should be outlined. This will largely build on the work of Step 2 (concrete experience), including the data from the care process analysis, shadowing, and discovering interviews, as well as aspects of Step 3 (reflective observation), including the formal consultation process, research, and causal modelling. Explaining the background to an intervention can help others to see which elements are essential rather than incidental. Of course, the initial challenge that inspired an arts in health intervention in the initial location may be different in other locations as demographics, situational factors, and topical issues change. However, in manualizing an intervention, the focus is on the current intervention; it will be up to future interventions or spin-outs of this original project to run a mini-version of this entire seven-step process to ensure that the intervention in its current form is still relevant or to identify which features might require some alterations.

3-4. What

This section should clarify the materials and procedures involved in delivering the intervention. This could involve materials provided to participants required for the running of the intervention or used in the training of intervention providers. If the materials used are described elsewhere, such as manufacturers' instructions or previous intervention protocols, these should be referenced. The original TIDieR guide refers to the materials as the ingredients in a recipe, and the procedures as the method. Procedures could involve the activities that occur during an intervention or processes used, including any supporting activities required in the background for the intervention to run smoothly. The more detail that can be provided here, the more useful the manual will be. However, if an intervention requires extensive tailoring to individual participants, there is space for this to be described later in the manual.

5. Who provided

For each staff member or facilitator involved in the project, their role should be described, including their own expertise, background, and any training they received specific to the intervention. Any other characteristics required in the facilitators, whether personality features or more practical things such as criminal record checks, should be identified. These may have come out from some of the evaluation work or through earlier consultation work too.

6. How

The modes of delivery should be outlined. Important features to mention include the contact time required and whether this is delivered in face-to-face interventions or via distance delivery. For face-to-face interventions, it should be clarified whether this involves delivery in a one-to-one or group setting and whether involvement requires either active involvement or a more receptive audience-style approach. Distance delivery can involve online programmes, apps, telephone contact, or more physical installations or media campaigns. In many interventions, there will be a number of modes involved, both in the initial recruitment of participants and in the subsequent running of the intervention and possible follow-up.

7. Where

Locations of the intervention should be logged, both for the initial recruitment and for the intervention itself. These might include hospital clinics, participants' homes, nursing homes, in-patient wards, community halls, or public settings. Locations can exert an influence over the nature of the intervention, either by providing a 'safe space' for participants or through more tangible infrastructure features such as disabled access, on-site nursing, or by offering concurrent treatment for participants. Knowing the location requirements can also help in future interventions when assessing the feasibility of replicating an intervention.

8. When and how much

The intervention schedule should be mapped out, including the frequency of intervention delivery, its duration, intensity, or dose, the overall length of the intervention, and the time of day. If participation involves any additional 'take-home' activities or participants are encouraged to engage in certain behaviours outside the immediate intervention, this should be catalogued too. The schedule of the intervention should also be mapped if appropriate. It is important to specify whether participants had to be at specific stages of health/treatment/recovery to participate so that the correct target group can be involved again in any replications of the intervention.

9. Tailoring

Building on the outline of the intervention given in sections 3-4, tailoring covers circumstances in which different participants receive essentially different versions of the intervention. In the case of one-to-one interventions, it may not be possible to log exactly what each participant received. However, the broad principles of what was adapted for different participants, why, and according to which guidelines should be explained. The ways of assessing participant suitability for different tailored approaches also should be outlined. It may be helpful to construct flowcharts to explain this process.

10. Modifications

If any changes were made to the intervention during its course, these should be catalogued, whether they were major design changes or simple alterations to enable the intervention to run better. This section will help ensure that future interventions do not revert to the less effective mode without realizing, or repeat unnecessary errors.

11-12. How well

These final two related sections assess how good intervention adherence or fidelity was for the intervention and what strategies were involved to support this. For example, if an intervention involves a 10-week programme but participants only routinely attend eight sessions, this is an important detail for future interventions so they can be assured that the intervention is still running well if they experience similar attendance rates. Any strategies for increasing adherence should be explained, both successful and unsuccessful. Participant experience of the intervention and any available evaluation data should also be logged so that future interventions can ascertain whether the project is being met with appropriate responses. Any problems or obstacles that were encountered, whether practical or emotional, also should be outlined, again to avoid unnecessary repetitions of such problems in the future.

Overall, the time investment required to construct a detailed manual will be important in preserving the detail about the intervention. The manual need not merely be a routine document but could be used as one of the outputs of the project along with evaluation results to promote the intervention and encourage others to replicate it or expand on its initial impact.

 More information about the TIDieR checklist including a video introduction can be found on the BMJ website: www.bmj.com/content/348/bmj.g1687.

Step 7: Reconnect

Step 7 is the final step in designing and implementing an arts in health intervention. By Step 7, an entire intervention will have been conceptualized, designed, implemented, and evaluated. It may well be running effectively and, following the financial models outlined in Chapter 7, have secured long-term funding or have been turned into a sustainable service. However, to ensure its ongoing success, there are three further processes that can help to support it.

Remap the environment

Step 1 involved undertaking a PESTLE analysis of the political, economic, social, technological, legal, and environmental factors that might provide a context for an intervention. Once an intervention is in place, reconnecting with these at both a micro (local organization) and macro (wider national or international) level could offer opportunities for the project. There may have been shifts in one or more of these factors that could now give a wider platform for the project. For example, there may be plans for a new political agenda around the health condition involved, a new funding stream may have opened, there may be campaigns to support certain demographics in an area such as a new local ageing programme, new technologies may have come to the market, safeguarding procedures may have changed, or it could simply be a new time of year. Now that there is not just an idea for an intervention but an existing intervention with a range of evaluation data, gaining organizational or wider recognition may be possible. People who may have been sceptical about an idea initially may be convinced now and be able to offer support or other opportunities. Alternatively, there may be new challenges on the horizon that should be planned for accordingly. Regular PESTLE analyses undertaken in the background will help to ensure a smooth path for the project ahead.

Assess the feasibility of expansion

Once an intervention has reached Step 7, there may well be discussion as to whether it can be rolled out to further settings. The UK's National Institute for Health Research 'Collaboration for Leadership in Applied Health Research and Care' team (CLAHRC) is developing a tool to assess the potential of an intervention for roll-out across different locations. They have identified and presented 12 criteria that were found in the majority of successful roll-out interventions explored. They have also developed a 5-point scale from 'very good' to 'good', 'fair', 'poor', and 'very poor' for each of the 12 criteria. Projects that scored fair or higher on each criteria were the ones that most often translated into expanding long-term interventions. The twelve proposed criteria are:

1. Commitment to the project—there is a shared understanding of what the project is trying to achieve from stakeholders

2. Involvement—there is a wide breadth of involvement from stakeholders and partners in relevant areas

3. Skills and capabilities—staff involved in the project have appropriate training, skills, and development opportunities

4. Evidence of benefits—evaluation and possibly research results are available and widely circulated, showing the value of the project

5. Leadership—there are supportive and respected project champions who can advocate for the project

6. Team functioning—there is a team that works well together and shares work effectively

7. Resources in place—there is appropriate financial support, staff time, and infrastructure

8. Robust and adaptable process—the project can adapt to local needs and settings and still be successful

9. Progress monitored for feedback and learning—monitoring systems are in place for the collection and reviewing of data

10. Alignment with organizational culture and priorities—the project meets the strategic aims of the organizations involved

11. Improvement infrastructure—continuous improvement is a priority for the organizations involved (see 'Innovate' below)

12. Alignment with external political and financial environment—the project is supported by its wider context

Charting an intervention using the 5-point scale against each of these criteria prior to planning a roll-out to further locations can show areas that may need to be worked on to give an intervention the best possible chance of success. Projects with the highest chance of development are those that have high scores across all of the 12 domains.

 The CLAHRC Long Term Success Tool is still under development. Further information can be found on the project website www.clahrcprojects.co.uk.

Innovate

Even the most successful interventions will require regular innovations to ensure that they maintain interest from the target group and stay current. Google have proposed eight 'pillars' of innovation that outline the company's approach to growing while staying innovative. These pillars could help arts in health interventions to stay relevant:

1. Have a mission that matters

If the original reasons for the intervention shift, it may mean that the intervention has to undergo a process of redevelopment. This may require simply rebranding the intervention and changing its aims, or it may mean altering the entire intervention. For example, if an intervention involves recorded music in a pre-surgical area as there are no distractions for patients, a change in the process meaning that patients wait somewhere else before the surgery or the provision of television screens in the waiting area may mean that the old intervention no longer has the same need. The innovation will then involve finding the new 'mission that matters', such as moving the music to a different waiting area, or developing an intervention for the television screens.

2. Think big but start small

Spin-offs of the original idea or add-ons to the project could be developed on a small scale to complement the main intervention. These could be scaled up over time if successful.

3. Strive for continual innovation, not instant perfection

It may take time for an intervention to settle completely into its rhythm. Small flaws may keep emerging. However, as long as the project is continuously re-examined and adapted as necessary, innovation will provide protection from problems. This iterative process is akin to the continuous care quality improvement model that is the foundation of many healthcare systems.

> **Q** For more information about care quality improvement, *Continuous Quality Improvement in HealthCare* by Curtis P McLaughlin and Arnold D Kaluzny (2006) provides an in-depth guide.(9)

4. Look for ideas elsewhere

Returning to the ideas of 'open innovation' from Step 4, ideas from elsewhere can help to keep a project up-to-date. This could involve visiting other similar projects or staying abreast of research developments. Often, innovation in arts projects comes from seemingly unrelated experiences. So ensuring that fresh arts ideas are incorporated into the original intervention will help with continued engagement of participants.

5. Share everything

Staff and participants involved in a project should make sure they report even seemingly insignificant details, whether these are reports on problems noted or fresh ideas. If these are small, they could simply be logged and read through on a monthly basis. If they are larger, there may need to be a more formal process to deal with them. This is discussed further in Chapter 8. One staff member or participant may have an idea that could improve the project, or vague observations could, when combined, point to new avenues for exploration.

6. Spark with imagination, fuel with data

Evaluating an intervention should not be a one-off event but should happen periodically, either as fresh evaluations or as audits (discussed further in Chapter 9). The data from this will ensure that the project stays on target. However, evaluation is also an opportunity to test the feasibility of new ideas. Participants could be asked what they feel is lacking, or questions could be incorporated that explore new problems or challenges that the intervention could be adapted to encompass. Collection of data is a way of testing intuition.

7. Be a platform

Interventions should be broadcast to as many people as possible. Sharing ideas with external parties can in turn become a source of innovation through ensuing discussions and exchanges of new ideas. External parties may have suggestions for innovation.

8. Never fail to fail

Innovation brings with it the risk of potentially worsening a project. Of course, this should be planned for to ensure that it does not put patients at risk or have a negative consequence for those involved. However, with an attitude that mistakes will happen and appropriate safeguards in place, more innovative ideas may be incorporated even if it emerges that they do not improve the project in the way initially planned. It is only through testing that the successful ideas will also be found.

> Q To find out more about Google's eight pillars of information, visit the Think With Google website www.thinkwithgoogle.com.

Summary

Overall, this seven-step process is by no means intended to constrain projects nor add unnecessary burden to the design and delivery. Indeed, often the ideas for arts interventions come about through the interests of the people involved. The artistic idea may already be quite advanced and funding may even have been sourced before this seven-step process is considered. In this instance, pretending not to have an intervention and starting from scratch could waste time and lose the project momentum. Nevertheless, as preparation for the project, it may be valuable to go back using these steps and check that the assumptions made so far fit with the requirements of the setting and participants. Certainly, undertaking each of the steps in this process can be a fast process if done efficiently. For example, Steps 1 and 2 could be accomplished within a week if staff time is available: PESTLE and care process analysis could be undertaken intensively in 2 days, shadowing could be planned for half a day, and discovery interviews could be carried out with a dozen people involved over two differently timed clinic sessions during the week. Similarly, Step 3 could be carried out the following week with 3 days of consultation followed by an analytical process. Step 4 could take place immediately after and a pilot could be up and running within a month. As most projects require at least a month to engage staff, it is sensible to put this time to use in gathering the data involved in these steps. Of course, this might not provide as much in-depth knowledge as when more time is taken, and certainly larger projects, or those that are more ambitious, complex, or involve more vulnerable participant groups will need significantly more time spent on their development. However, some interventions are simpler to design and carry out than others, and this should be a factor in terms of how much time is spent on the planning.

It may also be decided that a step or substep in the process is not necessary, perhaps because the staff involved have already gathered prior data that can answer some of the questions, or because it is deemed that one step is not a requirement to the success of a project. At least in this instance, the decision not to undertake a step will be a conscious one rather than arising from not having prior experience in the field, making it less likely to affect the outcome of the intervention.

It was also discussed at the start of Chapter 5 that not all arts interventions have the explicit aim of solving a challenge within health. Museums, for example, deliver a range of exhibitions with no explicit health purposes. However, simply visiting these exhibitions can have health and social benefits. Consequently, the full seven-step approach may not be relevant for all arts interventions, especially those that have health effects as secondary or even unconscious aims. Nevertheless, if an organization decides to undertake a new programme of work or wishes to expand its reach into health (such as a museum deciding to start up Friday morning object-handling sessions specifically for people with Alzheimer's disease), these steps could be of value in that process. Furthermore, experience within healthcare contexts has demonstrated that the projects that operate within specific healthcare institutions or that want to be included within public health agendas need to have defined visions and be meeting some kind of 'need'. Such interventions are precisely those for which this seven-step process will be most important.

In Chapter 7, we turn to the delivery of arts in health interventions, considering how artists and arts organizations can work in partnership with healthcare organizations to deliver successful interventions.

References

1. **Fancourt D, Poon M**. Validation of the Arts Observational Scale (ArtsObS) for the evaluation of performing arts activities in health care settings. Arts Health. 2015 Oct 29;0(0):1–14.
2. **Chevalier JM, Buckles D**. Participatory Action Research: Theory and Methods for Engaged Inquiry. London and New York: Routledge; 2013. 498 pp.
3. Arts for health and wellbeing: an evaluation framework [Internet]. London: Public Health England; 2016 Feb [cited 2016 Oct 31]. Available from: https://www.gov.uk/government/publications/arts-for-health-and-wellbeing-an-evaluation-framework.

4. **Doran GT.** There's a SMART way to write management's goals and objectives. Manage Rev. 1981;70(11):35–6.

5. **Womack JP, Jones DT, Roos D.** The Machine That Changed the World: The Story of Lean Production-- Toyota's Secret Weapon in the Global Car Wars That Is Now Revolutionizing World Industry. Reprint. New York: Free Press; 2007. 352 pp.

6. **Graban M.** Lean Hospitals: Improving Quality, Patient Safety, and Employee Engagement, Third Edition. 3 edition. Boca Raton: Productivity Press; 2016. 354 pp.

7. **Chalice R.** Improving Healthcare Using Toyota Lean Production Methods: 46 Steps for Improvement. Milwaukee: ASQ Quality Press; 2007. 324 p.

8. **Hoffmann TC, Glasziou PP, Boutron I, Milne R, Perera R, Moher D**, et al. Better reporting of interventions: template for intervention description and replication (TIDieR) checklist and guide. BMJ. 2014 Mar 7;348:g1687.

9. **McLaughlin CP, Kaluzny AD.** Continuous Quality Improvement in Health Care: Theory, Implementations, and Applications. Jones & Bartlett Learning; 2006. 706 pp.

Chapter 7

Partnerships and funding

One of the many beauties of the arts as a field is their variety. Not only are there a myriad of different art forms and a multitude of different ways of engaging in an arts activity, but types of art and engagement also vary between countries and cultures and evolve over time. However, as well as being a thing of beauty, this variety can also present a challenge in developing an arts in health intervention: even if it has already been decided what sort of arts intervention is going to be used (e.g. a crafts workshop), the precise types of crafts, the way they are put to use in the workshop, how participants engage with them, what they learn about them, and the outputs they produce could be completely different depending on which individual artist leads the workshop. Consequently, a major decision in delivering an arts in health intervention is identifying suitable artists or arts organizations to lead the sessions. Indeed, the quality of the art and the imagination with which it is developed into an intervention can make the difference between a truly effective and inspiring arts in health intervention and merely a nice experience. Consequently, this chapter focuses on how to develop successful partnerships between arts bodies and health bodies, including how to pitch a proposal, develop a brief, select appropriate partners to deliver projects, draw up contracts, identify funding streams for an intervention, establish appropriate training or induction programmes, and design monitoring and feedback systems to ensure those involved feel supported and gain the most they can from their experience in a project.

Developing partnerships

Partnerships can be instigated by people from both the arts world and the health world. For example, artists or arts organizations themselves may develop their own project idea independently of a health organization and then seek to identify a health partner. In such instances, it is important to be able to demonstrate a thorough understanding of the field of health in which the artist/organization wishes to work. One of the strongest ways of doing this is to prepare a case for support document (see Chapter 6). Within this document, it is recommended that the 'arts-based solution' model outlined in Chapter 5 is highlighted, whereby the artist identifies a specific health challenge and demonstrates how the proposed intervention or arts practice could be of value as a solution to this challenge. This is normally the strongest way of appealing to a health organization as it demonstrates how partnership working could be of benefit to that organization's core mission. Identifying health organizations for which the challenge identified is a priority or area of strategic interest can enhance the chance of partnerships developing. In some instances, it may have been possible to undertake a significant amount of consultation work prior to writing the case for support to identify the health challenge and how the arts could support this, leading to a comprehensive case for support that outlines in some detail what could be achieved. But more commonly it is difficult to undertake a full consultation without the support of a health organization, for example to provide information on patient care processes or to facilitate shadowing opportunities and discovery interviews. Furthermore, having everything mapped out in advance can actually be a barrier to healthcare professionals who may have their own thoughts and ideas to feed into the design. So the alternative approach is to prepare a summary case for support initially, outlining the broad challenge identified and summarizing how the art form proposed could be of support, with the suggestion that a larger consultation to assess whether an intervention could be viable is undertaken. Given that even well-formed project ideas often change through full consultation processes, this approach of seeking to establish a partnership early on and then develop the full project idea can be a strong method of working.

The other way in which partnerships can develop is that health organizations or research teams seek to partner with an artist. As a variation on this, it is also possible for arts organizations or charities who are already working with health partners to seek additional artistic input or a facilitator to run a project. In both of these instances, there are four main ways that partnerships can develop:

1. Collaborative design—an arts organization and a healthcare organization may have partnered early on with the aim of planning and delivering a project together. This is particularly common when two organizations have worked together previously

2. Direct approach—an artist who is already known, either as an existing partner or through their reputation for the type of work they do, may be approached by an organization looking to develop an arts in health intervention, provided with the brief, and invited to be part of the new project

3. Limited competition—an organization looking to develop an arts in health intervention may draw up a shortlist of potential artists or arts organizations, either through identification of artists who have worked on similar

projects, using advice from local or national arts bodies such as arts councils, or the use of databases such as national artist databases or community artist databases. Those included on the shortlist will be contacted with a brief and invitation to apply as part of a tender process

4. Open submission—an organization looking to develop an arts in health intervention may make advertisements about the project publicly available. Artists and arts organizations who are interested will then be sent the brief and an invitation to tender

There are pros and cons to all four of these ways of developing partnerships. On the one hand, working with existing partners can help strengthen collaborative working and lead to strong long-term partnerships. On the other hand, adding in the element of competition through a tender process can help to identify fresh ideas and younger companies or individuals who might not have been considered before, and it can also be a way of ensuring that a good price has been agreed for the project. However, if competition is involved, it is good working practice to ensure that applications are judged fairly and impartially. One way of achieving this is to undertake a tender process.

The tender process

Before the tender process begins, it is essential that a committee is in place to oversee the process, and the wider project. A committee is an opportunity to invite important stakeholders to be involved and can have wider benefits for the project. For example, inviting clinicians and other healthcare professionals to join a committee can increase their buy-in and involvement in the project; inviting communications teams can support early development of marketing strategies and publicity opportunities; inviting finance or fundraising staff can bring in support for identifying future funding; inviting patient representatives can help ensure that the project ideas are going to be suitable for the target group; inviting artists who have experience of similar work can help assess the quality and suitability of applicants for the role; and inviting a senior member of staff from the organization can ensure that the project has high-level support.

A typical challenge with a committee is bringing everybody together for meetings. Such meetings can be valuable, especially at the start of a project to ensure that different potential challenges or barriers have been identified and the project is being planned to meet the needs of the organizations involved. However, if meetings are a barrier to people participating in the committee, people can also be consulted on a one-to-one basis as the project is shaped.

Developing a brief

Once it has been decided that a tender process is to be undertaken, the most important step is developing a brief. Most typically, a brief is developed by an organization that has an idea for a project and is looking for an artist to lead it. The brief or specification is a document that sets out what the project is and what is required from the artist or arts organization. Even if a project is being developed collaboratively with an artist/organization rather than through a tender process, a brief can be a simple and effective way of ensuring that all parties share an understanding of what is going to be required in the project.

A key decision when recruiting an artist is at what stage in the process they should be involved: should a brief be developed and an artist identified right at the start of a project when the idea is first conceived, or later down the line once a fuller picture of what the intervention is going to involve has been formed? On the one hand, it may be helpful to integrate the artist with the conceptualizing and planning of the project so that project ideas are developed in tandem with the consultation process. This can be a strong method of working to ensure that the artist is aware of all of the sensitivities and complexities and the project is very closely tailored to the needs of the target participants. However, this may also be time-consuming and costly, and it may not be necessary to the development of a successful project. An alternative approach is to bring an artist in later in the process: either for the pilot or, if a pilot has taken place in a separate location and the project is now expanding to more sites, for the larger-scale implementation of a project. If this approach is taken, it is critical that a detailed brief is developed and helpful if the successful candidate is then able to access paperwork from the earlier consultation and piloting work to help him/her understand the intricacies of the project. It may be helpful too for the artist to undertake short shadowing exercises and focus groups with the target participants and staff to help orientate them to the project.

The brief itself will vary depending on the type of project. However, there are several important components that should always be included:

♦ The aim and objectives of the project—these can be drawn from the case for support (see Chapter 6) and demonstrate what the project hopes to achieve. These will be something to which an artist/organization can return throughout designing of the intervention to ensure that their ideas stay on track with the project aims

♦ The background to the project—why it is a priority, what the current situation is, and what evidence there is that the proposed project could be of value. Again, this may be drawn from the case for support

- Who the target participants are—key demographic characteristics (such as age-group), important information related to the health conditions involved that may affect the project design (e.g. whether participants will be taking part from their beds or whether some participants may have limited hearing or eyesight), and whether there will be other people involved such as carers or staff

- The scope of the project—what is expected, for example the length of each workshop, the length of the project as a whole, the numbers who will be involved, the location, etc. If the brief is being developed for the inclusion of an artist in the roll-out of an existing intervention and a manual of activity already exists (see Chapter 6), key information can be drawn from this for the brief

- Details of resources—this can include the budget available to an artist/organization, which other members of staff or other artists are already involved and how they will interact with the project, and whether there are any facilities or equipment available already (such as access to a piano or sound equipment)

- Timetable—the timeline for the project including key dates for project meetings and important milestones

- Evaluation—how the project will be monitored and evaluated and whether there are specific targets for the artist/organization as part of their involvement

- Details of selection process—deadlines for tenders, what should be submitted, how the submission will be judged, potential interview dates, and a date by which applicants will know the outcome

- The fee available for the work

When costing a project, an important consideration is that a professional is not underpaid for their work. One way to assess costing is to discuss with similar organizations what rates they have used with professionals undertaking similar roles in the past. Alternatively, there may be guidelines within a country set by unions for the amount that is expected to be paid per hour of work. Another approach is not to set an amount but to ask as part of the proposal for applicants to set their rates. Ways of prioritizing competitively priced bids are discussed in 'Evaluating tenders' later. In contrast, if there is already a set amount of money available for a project, applicants could be told what this is and then asked to propose what they could offer for that amount of money. However, the strongest projects are often those that have not had to compromise too much on what the project is going to entail and have some flexibility to develop the intervention without too strict a limit on resources, so a range of funding options are discussed in 'Funding a project' later in this chapter.

In addition to the core sections outlined above, if there is a technological component to the project, such as a website or app development, a further section will need to be added detailing what is feasible within the confines of the project (e.g. whether mobile phones have a signal within a hospital to download apps, on which operating platforms an app would need to be available, whether the budget available is just for development or whether it needs also to cover future updates, etc.) Sometimes in technology projects a tender process is split into two, with a parallel search for both an artist and a technology company carried out and targeted briefs developed for both.

Submissions

Once a brief has been developed, submissions for tender can be invited. The aim of the tender process is to select the applicant who will give the best quality of work at the best cost. As a result, tenders have to balance the proposed cost, quality, delivery, and risk. If a tender process is being used to select an artist/ organization (rather than an existing partner being invited to join a project), then it should be carried out fairly, without advantage given to other applicants. For example, the level of additional information given should not become disproportionate for one applicant over another. And if one applicant wishes to see the site or meet a member of the team, this should be offered as an opportunity to the other potential applicants too. The way that the brief is advertised also should be fair, especially for open submissions, ensuring that it is circulated on a variety of mailing lists or websites and there is ample time for organizations or individuals to find out about it and submit an application.

Tender processes may be split into two stages of application: an expression of interest or pre-qualification stage, followed by a full application stage. This is often only necessary for projects in which a large number of applicants are anticipated. The pre-qualification stage can be used to see whether applicants meet specific criteria (such as whether they are based in the appropriate country, have any relevant experience, and work with the art form being sought). If specific criteria are being used, these should be listed in the brief so that applicants have the opportunity to demonstrate how they meet these criteria. Sometimes this stage is also used to get a flavour of the type of activity the applicant is proposing. For example, if applications are being sought for a mixed arts workshop for older adults, there are a wide range of options that could be pursued. An expression of interest form could be used to get a short description of what the individual/organization would deliver to assess whether it is along the right lines and therefore of interest for a full submission.

In the application form, the actual questions will vary depending on the type of project. Often, it is helpful to ask applicants to summarize their knowledge of the area. For example, if the project involves working with adult mental health service users, the application form might ask them to outline some of the current key challenges in mental health and why there could be a need for a new project. Although some of this information will have been included in the brief as an overview, this can be a way of assessing how well acquainted an artist/organization is with the field, or how much work they are willing to put in to learn about it. Application forms often also ask for a summary of a participant's experience or a CV to see whether they have carried out similar work before. To ensure that people who are new to the field or who are transferring their skills are not disadvantaged (as many artists may not have worked in health before but may have an inherent sensitivity to the type of work and a wealth of fresh ideas), it may help to ask what applicants feel they can bring to the project or what other experiences have prepared them to undertake this project. If the project involves a vulnerable population or particular sensitivities, it may also be revealing to ask the applicants to consider these sensitivities and discuss how they would approach them. This can be a way of assessing whether the applicant has an appropriate understanding of the project environment.

A central part of the full application is usually a description of how the applicant would approach the brief. For example, if the brief asks for workshops for young children, what would they propose doing in those workshops? Or if the brief is for a resource website to connect people who have been bereaved in an online book discussion group, applicants could outline the structure of the website, what sort of design they envisage, the tone of the language, and any special features. In many instances, the arts committee may already have a relatively advanced idea of what an intervention will involve. This may have been carefully developed as part of the consultation process (see Chapter 5). However, asking for a proposal is still sensible for several reasons: (i) it is a way of assessing the creativity of applicants and their ability to work to a plan. It can be helpful for separating out applicants who are willing to develop something new from applicants who may merely be looking for avenues to set up their own pre-conceived project with limited flexibility to adapt it; (ii) the proposals may bring to light new ideas that have not yet been considered for the intervention that could strengthen the project; (iii) if the project has so far been developed with limited involvement from artists, it is important to make sure that artists have had a chance to input their expertise to ensure that the project is feasible and makes the most of artistic opportunities. Finally, the application may ask for a breakdown of how the artist/organization would spend the money. This is discussed further in 'Evaluating tenders'. To ensure that applications do not become too long, word counts for individual questions or a set page limit for the entire application are advisable.

Evaluating tenders

There is a broad range of ways in which tenders can be evaluated and successful candidates selected, varying in formality and complexity. Often evaluation involves numerical rating of the tender against certain set criteria. These criteria will typically exemplify the most important aspects of the project, such as whether the applicant has relevant experience, whether they are able to deliver the project within the timescale proposed, how high is the quality of their work, and whether they have demonstrated awareness of the key sensitivities surrounding the project. Often, these criteria will be matched with specific questions asked on the application form. Sometimes, certain criteria are weighted higher than others to reflect their importance in the decision-making process. For example, if the most important element is the project proposal from the artist/organization, this may be assigned a 40% weighting, with the remaining 60% weighting divided among the other elements being assessed. A further complexity in rating can be in regards to price. Some tenders do not ask for negotiation on price. Others outline an upper limit but allow for applicants to propose a lower amount of money. Often in this process, the lowest costing project is assigned the maximum number of marks available for that section of the application form, with subsequent bids being assigned lower marks as the cost increases, sometimes with the number of marks deducted proportionate to the amount of extra money requested above and beyond the cost of the cheapest project.

The rating of tenders could be carried out by members of the arts committee independently, with scores then aggregated and combined, with the highest scoring tender being selected. This system has several benefits, most obviously transparency, as it will then be very clear why a bid is successful and where other bids have fallen down. The involvement of multiple points of view and skill sets through the arts committee can also help to ensure a rounded assessment of the proposals, which considers the suitability of the potential partners from the points of view of managers, clinicians, and target participants.

Sometimes, instead of working with a detailed formal numerical assessment of applications, a simpler assessment may be made to shortlist the most promising tenders and invite those on the shortlist for interview. For projects in which interpersonal skills are particularly important, this may be more valuable than conducting the whole selection on paper. For the interview, as with assessments, the involvement of a varied range of stakeholders is important to confirm whether the artist/organization meets the approval of managers, clinicians, and participant representatives. The interview is an opportunity to continue assessing whether the applicant meets the brief and also explore the proposed project ideas in more detail. Sometimes it may be appropriate to have a short taster session as part of the interview. For example, if interviewing for the post of a music leader for a workshop with mothers and new babies, applicants could be asked to demonstrate a sample song or activity they may use, and some hypothetical scenarios (such as a baby crying and the mother getting distressed) could be proposed, either through role-play or as direct questions to see how the artist would respond. Another important element of an interview is that it gives the artist/organization an opportunity to find out more about a project and ask their own questions. It can be challenging to work in certain areas within health (as will be discussed further in Chapter 8), so artists may wish to find out more, identify whether their artistic practice is indeed suited to the setting, and ascertain what support will be available for them.

Drawing up contracts

Once an artist/organization has been selected, it is important that they are properly contracted to carry out their work. The majority of healthcare organizations or charities will have their own template contracts to be used for any projects delivered in partnership with them. However, contracts still need to be tailored to fit the needs of the programme. For example, a contract for a musician coming to give a one-off performance in a public space in a hospital may be short and relatively simple, whereas a contract for an artist-in-residence to work with children in hospital over a 6-month period will be more complex because of the longer timeframe, more formal role, access to sensitive areas of a hospital, and involvement with young people. Either way, there are several essential components of a contract:

1. The artist's brief—this may be taken directly from the original tender notice or rewritten following the selection process and discussion with the chosen artist/organization. This will outline what is expected of the artist in their time working on the project

2. The agreed fee and payment stages, including what the fee is expected to cover, and whether there will be additional payments for other aspects of work or the opportunity to renegotiate at a point in the future

3. The dates and length of the programme, to confirm that both parties can commit for the duration

4. Any specific information or arrangements, such as access to equipment, points of contact for the artist during the project, reporting requirements

5. Responsibilities—it is important to ascertain who bears responsibilities for certain aspects of the project, in particular the costs incurred from the project, any insurance or liability, the reporting of any incidents or causes for concern that arise across the course of the project and applications for

any licences or permits that may be required to carry out the project. More details on reporting incidents and causes for concern are given in Chapter 8

6. A cancellation or termination clause, giving a notice period for both parties and outlining the arrangements

If there are specific codes of ethics, guidelines, or expectations for working on the project, or health and safety regulations, these should be attached to the contract, to ensure that they are acceptable to both parties prior to the project commencing.

If a project involves tangible artwork, a new composition, the development of technology, or potentially commercializable outputs, a contract also must outline with whom copyright, intellectual property, patents, and licences will lie. For a new project, issues around who will 'own' the project idea also should be discussed. For example, if an artist is involved in developing the concept of a project, can that artist subsequently deliver the project in another setting? Or can the health organization hire another artist in the future to deliver the same project? Normally organizations will have their own regulations for such situations, but where multiple partners are involved in a project, this must be carefully negotiated up front before any project activity starts. Contacting organizations or individuals who have led similar projects in the past can be a helpful way of ascertaining any precedents.

> Websites such as www.artistsnetwork.com and www.graphicartistsguild.org give advice to artists on contracts for projects. Legal advice may be required if substantial changes are made to an organization's standard contract, which should be carefully considered as this may affect project budgets.

If the project is short term, sometimes a memorandum of understanding (MOU) is drawn up rather than a full contract. An MOU may be very similar in language and content to a contract. However, unlike a contract it is not legally binding. Whereas a contract creates an obligation and an enforceable agreement, with potential penalties if it is breached, an MOU does not contain legally enforceable promises. This can make it a more suitable option if, for example, an organization is providing support in kind, helping to outline what that support is to ensure that both parties understand what has been proposed and agreed, but not containing any formal legal terms.

> A template memorandum of understanding is available through the Australian Department of Education and Early Childhood Development website www.education.vic.gov.au.

Preparations and support in delivering a project

Once an artist/organization has been selected, it is also important to ensure that those involved in delivering the project are well prepared. There are a number of ways that this can be facilitated.

Preparation booklets

These can contain core information about hospital regulations, patient safeguarding, and health and safety, as well as giving guidance for artists/organizations on what to expect when working in the environment they are going into. For example, working in certain acute hospital settings, they may be exposed to upsetting scenes. It may also be helpful to include details about who the point of contact is if an artist has any queries at any point. Prior detail to prepare individuals can facilitate smooth working in that environment. The benefit of a preparation booklet is that it can be continually referred to by the artist/organization if they have queries during the project.

Induction days

A formal induction or orientation should always be offered to artists/organizations working in new settings too, so that they can see the spaces in which they will be working prior to their first session. If there are other people involved in the project, such as supervisors (see 'Supervisors' below) or healthcare professionals, introducing the artist in advance can prepare for the first session.

Shadowing sessions

It may also be helpful for artists to shadow a similar project prior to commencing their own so that they can see what is expected. This may give them an insight into how to deal with common situations and help to normalize the environment.

Training programmes

It may also be of interest to develop a training programme, so that, in addition to a main professional leading sessions, there could be another artist or a student shadowing and learning how to deliver the sessions. Such training programmes could be set up with local arts colleges or music and dance conservatoires, with bursaries offered to students while they are training and more responsibility allocated to them by the professional in the sessions as they gain experience. These training programmes can be helpful to the development of the project, so that there are more artists ready to lead sessions if the project grows. If the leader is ill or unable to attend a session, the trainee can also deputize, helping to ensure the project is delivered regardless of external factors.

Supervisors

When a new artist/organization starts work in a new setting, much can be gained from having a supervisor to support their work. Especially in healthcare environments such as hospitals, the supervisor can form the bridge between the healthcare professionals and the artist. For example, if a musician is performing in the day room of a patient ward in a hospital, the supervisor can ensure that the volume is appropriate, that the music is not disturbing any clinicians or patients who might be sleeping, and that those who want to come to the day room are aware the session is running and can join in. This bridge role can allow the artist the freedom to work in the moment with those who are in the session, without worrying about some of the external factors. If there is a project coordinator for a project, this may be a natural role for them. Alternatively, there may be a specific healthcare professional who wishes to take on this role. However, in settings that involve shift work or acute environments where this person may get called away, another supervisor may provide more consistency, with support from other individuals drawn on when they are available. A supervisor role could also be taken on by volunteers. Many hospitals and care homes have 'friend' or volunteer schemes with people undertaking training and then supporting projects on wards. If 'friends' or volunteers are involved in the project, this could mean that the supervisor role does not add further to the project budget. In some settings, it may not be permissible for an artist to be left alone with vulnerable participants or those with complex needs, or more complex police checks may be required, in which case a fully vetted and trained supervisor is essential. More details on this topic are provided in Chapter 8.

Feedback

Provision of feedback can be helpful when working with artists and arts organizations. In particular, if an artist/organization is involved in the early stages and piloting of a project, there may be evaluation data gathered to support project development. Involving the artist/organization in the evaluation and jointly considering the feedback can help the project to evolve. This may also give the artist/organization the opportunity to test different approaches to ascertain which work best with the target participant group. This form of evaluation should not be one way: artists/organizations also should be encouraged to feed back on their experiences of being involved. This could take the form of a personal diary kept by artists leading the sessions to detail how workshops have gone and how they themselves have found the experience. In keeping such diaries, care should be taken to ensure that participant confidentiality is maintained and nobody involved in the project is identifiable (see Chapter 8 on confidentiality). If a process evaluation is being carried out as part of project development (see Chapter 6), it is important to include the artist's/organization's experience of working with management teams within the healthcare setting, to ensure that it is a supportive and smooth process.

Monitoring and evaluation

Monitoring and evaluation can help artists/organizations who join a project later in development to adjust to the setting and participant group. It is anticipated that projects may take a while to settle in and adapt to the particular needs of those involved. Such monitoring and mutual feedback can enhance this process. Initially, this could take the form of short focus groups or interviews with people involved in the project and its delivery (whether participants, healthcare professionals, or management staff) to ascertain what is working well and what can be developed further. If there is a project manager or healthcare professional in charge of the project, they could shadow a session and hold a debriefing sessions afterwards so the artist has an opportunity to discuss their experiences of leading and gain immediate feedback. Once the artist is settled in, small elements of a previous evaluation could be repeated, to ensure that the project continues to meet its aims, or the artist/organization could be involved in future audits or research projects. Across the life of a project, there should remain an open line of communication between artists/organizations and those managing or supporting the project. This provides an opportunity for both sides to be made aware of positive feedback, reinforcing the impact that the project is having, and for any potential criticisms or negative feedback to be fed back and, where possible, the problem rectified.

Funding a project

One of the greatest challenges in running an arts in health project is funding: no matter how beneficial and necessary a project may appear to the team behind it, translating this importance and need to a funder can be difficult. Consequently, plans for how to fund a project and the partnerships required for this to succeed should be considered early in development and adapted as the business case for the project develops. Often it can help to develop a specific funding strategy, splitting the lifecycle of the project into four distinct stages.

◆ Pilot—referring to the initial testing of the project to assess its feasibility, as discussed in Chapter 6

- Establishment—referring to the more formal embedding of a project following its piloting
- Long-term plans—for once the project has been established and is looking for sustainable ongoing funding
- Roll-out—if the project is being spread to other locations

Each strategic stage will require different levels of funding (generally growing in size through the stages) and is likely to be of interest to different funders.

When costing projects, there are a number of things to consider. First, costs can be broadly split into:

- Directly incurred costs—those that arise directly as a result of the project such as the cost of artists to deliver a workshop that would not have been incurred otherwise, or the purchasing of musical instruments for a music workshop
- Directly allocated costs—the costs of resources used by a project that are shared by other activities, such as staff who are already employed but will be spending time on the project or the cost of office space and IT systems that form a necessary backdrop to an activity
- Indirect costs—non-specific costs that are not directly involved in a project but still important to it, such as the cost of staff members not directly involved in the project but still important to its running, for example HR or administrative staff or other core costs such as organizational insurance

Some funders will specifically only fund directly incurred costs, and often with general fundraising, funders want to know what percentage of their donation will go on directly incurred costs (in other words directly to the delivery of an arts in health project). Others will be happy to fund directly allocated or indirect costs, and may even specialize in this, for example as a way of supporting emerging organizations. Consequently, to fund directly incurred, directly allocated, and indirect costs across the four possible levels of activity outlined above, diversified funding strategies, which often draw on more than one approach, are vital. Important within funding strategies are realistic timescales, both for preparation of bids or fundraising activities and the time taken for decisions or to raise the money.

There is a range of ways of funding arts in health interventions. While specific funding bodies vary between regions and countries, they can be grouped broadly into different categories of funding. Some of these key categories are set out below.

Self-funding

The simplest funding model for an arts in health project is to self-fund the project. This may be provided by a healthcare organization, arts organization, or other organization involved in developing the intervention. This can be a very attractive option, especially for pilot projects in which only a small sum is required as it can help a project to get off the ground quickly while momentum is high. This can, in turn, provide important evaluation data (see Chapter 6) that can be used to put together a strong case for support for future funding bids. However, self-funding is rarely effective as a long-term strategy unless it is combined with other funding models as it can quickly deplete resources. Furthermore, self-funding does not make the most of some of the benefits that other funding models can bring, such as increasing the investment of stakeholders or enhancing reach.

Participant funding

Another simple funding model is participant funding, whereby people involved in the project (e.g. older adults taking part in a dance workshop) pay to take part. Payment can either be on a class-by-class basis, for a programme of activity, via membership of the organization providing the project, or through anonymous donations in a collection bucket at the end of each session. However, participant funding has several specific requirements. First, the amount of money generated by participants must be sufficient to cover the costs of running the project. This can be complex if participants can simply drop in and out, as it could lead to some sessions being under-attended and a loss being made. Sometimes, projects will calculate the cost of running a block of classes and ask participants to sign up and pay up-front for the entire block. Only if enough people sign up will the project be offered. This can have the advantage of encouraging a proper buy-in from participants and reducing drop-outs over the course of the project. However, it can be disappointing for potential participants if the minimum number is not reached, and can be hard for freelance artists involved if they are unsure of whether they will actually be required for the work or not. Also, it may not always be appropriate for participants to pay to take part, for example if the intervention does not have set times (such as a musician performing in a waiting area across a day, or an art installation in a public area). Participant funding may preclude certain people from lower-income backgrounds from taking part. Successful participant-funded projects often combine small fees with in-kind support (such as a free venue) and alternative modes of funding, rather than relying solely on participant funding for the project to go ahead.

Fundraising

A third way of funding a project is to plan fundraising events. These can range from small-scale activities such as bake sales or sponsored runs though to larger activities such as social media campaigns or fundraising auctions or dinners.

As such, the amount of resource needed for fundraising can vary enormously. Fundraising events often require an initial financial investment for them to run, with plans that the event will recuperate the initial investment and also raise additional funds. However, this initial investment can add an element of risk to fundraising activities. In-kind support with the running of events or sponsorship that covers the up-front cost of the event can help in reducing this risk. If a fundraising campaign becomes big enough, it can be a viable way of providing ongoing support for a project. In addition, if participants in a project become particularly involved, they can set up their own spin-off fundraising activities for the project. However, the amount of resource required to plan large-scale fundraising events and to maintain fundraising activity long term, mean that fundraising is often best when used in combination with other ways of sourcing money such as grant funding (discussed later in this chapter).

Crowdfunding

A variation on standard fundraising events is crowdfunding, which is becoming a high-profile form of alternative finance. It enables projects to take place via large numbers of small contributions through online platforms such as 'Crowdfunder' and 'Kickstarter', which host pitches set up by individuals or organizations for funding and connect them to potential supporters/funders. A key component of the campaign is setting fundraising targets and timelines. Often, the project only receives the money if the target is met, but if it is not met, the individuals who pledged are not charged (although there are some other models available on certain online platforms). Crowdfunding has a number of different models for rewarding people who invest, including the following:

- Donation-based models (e.g. Chuffed, GlobalGiving, and JustGiving) collect pure donations for causes or projects
- Reward-based models (e.g. Crowdfunder, Kickstarter, and Wefund) allow contributors to receive non-financial rewards in return, often using a tiered system with larger rewards for larger contributions. These rewards are set by the project team and can include copies of annual reports or access to newsletters, free tickets to events or performances, or merchandise
- Lending-based models (e.g. Funding Circle and Kiva) are for projects that are seeking loans but that intend to repay the money
- Equity-based models (e.g. Crowd2Fund and Microgenius) enable people to invest for equity or profit/revenue sharing in projects

Crowdfunding has many benefits, including engaging new supporters, creating new advocates, extending the reach of a project, and drawing in match funding that could support other funding applications. However, successful campaigns require careful strategies and strong marketing as well as contingency plans.

 For more information about crowdfunding models, each of the organizations named above has its own website containing further details and examples of projects.

Volunteer programmes

It is also possible to run projects that are led by volunteers, such as artists or musicians donating their time. Volunteer programmes can be highly effective as they can cost very little to run, bring the cause to the attention of a wider audience, and sometimes lead on to other fundraising efforts through the volunteers involved. However, if a volunteer is going to work in a healthcare organization, they must be carefully vetted, including potentially going through criminal record checks and health and safety checks (see Chapter 8). If they have not had prior experience, they may also require a training session and careful supervision. Furthermore, volunteer programmes are not always appropriate. For example, a project that involves one-on-one music interaction with premature babies in intensive care would require the specialist knowledge and training of a professional who has experience working in that setting. Not only might a volunteer not know how to deliver a suitable activity in that environment, but also they may not know how to deal with the situation themselves and could find it distressing. Consequently, volunteer programmes should be used carefully, not merely as a way of avoiding the cost of a professional, and should be combined with thorough preparation and monitoring of the volunteer.

Musicians on Call in the US is a volunteer programme where professional and amateur musicians donate their time to perform for patients in hospitals: www.musiciansoncall.org.

In-kind support

Similar to volunteer programmes are programmes with in-kind support. In-kind support comprises non-cash contributions to a project, either by things being provided free of charge or at a reduced rate. This can include waived or reduced rates on tangible items such as venue hire, equipment, or marketing materials, or waived or reduced rates for somebody's time, such as an artist, documentary-maker, clinician, or consultant. Many projects contain in-kind support without being aware of it, through the support of volunteers, through advisors or consultants, or through organizations or individuals providing help above and beyond any charged hours. Identifying and logging this support can be particularly helpful when seeking other funding as it can demonstrate buy-in from key stakeholders and help to provide a case for match funding, showing that a percentage of the overall cost of a project is already in place. Sometimes, organizations and individuals can provide their services in kind for a pilot project if it will help to leverage interest and evaluation data that will then allow larger funds to be accessed. However, in-kind support cannot be expected in projects, and is normally insufficient on its own to allow a project to go ahead, especially beyond the pilot stage, so in isolation it is not a reliable way to set up an intervention.

Grant funding

One of the main ways of funding arts in health projects is grant funding. Grants can be made from a range of sources including governments, arts councils, local authorities, and charities. They have the benefit of not needing to be paid back but the project itself must fit the specific grant stream or call to be considered and many grants are very competitive. Grant funding works well with in-kind support or match funding as these can show what support and resources are already in place for a project, which can increase the perceived need for it, reduce the perceived risk, and confirm that necessary partners are involved to deliver it. Grant funding can work well in helping a project to establish itself more firmly once an initial pilot has been run. However, some grant funders prefer only to fund projects that are relatively new, so it can be more challenging to identify grant funders who will fund the long-term continuation of a project. Many grant funders require lengthy paperwork for a project to be considered, as well as financial details about the organizations involved in the project, and some also request specific evaluation or monitoring to help them identify whether their money has been well spent. The time required to put together an application and undertake the reporting back can therefore be significant and needs to be considered as part of the funding strategy. Nevertheless, grants can range from small to very large sums of money so are suitable for a wide range of projects.

Private or individual sponsorship

Another funding model is to seek private or corporate sponsorship. This can include support from a broad range of organizations such as banks or law firms, from health-related organizations such as private healthcare companies or pharmaceutical companies, or from individual philanthropists. Sponsors are often interested in projects to which they can feel connected, such as projects happening locally to them, or projects that involve the same target demographic as their work. Some sponsors have specific schemes for selecting organizations they wish to sponsor or set amounts of money available. For others, personal relationships can be key to gaining initial interest. Where there is no set application route for sponsorship, potential sponsors often wish to see the case for support (see Chapter 6), along with an explanation as to why they are appropriate sponsors and what they could gain from being involved. For organizations, this could range from building the profile of their name or brand, to helping them reach new audiences, improve their corporate image or achieve their charitable goals. If it is a large project, it may be advisable to create sponsorship levels (such as bronze, silver, gold) with different rewards for different levels of sponsorship, ranging from simple rewards such as social media or distributing fliers on behalf of the sponsor, to larger rewards such as tickets to performances or a drinks reception to recognize support. Sponsors also may wish to have their branding or company logo on project materials.

> Q Tenovus Cancer Care in Wales have developed choirs for people affected by cancer involving sponsorship as one of their forms of funding. Their choirs have received sponsorship from pharmaceutical companies including Novartis Pharmaceuticals UK Ltd and Astellas Pharma Ltd. These companies have, among other things, had their branding involved in publicity and the choirs have sung at their conferences to demonstrate the impact of their generous support. More information is available from their website www.tenovuscancercare.org.uk.

Research funding

Another possibility for funding arts in health projects is via research funding. This option will only be appropriate if there is a distinct research question that is worthy of being posed (see Chapter 10). For research funding, the principal applicant is normally a university or research organization and the principal costs are research costs. However, some research funders will also fund the cost of the intervention being researched. This could provide funding for an arts organization or individual to deliver their work over a period of months or even years depending on the research design. However, there are a number of restrictions that research funding can carry with it. First, the intervention must fit within the research design, which could mean that participants have to meet eligibility criteria, the amount of time for which the intervention can be delivered is limited, and the intervention itself has to follow strict guidelines to ensure that it is consistently delivered. These elements may remove some flexibility and freedom from the intervention delivery. To avoid a conflict between artists and researchers in research funding, the most competitive bids are built up from strong partnerships and a shared interest in the research findings. As such, research funding should not be seen as a substitute for alternative ways of funding an intervention, but should instead be viewed as an opportunity to understand the impact of an intervention and to strengthen the case for support for approaching other funders.

Social investment

An alternative to grants and sponsorship is social investment. This is a cross between traditional investment (where investors expect a financial return on their investment) and grant-making (where the social impact is targeted, with no expected financial return). Social investment can include a wide range of models, including loans, grants, and social impact bonds. Within a social impact bond, there are typically three parties: investors, service providers, and commissioners. The investors pay a service provider to deliver a programme. If the programme achieves its social aims, then the commissioner repays the investor their initial investment plus a return for the financial risks they took. If the social aims are not achieved, then the investor loses their initial investment. Social impact bonds can be valuable funding options as they open up more options for corporations to sponsor projects, reward effective interventions, and remove the risk from commissioners, as they only have to pay if the project is actually successful. They also inherently depend on rigorous evaluation, which means that the programme is carefully monitored from the outset. However, this dependency on social outcomes means that commissioners may only be interested in specific types of impact. Consequently, this funding option is most likely to be successful if it is led by the priorities of commissioners, with bespoke arts programmes designed to address their priority areas rather than an existing project that does not address one of their priority areas being suggested. It should be noted that social investment is not always available as an option to all organizations. In some countries, legal structures can affect whether an organization is allowed to access social investment, with social enterprises and companies limited by shares, commercial community interest companies, and cooperatives with investment from their members being the most common service providers involved.

Q For more information on social finance models including social investment and social impact bonds, *Social Finance* edited by Alex Nicholls, Rob Paton, and Jed Emerson (2015) provides a clear guide including insightful case studies.(1)

Per cent schemes

Further support has come through government-approved Per Cent For Art Schemes in certain countries around the world which provide a set percentage (often 1%) of the budget of capital construction schemes as ring-fenced for the arts. This option is often most appropriate for visual art installations or arts in the healthcare environment, either with money provided directly as part of core budgets for capital builds, for example, or with grants invited from other organizations up to the value of the 1%. Nevertheless, the principle could be applied to other types of arts interventions or used as the impetus for a fund-raising campaign when new buildings or wards in healthcare organizations are being built.

Q A prominent example of a Per Cent For Art Scheme comes from the Fiona Stanley Hospital in Australia, which has 10 individual Per Cent For Art commissions from prominent Western Australian Artists. More information about the project is available on the Government of Western Australia website www.finance.wa.gov.au and the hospital's own website www.fsh.health.wa.gov.au.

Commissioning

Finally, commissioning involves the awarding of contracts from healthcare organizations on a competitive basis to companies, charities, or social enterprises. Commissioners can, in different countries, include public health bodies, hospitals, private health insurance companies, local or national health boards, and social care teams, among others. Commissioning is very popular in many countries as a way of reducing the amount that a healthcare service has to deliver itself and instead bringing in external providers to deliver strands of work. As with social investment, commissioning depends on an arts intervention meeting the priorities and strategic needs of the commissioner. But unlike social investment, there is not normally a direct financial return for the commissioner. There are various models, including a single provider model (where an artist or organization is commissioned directly by the commissioner), a subcontractor model (where the artist or organization is contracted by another provider to deliver a strand of work as part of their larger programme), and a consortia model (where artists or organizations group together to provide a larger project, with peer learning and shared resources strengthening the bid). In some countries, there are also moves towards a personal health budget, whereby patients are allocated a sum of money proportionate to the complexity and severity of their health condition and they can decide what services they feel would best support their health and are the most important on which to spend their money. These services can include conventional treatments, psychological therapies, and others such as exercise programmes or arts workshops. Applications for commissioning are sometimes sought through a tender process. Alternatively, some commissioners operate a competitive dialogue approach, whereby ideas can be developed by the commissioners and potential partners together.

> Q In the UK, the NCVO has produced a series of guides on cultural commissioning, which are available on their website www.ncvo.org.uk.

Summary

In this chapter, we have discussed ways of identifying suitable artists and arts organizations to deliver interventions, appropriate ways of preparing them and providing support for them in their work, and considered 12 different models for funding arts in health interventions. What is evident is that there is no single or correct way of developing project or funding partnerships. The stage of development of each project and the type of intervention being planned will have a bearing on how partnerships come about and how well they work, as will the individual personalities and preferences of those individuals and organizations involved. However, although it is possible to be flexible in relation to certain aspects of projects such as those discussed in this chapter, there are other aspects of the delivery of arts in health interventions that do have more standard protocols. In Chapter 8, we will explore important issues around safeguarding, occupational health, and patient and public engagement; issues that could feed back into the selection of artists and in particular the preparations and type of support available for them in their work.

Reference

1. Nicholls A, Paton R, Emerson J. Social Finance. Oxford University Press; 2015. 672 pp.

Chapter 8

Working in healthcare

Working with the arts in healthcare can present a range of challenges. Although many of the issues that arise overlap with other areas of artistic work, such as projects in educational settings, there are also a number of issues that are of particular importance when working with people with health conditions. In general, each health organization will have its own set of policies and protocols for safeguarding patients and the public and reducing risk. However, there are still key essentials that can be transferred between settings and that should be considered both prior to an arts in health activity being delivered and across its duration. This chapter will cover crucial information for administrators, project managers, and practitioners that may also be useful for researchers before they design and lead arts in health projects.

Patient safeguarding

When delivering arts in health interventions, the most fundamental issue is that patients and the public engaging with the intervention are safeguarded. Safeguarding refers broadly to protecting individuals from harm and supporting their health, wellbeing, and human rights. The term is particularly used in the UK and Ireland, but the concept is global. Defining what safeguarding should entail when delivering arts in health interventions can be complex. As interventions are often provided alongside a person's usual care, issues such as who bears responsibility for an individual (whether the core health team or those involved in additional services) can come to the fore. However, to provide optimum protection for an individual, everyone who works with that individual should be concerned with their safeguarding and welfare. There are a number of ways that this can be achieved.

Working with patients and the public

The Scottish Executive has recommended a number of codes of conduct for working in healthcare, whether in healthcare settings such as hospitals or in the local community or participants' homes. These codes of conduct can provide a helpful guide for those involved in the delivery of arts in health interventions. They include:

1. Accountability—those delivering arts in health projects must ensure that their actions can be justified with sound reasons. Making a note of important conversations with participants can be a way of monitoring activities, especially when there is more than one person involved in a project for whom handover notes could be of value

2. Awareness—people involved in the delivery of interventions should be honest about what they can and cannot do, seeking help for things that are beyond their area of expertise

3. Integrity—those delivering interventions should always do what is right to protect participants, doing their best to ensure that anything they do does not harm participants' mental or physical health, or delay their recovery

4. Advocacy—in delivering interventions, workshop leaders and project managers should promote and protect the interests of participants, putting participants' needs first and acknowledging participants' equality and diversity

5. Sensitivity—those delivering arts in health projects should respect participants' feelings and emotions, always being polite and considering situations from participants' perspectives

6. Objectivity—all participants should be treated the same way. Personal feelings should not get in the way of delivering an arts intervention. Activities undertaken should reflect participants' needs, whatever their race, sex, sexuality, age, disability, or religious belief. Those delivering arts in health projects should also maintain professional relationships with participants

7. Consideration and respect—participants should always be treated with dignity, and thoughtfulness should be shown for participants' feelings and needs, protecting them if they are unnecessarily exposed to an embarrassing situation

8. Consent—workshop leaders should work in partnership with participants, explaining what activities are going to be undertaken and confirming they are happy to be involved. Chapter 12 explores consent in more detail as part of ethical responsibilities in research

9. Confidentiality—participants' privacy should be respected and confidential information requested or accessed only when absolutely necessary. This is explored more in the next section 'Patient confidentiality'

10. Cooperation—workshop leaders should strive to work effectively with colleagues as part of team, working to meet the shared goals of the project

11. Protection—participants and colleagues should not be made at risk of harm. This is explored more later in this chapter

12. Development—workshop leaders should look for ways to increase their knowledge and skills, such as through attending training sessions and refreshing knowledge of essential information

13. Alertness—workshop leaders should observe participants and report any important observations to an appropriate person to safeguard the best interests of participants

Q The Scottish Executive 'Code of conduct for healthcare support workers', which contains further details on working with patients and the public, can be accessed via the website www.healthworkerstandards.scot.nhs.uk.

In addition to certain recommended codes of conduct, there are also regulations that may need to be followed. For example, depending on the participant group and the setting of the project, it may be necessary for people involved to undergo police checks or criminal record checks. Although rules vary between countries, these are generally compulsory for work with children or adolescents, or work with vulnerable adults. Clarification will also need to be sought from the organizations involved as to whether checks are required for people shadowing a session or taking on any supervisory role. In addition to these checks, there may be other reference checks and mandatory training before an individual can commence working in a healthcare setting or delivering a project working with vulnerable people. It is important that all of these necessary checks are completed prior to a project starting, and that the time required for these checks to be undertaken and any associated costs are factored into project design.

Q For more information on criminal record checks, individual countries host their own webpages, such as www.gov.uk/disclosure-barring-service-check/overview for the UK.

Patient confidentiality

People working in healthcare also have a duty to protect the confidentiality of patients, and this applies to those involved in arts in health interventions too. The Caldicott principles were the result of a review commissioned by the Chief Medical Officer of England in 1997 to ensure that patient confidentiality was not undermined. Initially, the Caldicott Report high-lighted six key principles and made a further 16 recommendations.(1) The six key principles are:

1. **Justify the purpose**—for the majority of arts in health interventions, it may not be necessary to know confidential patient details. There should be a specific reason for a healthcare professional to pass any data across, and equally a specific reason to ask for this information directly from the patient. Every single proposed access to patient data should be clearly justified

2. **Do not use patient-identifiable information unless it is absolutely necessary**—if it is necessary, patients should normally be made aware that their personal details are being passed across and should give either verbal or written consent, with this consent process documented. This is especially important during research studies. When working with children, parental consent should be sought, but children under the age of 16 who have the capacity and understanding to make decisions may also be involved in this process depending on the nature of the project or research. When working with people who are unable to provide informed consent, such as patients with severe dementia, the legally responsible adult should be involved

3. **Use the minimum necessary patient-identifiable information**—if data are required, only the data that are actually relevant to the project should be passed across, rather than patient medical histories and notes being made fully available. If information is being requested from participants, their privacy should be respected and additional questions avoided unless they are crucial to the running of the project

4. **Access to patient-identifiable information should be on a strict need-to-know basis**—if there are multiple people involved in delivering an intervention, only those within the team who require the information should have access to it

5. **Everyone should be aware of their responsibilities**—individuals should respect confidentiality and not pass on any of the information to anybody else. This also applies to information that participants voluntarily or involuntarily disclose over the course of an intervention

6. **Understand and comply with the law**—all accessing of patient data should follow legal requirements as well as organizational protocols

Q The original Caldicott 'Report on the Review of Patient-Identifiable Information' published in December 1997 by the Health in Wales website www.wales.nhs.uk.

Flagging causes for concern

In 2012, a seventh principle was added to the Caldicott principles: 'The duty to share information can be as important as the duty to protect patient confidentiality'.(1) As mentioned in the Scottish Executive recommendations, individuals have a duty to protect participants they are working with, identifying people who might be in a vulnerable position and ensuring that they have support available to them. For short-term projects or those that take place in healthcare settings, there may already be a strong support network in place that a project can feed into. For example, a participant who has a mental health condition may already be under the care of an on-site psychiatrist who could be informed if the participant appeared to be in need of further advice or support. However, for projects that work in community settings or in individuals' homes, it may be necessary to develop a system for protecting participants and flagging causes for concern at the start of a project.

There are a number of potential causes for concern that should be monitored over the course of a project. If a project is short term, such as a single music workshop, separating a cause for concern from an accident or simply an aspect of an individual's personality or history may be extremely hard to do. However, if a project is longer term, patterns of behaviour may emerge, such as:

1. Signs of physical abuse—these could include bruising, burns, scars, fractures, or other evident injuries

2. Signs of neglect—these could include physical injuries, other signs of poor physical health, or unusual behaviours that seem out of place

3. Signs of emotional abuse—emotional abuse can manifest itself in low self-esteem, withdrawn behaviours, insecure attachment behaviours, challenging or out-of-control behaviours, self-harming, severe mental health conditions, impaired family relationships, and alcohol or substance misuse

4. Signs relating to a health condition—these could include a participant mentioning new health symptoms they are not reporting to their healthcare professional, disclosing an intention to harm themselves, or the results from psychological or physiological testing as part of a research project or evaluation that give cause for concern

5. Moral or legal information—this could be information disclosed by a participant regarding a previous crime they may have committed, an intention to commit a crime or to harm another, or another illegal or immoral activity

Before a project starts, a system should be put in place for how to flag causes for concern. In the first instance, this may involve all individuals leading a project undergoing training with a healthcare professional on what behavioural and physical signs to look out for over the course of the project. If an individual spots these signs, a second stage may be for them to have a point of contact to whom they should report these, such as the project manager. The project manager could then assess whether the concern is mild, moderate, or severe, based on what has been reported, how many people have noticed it, and whether any similar signs have been reported before. Mild signs may simply be recorded locally to ascertain whether a pattern emerges. Moderate concerns may be passed back to a health or social care professional who has been lined up in advance to act on information passed from the project team. Severe concerns of a time-sensitive nature may need to have a fast-track process to ensure that a professional is able to deal with the situation quickly and protect the participant involved. Decisions should also be made at the start of the project regarding whether participants themselves will be told if information has been passed back to a professional.

Q For further details on how to recognize signs of abuse and neglect and protect adults and children involved in projects, the UK Social Care Institute for Excellence provides a number of resources in its 'Safeguarding' pages www.scie.org.uk.

An important issue in reporting such concerns is maintaining participant confidentiality. In particular if a project involves working with a vulnerable group, it is advisable that participants receive an information sheet about the project, explaining what to expect. Particularly for projects that involve monitoring of physical or mental health symptoms, this information sheet may explain that a professional will be notified in the event that a member of the project team has any concerns for the individual's welfare. Depending on the type of project, participants may be asked to sign a consent form confirming that they are happy with this. Participant information sheets and consent forms are discussed further in Chapter 12.

To maintain a balance between respecting participant confidentiality and protecting participants, projects should consider issues around reporting right from the outset, consulting widely with health and/or social care professionals as well as potential participants to assess what the risks are and how participants can be best protected (see Chapter 10 for more on patient and public involvement).

Q The British Medical Association has published a toolkit entitled *Safeguarding Vulnerable Adults* (2011) which is available as part of the 'Ethics: A-Z' on its website www.bma.org.uk.

Photography and filming

The same confidentiality rules for patient data apply to photography, filming, and audio recording. These should be used only when there is a justified purpose, with the minimum amount of information about those involved as participants used in conjunction with the photograph, video, or recording, and participants should consent to this happening in advance. Consent forms for photography and filming are often already available from healthcare organizations; however, if they are being developed specifically for a new project, the following issues should be considered and outlined in the consent form:

1. Where the photograph may be used and in what context, in particular if it will be used on social media. Often, if the exact outlets have not been decided, the consent form will cover multiple purposes (such as print, web, digital display, and all other forms of media)

2. Whether the individual will be identified by name or as having a specific health condition as part of this process (e.g. if the photograph will be used as an example of a music programme on an HIV ward)

3. Where the photograph will be stored and who will have access to it, to ensure its security

4. Whether the individual will receive any right to the photograph or reimbursement or, if not, who will own the photograph

5. Whether the individual will be contacted when the photograph is used

6. Whether the individual will receive a copy of the photograph

7. Whether consent will be sought again at any point or under any circumstance or whether this consent is intended to cover future uses

Individual organizations may have their own policies on issues such as whether cameras on mobile phones can be used for photographic purposes or whether this is not secure enough. As outlined in Chapter 12, if participants are signing a consent form as part of their involvement in a research project around an arts in health intervention, optional additional boxes covering filming and photography could be included on the same form to reduce the amount of paperwork with which participants have to engage.

Healthcare organizations may also have their own policies on receiving permission from communications offices and media departments prior to any external parties coming in to film or take photographs, or prior to the organization itself being named in any external press. In particular, filming should be organized so as not to interfere with any treatment or care within a healthcare setting or intrude on other patients in the vicinity. Special care should be taken that patient medical notes or observation charts are not caught on camera as this could compromise patient confidentiality.

Health and safety

Another fundamental issue in the delivery of arts in health interventions is health and safety. This not only affects patients and the public involved in projects, but also those delivering interventions, whether in healthcare, community, or private settings. Health and safety covers a broad range of activities, with two of the most important being infection control and risk assessments.

Standard infection control precautions

Nosocomial infections (also referred to as hospital-acquired infections) are infections that are not present when a patient is admitted to a healthcare setting such as a hospital but that develop over the course of their stay. There are two types:

- Endogenous infection, self-infection, or auto-infection—the cause of the infection was present in the patient at the time of admission (e.g. to the hospital) and during their stay the patient's altered resistance causes the infection to materialize
- Cross-contamination followed by cross-infection—during the course of the stay, the patient comes into contact with new infective agents, becomes contaminated, and develops an infection

We are exposed to infections on a daily basis, but healthy individuals have a general resistance to many of these. However, patients in hospitals, hospices, or care homes often have reduced resistance; particularly those with underlying diseases, newborn babies, the elderly, and those with injuries or wounds. As a result, people in healthcare settings are more likely to develop an infection after contamination.

In a healthcare setting, the sources of infection may be staff or visitors, other patients, or the environment. Consequently, anybody working in a healthcare setting has a responsibility to ensure that they reduce any risks of passing on infections through their activities. The most likely ways of spreading infections are through direct contact (such as hand-to-hand contact), indirect contact (such as touching door handles), or through airborne transmission (such as through sneezing or coughing). There are some simple guidelines that can be followed to reduce the chance of spreading an infection:

1. Many healthcare settings have a minimum amount of time that a staff member (or individual carrying out work in the organization) has to be free of symptoms such as a temperature, diarrhoea, and vomiting before they can

return to work. If an individual is unsure of whether their symptoms are contagious, infection control teams in hospitals or healthcare professionals in other healthcare settings can often make the decision as to whether an individual can come into the healthcare setting or not

2. Many healthcare settings operate a 'bare below the elbow' rule. This means that sleeves should be rolled up, any watches or bracelets or decorative rings removed, nails kept short, clean and polish-free (with no artificial nails), and any cuts or abrasions covered with a waterproof dressing

3. Items of clothing, long necklaces, or long hair that could trail or become a risk for indirect contact should be avoided or secured, such as hair tied back

4. Hands should be washed thoroughly before entering a patient area. Thorough hand washing with adequate quantities of water and soap can remove the majority of potential contaminants. Antimicrobial soap can remove further contaminants, and alcohol gel can further disinfect the hands. However, alcohol gel should not be used as a substitute for hand washing. Figure 8.1 shows the 11 steps for hand washing recommended by the World Health Organization. Importantly, hands also must be adequately dried using driers or disposable hand towels as wet surfaces transfer organisms more readily than dry ones. The World Health Organization recommends 'five moments for hand hygiene' when working in healthcare: (i) before contact with individuals, (ii) before a clean or aseptic procedure, (iii) after body fluid exposure risk, (iv) after contact with an individual, and (v) after contact with an individual's surroundings (such as their bed). Of these, moments (i), (iv), and (v) are especially important to those involved in delivering arts in health interventions

5. Equipment (including musical instruments and arts utensils) being used in any session should also be cleaned and sterilized before use. If equipment is directly touched by patients, it should also be cleaned between uses. Materials that are harder to clean (such as fabrics) should be discussed with a member of healthcare staff before they are used, and may have special machine-washing requirements. Some materials, such as latex, may not be allowed into certain areas

6. If a patient is being visited in isolation, there are additional precautions. These may include wearing protective gloves, gowns, and a mask. These should be put on immediately before entering the environment and removed and disposed of immediately afterwards

In addition to following guidelines such as these, many healthcare environments require people working on the premises to undertake occupational

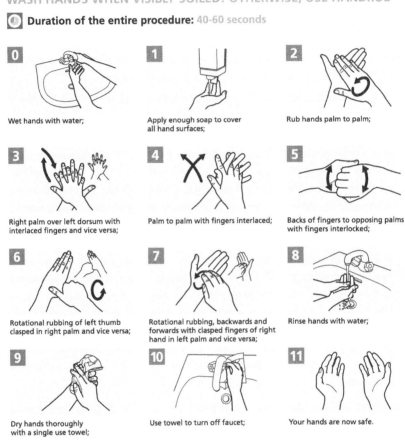

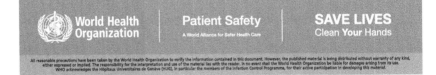

Figure 8.1 How to Handwash? Reprinted from The Infection Control Programme, Hôpitaux Universitaires de Genève, *How to Handwash?* [online poster] http://www.who.int/gpsc/5may/How_To_HandWash_Poster.pdf, accessed 9th December 2016, Copyright © WHO, 2009.

health checks prior to a project commencing to assess whether an individual has immunity to certain infectious diseases they may encounter in the health-care environment, and to determine whether the individual has an infection that could be transmitted to others. As part of this, an individual may be asked to provide a medical history and proof of vaccinations or agree to a blood test.

> Q The UK Royal College of Nursing has produced a guide entitled *Good practice in infection prevention and control* that provides more detail on hygiene and how to deal with accidental exposure to possible sources of infection. It is available via the NHS Wales website www.wales.nhs.uk.

Risk assessments

As well as infection control, there are other potential hazards and risks relating to the delivery of arts in health interventions that must be carefully considered. One of the best ways of identifying such hazards and risks is to undertake a risk assessment. Risk assessments can cover a very broad range of categories, such as financial risk, strategic risk, and operational risk. However, many of these high-level project risks should have been picked up as part of the consultation and piloting phases described in Chapters 5 and 6. Additional categories of risk that must be considered before a project is implemented relate to potential physical risks and hazards.

If a project is taking place within a wider organization such as a hospital or community centre, large-scale risk assessments for such physical risks or hazards will have been undertaken for this setting, in which case risk assessments for this specific project can focus on elements that are bespoke to the running of the intervention. Risks not just to project participants but also workshop leaders, friends, or relatives who may accompany a participant to a project, healthcare professionals who may be involved, members of the public, and any other people who may come into contact with the project should be considered. These could include, among other things:

* Venue—e.g. risks relating to furniture or carpeting in the room, or related to access, heating, lighting, and noise
* Equipment—e.g. risks relating to the use of musical instruments, electronics or amplification, technology, and arts consumables
* Personnel—e.g. risks that might arise because of insufficient training or experience of leaders and supervisors or events that may occur during a session related to participants' medical conditions such as risks of falling or requiring urgent medication

◆ Safety and security—e.g. risks relating to fire escape routes, alarm response procedures, or intruders

◆ Psychosocial—e.g. potential distress to participants or leaders (discussed further in 'Occupational health')

There are five stages to a risk assessment:

1. Identifying hazards and those at risk—the opinions of different people with varying perspectives on the project should be sought as to what might be the potential hazards and risks relating to an intervention. As part of this, the environment in which a project is going to take place should be visited. Screening lists exist for different types of risks and may be helpful in identifying some of the key ones, but each project should be considered individually to ensure that more unusual risks have not been missed

2. Evaluating and prioritizing risks—it is recommended that a prioritization scheme be developed to identify risks that are the most urgent and must be minimized for the project to run. For example, risks could be categorized by severity (e.g. negligible vs. acceptable for a short time vs. not acceptable) or by probability of accident (e.g. unlikely, moderate likelihood, and strong likelihood)

3. Deciding on preventative action—if possible, a risk should be avoided rather than reduced. Furthermore, there is a hierarchy of types of prevention and protection: technical solutions are best (e.g. the risk is physically removed), followed by organizational solutions (e.g. a way to avoid the risk is identified) followed by individual measures (e.g. individuals are pre-warned about the risk)

4. Taking action—a prioritization plan may be drawn up noting what the risk is, what prevention or protection measures have been decided on, who is responsible for these measures, the timeline for this activity, and the monitoring plan and review date

5. Documentation, monitoring, and review—the risk assessment should be carefully documented as it may be required at some stage in the project or become a part of an ethical review process. Monitoring should be documented also and the assessment reviewed at regular intervals to confirm that nothing has changed

If, despite the risk assessment, an incident does occur, it is important to have a system in place for how to report it to identify the cause of the incident, plan to prevent a similar incident occurring in the future, and to meet legislative requirements. Each healthcare organization will have its own system for reporting incidents. However, most systems require five key pieces of information:

1. A description of the circumstances of the incident
2. The cause of the incident
3. Who was involved and the impact on the individual(s) involved and the wider environment
4. Measures taken at the time
5. Steps to be taken to prevent future incidents

It is important that all incidents are reported quickly and follow-up actions taken to minimize the chance of future incidents occurring.

Q For further information on identifying risks, undertaking a risk assessment, and tackling risks, the Health and Safety Executive has a website containing a wealth of resources: www.hse.gov.uk.

For projects, it can be helpful to designate a health and safety officer who has overall responsibility for risk assessments. Different countries have various health and safety training programmes that could support this individual. Furthermore, although there may already be a plethora of trained medical staff available where a project is taking place (if that project is taking place in a healthcare organization), it is still important to know what the formal procedure should be in the case of an accident or incident that requires medical support. If a project is being carried out in a non-healthcare setting such as a community site, at least one member of the team who will be present at all sessions (or a rota of people if this is not feasible) should be trained in first aid. Copies of first aid certification and any additional health and safety training should be kept with other important project documents.

Occupational health

In addition to patient safeguarding, another crucial issue in delivering arts in health interventions relates to occupational health. Occupational health is a multi-disciplinary activity that aims to protect and promote the health of workers, develop healthy and safe working environments, enhance the wellbeing of workers, and enable workers to contribute positively.

Q The World Health Organization has produced a manual that explores some of the key topics in occupational health, entitled *Occupational Health: a manual for primary health care workers* (2011). This is available on its website www.who.int.

Working in healthcare, whether in a healthcare setting, in the community, or in a private space, can be demanding, so it also important that those involved in the delivery of arts in health interventions safeguard their own wellbeing. There are various types of negative impact that an environment could have on an individual, including:

◆ Physical stressors—e.g. poor lighting, noise, and physical exertion

◆ Environmental psychosocial stressors—e.g. work overload, witnessing distressing events, and emotional stress

These stressors may affect people differently depending on their personality type, individual susceptibility and the level of support they receive from their team.

Responses to these stressors in the short term can include fatigue, anxiety, dissatisfaction, and psychosomatic symptoms (such as headaches, backache, and disturbed sleep), with potentially higher absenteeism, reduced productivity, and decreased group cohesion. In the long term, they can lead to depression, aggression, and burnout. As such, it is important to try and prevent stressors occurring or, where they are unavoidable, put in place systems to provide support. There are three main ways this can be undertaken:

1. Primary prevention—prior to an individual (such as an artist, project manager, or researcher) becoming involved in a project, steps should be put in place to ensure that the individual receives appropriate preparation for the type of work they will be undertaking. In Chapter 7 we discussed the value of shadowing a project to become accustomed to the environment, having a supervisor to help provide support while a project is under way, and using diaries or feedback sessions to allow individuals to discuss what they have experienced, ask questions, and receive advice on how to manage different situations. Having this structure in place at the start of a project can be an effective way of making sure an individual feels supported and is prepared to deal with the environment. Including stressors within the general risk assessment can also help to identify them in advance, enabling advance planning

2. Secondary prevention—if an individual identifies that they are beginning to find any aspect of the project demanding, there should also be a system in place for them to raise this before it becomes a bigger issue. For small projects, having a main point of contact for those involved in the delivery of an intervention can help to provide continuous support. For larger projects, having drop-in sessions on a regular basis for people to come and discuss any issues can help to identify problems before they become too big. Once the problem has been identified, it may be possible to put in place more

support for the individual, to plan a change in rota to provide them with more time off, or to refer them to somebody who can provide further support for them. Team away days, social events, and project celebrations can also help to bring those involved together to relax and appreciate the positive impact of a project too

3. Tertiary prevention—there should also be a plan in place for what happens if somebody needs immediate support, for example, if there is a distressing incident that occurs during a session, or an individual is affected by something they have witnessed while in a healthcare environment. If there is a counselling service in the organization, individuals could be provided with the details of how to access this for confidential support. Often identifying tertiary support will involve working closely with the healthcare organization involved to see what is offered to other staff and whether this can also be made available to those involved in the project. If an incident does occur, it is important to review the situation and assess whether anything could be changed in the future to minimize the chance of the situation occurring again

Q The European Union Programme for Employment and Social Solidarity (PROGRESS) developed a guide entitled *Occupational health and safety risks in the healthcare sector: guide to prevention and good practice* (2010), which identifies a wide range of individual risks including psychosocial risks and considers how to manage them.(2)

Engaging patients and staff

One of the most important elements of an arts in health project is to engage participants and help them to feel comfortable and relaxed. However, this can also be challenging, especially when working in a healthcare setting or with a vulnerable group who is new to an activity. Advice on how to deal with different situations varies according to the location, participant group, and type of activity. However, there are often common themes that run between different arts in health projects. Below are a list of common questions relating to working with participants and with healthcare staff. These are not intended to be hard and fast rules for project success but may help in preparing an arts in health intervention. These questions cover four common themes that can emerge during arts in health projects: creating rapport, respecting participation and privacy, communicating with staff, and what to do in an emergency.

- When working in a healthcare setting such as a hospital with multiple beds, what is the best way to engage participants in an activity?

Entering a healthcare setting and trying to engage a group of people who may not necessarily have opted to take part in an activity (such as a public performance) can be challenging. First, any artist or individual involved in a project should introduce themselves to participants and say a little about the type of arts activity they are involved in and what they are planning for the session they are about to lead. If appropriate and if the group is relatively small, it may help to ask the names of the people nearby and draw them into the activity by asking them some simple questions, such as have they ever taken part in the arts activity before. As the activity gets going, participants may naturally become more involved or they can be encouraged to give their opinions from an observer's perspective. Offering choice can be really key in this. For example, a musician could offer to take requests from participants, by taking open suggestions, providing participants with a list of their songs from which to pick, or simply giving people binary choices, such as 'an upbeat or a relaxing piece' or 'classical or jazz'. The selection process allows participants a choice, which can be empowering in a setting where they may feel some of their independence has been removed, and can draw them into being more engaged.

◆ What is the best thing to do if a participant starts describing their health condition or asking for help?

Some people are very open about their mental or physical health, whereas others are much more private. Sometimes a participant may use an arts activity to open up about their condition. Simply listening may be enough to help that person feel supported. However, asking questions should be sensitively handled, preferably with a project policy determined up front as to whether individuals should ask any questions or not, especially if this is not essential to the running of the project. Offering medical advice should be completely avoided for those outside the care team. If a participant says they are feeling unwell or asks for a medical professional, the first aider in the project team should be called or, if the project is taking place in a healthcare setting, the patient's call button should be pressed for them or a healthcare professional alerted. Again, decisions as to who should be alerted (whether a nurse or other member of staff) should be made in collaboration with the care team on site up front so the project team know what procedure to follow.

◆ What should be done if one patient in a healthcare setting (such as on a hospital ward or in a care home day room) is sleeping or speaking with a healthcare professional when an activity is scheduled to start?

An arts activity should never disrupt the ongoing work of a healthcare organization. If it appears that a medical consultation is in process, it may be advisable to ask another member of healthcare staff whether an activity can commence or whether it should be delayed until the consultation is over. If the activity is planned to move around different areas of the healthcare setting, it may be preferable to return later when people are awake and free, but alternatively it may be possible to start quietly with a subgroup of people in the ward or room. However, if a sleeping participant wakes up and asks that the activity be stopped to allow them to continue sleeping, their wishes should be respected.

- What should be done if one participant in a group setting asks for an activity to be stopped?

This can be a challenging issue if the majority of participants are enjoying the activity. This is where a project supervisor can be of support. He or she can ascertain whether the participant wants the activity to stop altogether, or just a component of it (such as a new song to be played as they simply do not like one particular song). If the participant is not enjoying the activity at all, he or she could be helped to move elsewhere (such as out of day room) or, if the activity is happening in a hospital ward and the participant cannot move, the supervisor could ask if it is OK for the artist to finish what they are currently doing and then move away. If a participant gets distressed or angry because of an activity and is unable to move elsewhere, the activity should be quickly brought to a close to prevent causing any further problems.

- How much should healthcare professionals be involved in activity sessions?

This will depend entirely on the activity and what has been planned with the healthcare professionals involved. Some projects may have a dedicated professional in the sessions either to provide support or to take part themselves. However, other projects may be partly designed to reduce the burden on healthcare staff and entertain patients, giving staff more time to undertake other activities. In this instance, it can be helpful to designate in advance of the project a member of staff who can be the point of contact: somebody the project team can report to when they arrive, liaise with about any issues or sensitivities on the day of which they should be aware, and approach if they have questions. In this case, asking for support or advice from other staff should be avoided unless essential so as not to add to staff workload.

- What is the best thing to do if a participant tries to give money to the artist?

As discussed in Chapter 7, different projects have different funding strategies. For some projects, this may be a viable part of donations processes with designated donations buckets, or participants may be directly invited to pay or make a contribution to their involvement. However, for other projects it may be unexpected and not formally part of the funding strategy. In this instance, participants should be notified that the project is already funded and they have no need to make a contribution, so as to stop others in a group also feeling they need to pay. If the participant is still keen to make a contribution, there should be a planned system in place, for example with any additional money going towards the wider fundraising efforts of the organization delivering the project or being donated to a charity involved. Participants who wish to make a donation should then be informed as to where their money will be donated.

◆ What should be done if an alarm goes off?

If it is an alarm on a patient machine, the patients themselves may know what to do, or the supervisor can help them to press a call button or ask the patient if they would like them to fetch a healthcare professional. The activity may be able to continue if this is a routine occurrence. If it is an emergency alarm and the activity is happening in a healthcare setting, the artist should immediately stop and move out of the way to allow the healthcare professionals to follow their regular procedures. This is the same procedure as for a patient requiring urgent medical help.

> Q For more on guidelines for delivering arts in health interventions, the Health Service Executive South (Cork) Arts + Health Programme and the Waterford Healing Arts Trust in Ireland commissioned guidelines for good practice available via www.artshealthandwellbeing.org.uk.(3)

Summary

This chapter has outlined some key issues pertaining to working in healthcare, including aspects of safeguarding, health and safety, and how to engage patients and public. Its aim has been to provide those who are planning on working in healthcare with a foundation in understanding some of the most important issues that may arise and how to prepare for them; a foundation that can be built on by becoming acquainted with the institutional guidelines specific to each project.

So far, this book has explored the context for arts in health interventions and their design and delivery. One of the key themes that has emerged across the chapters is the centrality of research in arts in health, as a way of supporting the design of new interventions, ascertaining whether an intervention can deliver key health benefits (sometimes as an extension of earlier evaluation activity), helping to build the case for support and providing a stronger rationale for roll-out. In Part IV, we will turn to research in more detail, considering how a promising intervention can be taken forwards into a research project, the benefits of doing so, and the potential ways this could be carried out.

References

1. **Department of Health**. Report on the review of patient-identifiable information [Internet]. London; 1997 Dec [cited 2016 Nov 2] p. 137. (The Caldicott Report). Available from: http://webarchive.nationalarchives.gov.uk/20130107105354/http://www.dh.gov.uk/en/Publicationsandstatistics/Publications/PublicationsPolicyAndGuidance/DH_4068403.

2. **European Union Programme for Employment and Social Solidarity (PROGRESS)**. Occupational health and safety risks in the healthcare sector: guide to prevention and practice. Luxembourg: European Commission; 2010.

3. **White M, Robson M.** Participatory Arts Practice in Healthcare Contexts. Waterford Healing Arts Trust and the Health Service Executive South (Cork) Arts + Health Programme: Centre for Medical Humanities; 2010 Oct pp. 1–13.

Part III

Researching arts in health interventions

Chapter 9

An introduction to research

Why research?

In 2011, journalist Eryn Brown wrote an article in the *Los Angeles Times* entitled '"Duh" science: Why researchers spend so much time proving the obvious'.(1) She discussed the issue of why medical researchers who have unlocked the human genome and wiped out smallpox also engage in 'the practice of hypothesising, testing and publishing the seemingly obvious'. Similar to the examples Brown cites in her article, many research questions in arts in health might appear to have answers so obvious they need not be researched: of course relaxing music calms anxiety in pre-surgical patients; it stands to reason that providing artwork in waiting areas can help to alleviate boredom; and it's clear that weekly dance classes lead to improved strength in older adults. However, as Brown acknowledges, research is vitally important even for seemingly obvious research questions for a range of reasons, including:

1. **Confirmation**—However obvious something seems in theory or anecdote, it may not be true in practice. A study published in the journal *Injury Prevention* in 2000 looked at whether toughened glasses led to reduced injuries in bars.(2) On the surface, stronger pint glasses logically sound a sensible idea as they will be less likely to smash. However, the study found that people were less careful with toughened glasses and there were in fact nearly double the number of injuries; the exact opposite of what the researchers had hypothesized. This example illustrates how perceived truths or anecdotal reports are insufficient in determining whether an effect is likely to occur and research is needed, even on apparently obvious questions

2. **Influence**—To influence perceptions and policy, there not only has to be proof but repeated proof, again and again. A famous example is the number of studies linking smoking and lung cancer that had to be published before there were significant changes in smoking legislation and public activity. To convince healthcare professionals, funders, and the public of the benefits of the arts, repeated research studies are needed to achieve a

general scientific consensus. These may take the form of replications of previous studies to confirm findings, extensions of previous studies with larger groups or in different settings, or studies that approach the same question from different angles

3. **Mechanisms**—Even if the answer to the research question might appear simple, the mechanisms by which this effect is achieved can be complex. For example, for relaxing music to calm anxiety in pre-surgical patients, a cascade of activity must place, including activation of various parts of the brain, and release of a number of hormones and signals across vast networks of nerve cells. The resultant effect is also not confined to a feeling of lower anxiety but involves altered activity within certain organs such as lowered heart rate alongside changes in levels of biomarkers of the endocrine and immune systems.(3) There may be other implications too, such as changes in the levels of induction agents needed for the anaesthetic or reduced quantities of analgesics after surgery. Consequently, research turns the initial simple question as to whether music can reduce pre-surgical anxiety into a much richer topic and has the potential to demonstrate an even greater effect on patient care than initially anticipated

4. **Variation**—It is also important to take into account variation. Artistic experiences are individually, socially, and culturally informed, so a single intervention could have different effects on people of different ages, cultural and socioeconomic backgrounds, and health status. Again, research is vital for characterizing this variation both to understand how the arts can be best tailored to suit different populations and also to be realistic about the impact the arts can have with different participant groups

Consequently, sometimes arts in health research may on the surface address some quite basic or 'common-sense' questions. However, systematically investigating arts interventions through research is essential to understand the extent and nature of these effects, produce generalizable knowledge, and engage stakeholders, especially those who may be more cautious as to the potential benefits of the arts for health. Furthermore, not all questions are common sense. Many of the greatest strides forwards in the field have come about through research that has demonstrated benefits of arts engagement that had not previously even been considered to exist. So research can be one of the most powerful ways of supporting development in the field.

Is it research? Evaluation versus research

Following on from the discussions in Chapter 6 about evaluation, an important question is how is research different from evaluation? There is often confusion around the two terms, partly because many aspects of the methods used in research and evaluation are very similar, if not the same. For example, both research and evaluation draw on qualitative methods, such as interviews, focus groups, and observation, and quantitative methods, such as questionnaires and ratings. Although certain specific research methods and types of analysis are more common in research than evaluation (and vice versa), setting clear boundaries between the two can be difficult. Indeed, in an online discussion on the topic led by the American Evaluation Association (EVALTALK), one of the founding theorists of evaluation, William Trochim, argued that in terms of methods there is no difference between research and evaluation:

> 'What we do in process-programme-formative-summative evaluation … is virtually impossible to distinguish … from what I understand as applied social research.'(4)

Consequently, instead of seeking to draw a distinguishing line between research and evaluation in terms of methods, a simpler way of understanding the distinction is to consider their history, purpose, process, and practicalities.

From a *historical* perspective, research is much older than evaluation. Our earliest recorded use of the term 'research' comes from 1577, from the Old French 're'+'cerchier' meaning to search or seek. The core aim of research across history has been to increase knowledge, either through establishing new facts or confirming previous ones, solving problems, and developing new theories. However, evaluation is a much newer discipline than research. Its genesis is often traced to the United States in the Elementary and Secondary Education Act (ESEA) in 1965, which required account of the use and impact of public funds. Initial efforts by researchers and educational psychologists, however, did not fully capture the effects that funding was having, missing some of the unanticipated but nevertheless valuable effects of funding. Consequently, from the late 1960s to the early 1980s, there was a burgeoning of activity around evaluation, with a reorientation of thinking around what it was important to measure to determine the effectiveness of interventions; something that was identified as being different from setting out to answer specific research questions.(5) This brings us to the issue of *purpose*. One of the founding theorists of evaluation, Michael Scriven, explained:

> 'Evaluation determines the merit, worth or value of things. The evaluation process identifies relevant values or standards that apply to what is being evaluated, performs empirical investigation using techniques from the social sciences, and then integrates conclusions with the standards into an overall evaluation or set of evaluations. Social science research, by contrast, does not aim for or achieve evaluative conclusions. It is restricted to empirical (rather than evaluative) research, and bases its conclusions

only on factual results—that is observed, measured, or calculated data. Social science research does not establish standards or values and then integrate them with factual results to reach evaluative conclusions. In fact, the dominant social science doctrine for many decades prided itself on being value free.'(5)

Other theorists pointed to the necessity of evaluation to consider factors both internal and external to an intervention (such as the sociopolitical landscape in which the intervention is delivered), as well as capturing how an intervention is oriented towards policy and funding.(5) Seeking to clarify this distinction, in the book *Fundamental Issues in Evaluation*, edited by Nick Smith and Paul Brandon, Sandra Mathison proposed six ways in which the purposes of evaluation and research are different (6):

1. Evaluation particularizes, research generalizes
2. Evaluation is designed to *improve* something, while research is designed to *prove* something
3. Evaluation provides the basis for decision-making; research provides the basis for drawing conclusions
4. Evaluation—so what? Research—what's so?
5. Evaluation—how well it works? Research—how it works?
6. Evaluation is about what is valuable; research is about what is

Of course, many of these distinctions can be debated, especially as they can become caricatured. For example, evaluation might well focus on the effects of a specific intervention, such as a dance class for older adults in a rural hospital, but the findings of the evaluation are often generalized in the decisions of funders to scale up projects. Equally, research may not be about generalizable findings, but may include specific case studies of individuals involved in an intervention. So while the distinctions relating to purpose can help in orientating the purpose of research and evaluation, they must be interpreted cautiously.

In terms of *process*, evaluation and research tend to happen at different stages in the development of an intervention. As shown in Chapter 6, evaluation can be used to assess an intervention's design and performance (a formative evaluation), explore the successes and challenges related to how it runs (a process evaluation), and ascertain whether the interventions shows signs of having the desired effects on participants (an outcome evaluation). Following this, research can form a valuable next step to ascertain in more detail the depth and breadth of impact. But equally, if the impetus for a project is an initial research question, it will still be necessary to take some steps backwards to conceptualize, design, and pilot the intervention to ensure it is appropriate to answer the research question (Chapters 5 and 6). If evaluation is not carried out prior to the start of the research project (perhaps because of financial or timing constraints), it is recommended that evaluation questions be included within the research design. This way, if hypothesized results are not found, it will be clear whether this is because they are simply not caused by the intervention, or because the intervention was not received in the way it was intended to be.

Finally, in terms of *practicalities*, an important distinction between research and evaluation is that research projects normally require ethical approval. This is covered in more detail in Chapter 12. However, the UK Medical Research Council has a useful tool for determining whether a project is research or evaluation. The tool asks the following questions:

1. Are participants randomized (allocated not on the basis of their own choice) into different groups?

2. Does the study involve changing patient care or treatment from the accepted standards of any participants involved? (This is as opposed to adding an intervention to usual care)

3. Are your findings going to be generalizable? (In other words, will the findings be extrapolated from participants in the study to apply to a broader participant population, a different setting, or a different project run elsewhere?)

If the answer to any of these questions is 'yes', then the project counts as research. However, if the answers to all the questions are 'no', the project is not deemed, at least in terms of ethical standards, to be research. Consequently, although separating evaluation and research on the basis of purpose, process, and practicalities might miss the nuances of the theoretical debates around evaluation versus research, it can help when making a decision regarding which is more appropriate during a project.

Evaluation and research versus audits

In addition to questions around the distinction between research and evaluation, it is also important to distinguish both of these terms from audits. In Chapter 5, we discussed the contributions made by Florence Nightingale to healthcare during the Crimean war, including her development of interventions to support health and establishment of a system of auditing these interventions. Since then, audits have been used in healthcare, with increasing consistency since the late twentieth century.

The UK Health Research Authority defines clinical audits as 'a quality improvement process that seeks to improve patient care and outcomes through systematic review of care against explicit criteria'.(7) Audit cycles involve agreement of standards of best practice up front (before data are collected). These standards may be based on previous evaluation or research data for specific projects (as discussed in Chapter 6), or may be national or international standards. Data are then collected on current practice and compared with the standards. If current practice is found to fall below the levels set by the standards, this can then be investigated and changes planned and implemented. Audits typically take place on a planned regular basis (such as annually).

Audits have enormous value in confirming that best practice is being followed and standards maintained. In addition, they can prompt concerns, complaints, or other views to be aired. They also have quite a distinct role from both evaluation and research. As discussed in Chapter 6, the evaluation of a programme can lead to some expected standards being set. An audit can then be used to check that an intervention is still meeting these expected standards. This process of checking will not normally involve any kind of control group or new intervention, but rather test what is already available and running using pre-set questions. This process of checking standards provided by audits can be helpful alongside research studies too. For example, if a research project contains multiple sites, audits can be used to assess whether interventions are running as planned at each site, meeting the standards expected. This can confirm whether the data being collected from the different sites are going to be comparable.

Consequently, audits are not as exploratory as evaluations, and do not produce completely new knowledge such as can be produced in research. What audits can do is reveal important information on how programmes are running in practice, ensure that new branches of programmes continue to adhere to the core central standards, and flag problems early to ensure programmes operate as planned in meeting the needs of participants. Perhaps most importantly, audit data can be linked straight into an improvement cycle, so that changes can be implemented to bring programmes back up to the expected standards. So audits, evaluation, and research should sit comfortably alongside one another, each with different purposes and implications for programmes.

Q For more information about clinical audits, Robin Burgess' *New Principles of Best Practice in Clinical Audit* (2011) explores how to undertake an audit and implement sustainable change.(7)

Arts in health 'exceptionalism'

Another issue surrounding arts in health research is how it is positioned in relation to wider health research. Although people generally recognize that arts in health interventions must be rigorously researched to demonstrate their value, what this research looks like and what types of evidence it needs to produce to count as 'rigorous' have been hotly debated. In particular there are concerns around experimental scientific methods being used to assess arts in health interventions such as randomized controlled trials (RCTs). RCTs are experimental designs that minimize bias through allocating participants to either the intervention being studied or some form of 'control' group (such as either no intervention or a comparison intervention) based not on participant preference but on chance (a process known as 'randomization'). RCTs are one of the most favoured models in medical research. However, some have questioned whether they are suitable for capturing the multi-faceted effects of arts in health interventions. For example, are arts interventions too complex to be captured with experimental scientific methods? Does the use of biomedical models (such as RCTs) to compare arts interventions and biomedical interventions lend bias in support of the biomedical interventions? And do these methods set up standards that are 'impossible' to achieve through arts interventions, meaning that they can only fail and biomedical interventions surface as the only possible option for patients? Can arts in health truly be categorized along with other health interventions or are they not unique or 'exceptional'?

These questions have been discussed at conferences, roundtable events, at research, funding and grassroots levels, and, perhaps most publicly, in online blogs. As examples, two leading researchers in arts in health have published on their concerns about experimental methods in arts in health research. Dr Mike White, who was a researcher in the Centre for Medical Humanities at Durham University, wrote a high-profile blog for the Centre which included an entry entitled 'RCTs—The Holy Grail of Arts in Health?'.(8) White had concerns that the emphasis on RCTs within medical research could lead to the application of a 'one-size experimental design in arts interventions in non-clinical settings'. He wrote:

> 'We must not stifle that emergent vision and potential by only seeking a proven evidence base for arts in health that is narrowly defined through "control" based interventions. It reduces the whole arts and health field to being some kind of ancillary treatment in healthcare.'

White was not against experimental models, accepting that 'rigorous evidence gleaned from RCTs of course has a crucial function in convincing health economists and those holding the Treasury Green Book'. But he disliked the idea that there could be a pre-determined 'common research design for a very diverse field'. Instead, White called for research that integrated experimental models from the medical field with other non-experimental models such as case studies. A similar position to White's is taken in another blog by Clive Parkinson, Director of Arts for Health at Manchester Metropolitan University. In his blog 'Fiction-Non-Fiction', he too opposed the idea of 'a standardised tool-kit where all the nuance and complexity of culture and the arts can be packaged into a small, instrumental, do-it-yourself kit. A one size-fits-all panacea that can be branded and sold on'.(9) He spoke against the idea that 'the arts/health movement somehow adopts the clinical objectivity of the pharmaceutical industry' as he saw this as 'reducing' our understanding of arts in health 'or replacing it with an explanation that omits human experience and its involvement in any understanding'.

However, although these concerns around striking a balance between scientific rigour and the flexibility and creativity essential to arts and finding ways of really capturing the range of benefits of the arts are valid, the field of arts in health is not 'unique' or 'exceptional' in having these concerns. These same problems are faced in broader fields of public health and social science on a daily basis, such as in testing the impact of new community exercise initiatives among teenagers on fitness and social integration or exploring whether one-to-one therapy sessions can enhance wellbeing and agency in people with chronic health conditions. These types of interventions, which involve several interacting components, are known as 'complex interventions'.

It is recognized that researching complex interventions can be challenging as they may have a range of possible outcomes, or there may be variability in the target population, or different participants may receive different tailored versions of the intervention. So in 2000, the UK Medical Research Council published a *Framework for the Development and Evaluation of RCTs for Complex Intervention to Improve Health*.(10) The aim of this was to provide guidelines for how to research interventions that needed robust evidence behind them but did not fit neatly into the normal medical models. The initial guidelines were subsequently updated in 2008, entitled *Developing and evaluating complex interventions: the new Medical Research Council guidance*. (11) The guidelines refute some of the 'blanket' statements about medical research, such as the 'assumption that conventional clinical trials provide a template for all the different approaches to evaluation', and aim to tackle the lack of guidance on how to research interventions that are highly complex or come from outside the health sector, as well as placing more attention on the social, political, and geographical context in which interventions take place.

Arts in health interventions are classic examples of 'complex interventions'. As a number of people within the field of arts in health have identified, selecting a research design that allows for their complexity can be difficult; certainly RCTs may miss some of these features. This is where the UK guidelines are important, as they do not prescribe that RCTs have to be used. Indeed, they fully support decisions not to use RCTs. However, they call for care in deciding which study design to select and in making the decision to dispense with RCTs altogether, and crucially they take the time to dispel some of the 'blanket' statements around RCTs. For example:

1. **Blanket statement 1: some designs are not suitable for certain fields.** The guidelines warn 'Beware of 'blanket' statements about what designs are suitable for what kind of intervention (e.g. 'randomized trials are inappropriate for community-based interventions, psychiatry, surgery, etc.') A design may rarely be used in a particular field but that does not mean it cannot be used, and you should make your choice on the basis of specific characteristics of your study'(11)

2. **Blanket statement 2: randomization removes the essence of the intervention and is unethical.** 'You should always consider randomisation, because it is the most robust method of preventing the selection bias that occurs whenever those who receive the intervention differ systematically from those who do not, in ways likely to affect outcomes.'(11) At a simple level, randomization involves allocating people equally to experimental and control groups, which can lead to discontent among people who hoped to be allocated to a different group. However, there are randomization methods that can reduce potential discontent. The randomization itself can take into account different factors about a person, increasing or decreasing their chance of being in a particular group (see Chapter 11). Or the design of the study can be more sophisticated. For example, wait-list designs mean that everybody receives the intervention, but some participants are randomized to having to wait before receiving it (during which time they form the 'control' or 'non-intervention' group). Cluster randomized trials randomly allocate at a wider level, such as one hospital or community receiving one intervention and another receiving the control or comparison intervention, preventing jealousy among individuals in close communities. Stepped wedge designs combine wait-list and cluster designs, providing an intervention to all sites (e.g. hospitals or communities) but one by one. Randomization is discussed more in Chapter 11.

3. **Blanket statement 3: RCTs only allow for a single outcome to be assessed.** The guidelines actually clarify that RCTs do not limit outcomes to just one. 'A crucial aspect of the design … is the choice of outcome measures. You need to think about which outcomes are most important, and which are secondary, and how you will deal with multiple outcomes in the analysis … A good theoretical understanding of the intervention, derived from careful development work is key in choosing suitable outcome measures.'(11) While overloading a design with many measures might be unwise, RCTs can measure

multiple constructs within one study, allowing several different facets of an arts in health intervention to be explored.

4. **Blanket statement 4: If a chosen research design is an RCT, there can be no other design involved.** The guidelines speak of the value of other models 'nested within a trial'.(11) These can include process evaluations or assessments of cost-effectiveness, or can involve case studies and evaluations alongside the main research questions. This will be discussed more in Chapter 10.

The guidelines offer extensive advice on how to decide which design is best for a complex intervention. However, they also warn that if these more rigorous designs are not followed, reliable estimates of the effect of interventions will be very limited and not easily generalizable, and researchers will have 'to explain to decision-makers … the trade-offs involved in settling for weaker methods'. (11) Consequently, even if it is not possible to conduct an entirely rigorous RCT that controls for every possible variable in the study, the guidelines advise that "best available" methods, even if they are not theoretically optimal, may yield useful results.(11)

In truth, this brings us to the core of the issue around experimental designs for arts in health research. RCTs do not provide a perfect model for assessing the impact of arts interventions in health. In certain situations, they are actually very poor fits. For example, in trying to capture the essence of *why* engaging with a drumming group affects wellbeing, a stronger approach than designing an RCT might be to undertake in-depth interviews with participants involved in a drumming group. Decisions about which design is most appropriate for different research questions are explored in the Chapter 10. However, healthcare and medicine are founded on evidence-based models from predominantly experimental methods such as RCTs. Researchers and commissioners within healthcare and medicine will generally look to these experimental methods as the best form of evidence (and attempting to change that would require a seismic shift). This is not because of snobbery or a dislike of more complex interventions, but rather a desire to select the most effective and safe tools for patient care.

Consequently, if arts in health interventions are to be taken seriously within healthcare and medicine, they have to speak the language of health and follow experimental methods wherever possible. However, this need not be a case of 'either-or' and certainly should not mean that they restrict the language we use: experimental methods can sit alongside non-experimental methods; research projects can have multiple phases to answer different questions or explore the same question from different angles; and creative RCT designs and approaches to randomization can be employed. This really provides one solution to the RCT debate: it is not a case that an RCT comes at the expense of other methods, but rather that wherever possible, it too should be involved when researching an intervention. (Issues around designing such studies will be discussed further in Chapter 10). This approach is not novel but is followed by a vast range of other complex interventions including social interventions, public health interventions, and complementary therapies. Arts in health interventions are no different; they are not exceptional and we risk discrediting them if we suggest they are.

Q In 2015, a conference was held in Exeter in the UK entitled 'Researching Complex Interventions in Health: The State of the Art'. A broad range of topics relating to complex interventions was covered, including use of mixed qualitative and quantitative methods, carrying out pilot and feasibility studies, and use of non-standard experimental designs. The abstracts from the conference which summarize the presentations that were made are published in volume 16 of the journal *BMC Health Services Research* and are available online.(12)

Types of disciplinary working

This brings us to the critical question of *how* to speak multiple languages at once, incorporate different research designs and meet the requirements of perhaps not just one or two fields of research but many more. In 1992, PL Rosenfield proposed three types of disciplinary working: multi-disciplinary, inter-disciplinary, and trans-disciplinary.(13) These three categories have remained popular among researchers and have been further developed since. Historically, much arts in health research has been 'multi-disciplinary': teams from a variety of arts backgrounds and a broad range of health and science backgrounds have approached the topic of arts in health from their own areas of expertise. This has often resulted in research that only 'speaks' to the discipline from which it came. For example, rigorously controlled RCTs have been critiqued for missing out on the creative essence of arts interventions, whereas more flexible arts-based studies have not been seen as scientific enough to provide generalizable findings.

An alternative type of working is 'inter-disciplinary' working. This involves different disciplines providing experts to form a core study team, who then approach a research question in unison. This can help to remove some of the artificial gaps between the disciplines; furthermore such an approach can lead to answers to research questions that speak to both the arts and the health worlds, providing more comprehensive and meaningful data. An important point in this process is not merely to compromise on everybody's ideal research designs and methodologies but instead to develop more sophisticated methods, perhaps with multi-layered research tools or multi-phase studies to approach the question from different angles. This is likely to produce more thorough and in-depth answers that could have a greater impact on the field. However, it requires strong relationships within teams and an openness to ideas outside individuals' areas of expertise.

The third type of disciplinary working is 'trans-disciplinary'. This involves researchers being trained in multiple disciplines so that they contain within themselves the expertise from different fields. Historically, this has been difficult for researchers as many university degrees, especially in the UK, require a focus on one main subject. However, with new courses, especially post-graduate courses, being developed, it is now increasingly possible for researchers to have dual backgrounds, setting them up to develop fully integrated research studies across different fields. With trans-disciplinary working, it is important that researchers maintain strong links back to specific arts or health fields as well as to the field of arts in health, to ensure that research findings feed into new research studies and data continue to be of value to arts, health, and arts in health.

> Q Further details on types of disciplinary working in healthcare are given in a paper published in the journal *Health Services Research* in 2007: 'Defining inter-disciplinary research: conclusions from a critical review of the literature'.(14)

Summary

Overall, research is an exciting process for arts in health interventions as it can take a promising intervention to a new level, providing potentially compelling data, increasing the case for support for funding, and expanding the reach of the programme. It is also of vital importance. For although there is increasing research demonstrating clear and significant benefits of the arts within health, at the heart of the need for research and the need for using experimental methods in research is the core fact that not all arts in health interventions will have a tangible benefit for patient experience or outcomes. There is a strategic need to know which interventions work with which participant groups and why they work so that funding is put where it can have the greatest impact. While research may appear daunting because of the many legal, ethical, and methodological complexities, as well as the 'risk' that results will not be as promising as anticipated, it is only through research that arts interventions can be effectively and sustainably integrated within healthcare. Chapter 10 will take the form of a step-by-step guide through the research process to demystify some of the stages. However, before we embark on this step-by-step guide, some research tips and resources are presented below.

Research tips and resources

Top tips for research

1. **Know the literature**—One of the challenges with arts in health research is that, because of its multi-disciplinary nature, research can be published in hundreds of journals, including those relating to the arts, medicine, psychology, wellbeing, public health, etc. A question that often arises in the field is 'where is the research?'. In truth, it is scattered disparately, so the first challenge is to find it. If a particular study is being planned, searches of research databases such as Google Scholar, PubMed, ScienceDirect, PsychINFO, Web of Science, and ProQuest using keywords relating to the topic of interest can help to bring some of the key studies together. Often researchers specialize in one particular topic for a few years (or even longer), so if a good article is found by one researcher it can also be worth searching for the research listings of this researcher through the same databases, or through more general internet searches for their university homepages or through research repositories such as Research Gate or Academia.edu. It is also important to stay up-to-date with recent papers as studies can produce different findings

2. **Use systematic reviews to narrow reading**—For some topics, there may be an overload of relevant research papers. One way to reduce the reading is to search specifically for systematic reviews. These are comprehensive reviews of all papers relating to a specific topic and they often present data in accessible ways such as graphs or tables as well as summarizing common findings. However, systematic reviews date quickly, so they are best when combined with ordinary article searches

3. **Allow for different outcomes**—Many research studies start with very specific research questions or hypotheses. However, it is often advisable to think beyond a narrow scope and consider what other effects an intervention can have. For example, if you are researching whether photography could reduce anxiety in patients with an anxiety disorder, do not confine the study to the single measure of anxiety. It is quite possible that there may not be any significant changes in anxiety because the intervention is not effectively tailored to anxiety, or because the anxiety measure is not well suited to the intervention, or because the patient group chosen is not especially responsive. However, it may be that there are significant improvements in other related constructs, such as social resilience through connecting with others during the project. This could still be of value to people with anxiety in reducing parallel feelings

of isolation and helping to build up a social support network for them that could support their mental health further in the future. Previous related studies may give indications as to which additional constructs could be tested. However, it is equally important not to overload a study with measures. This can lead to overburdening of research participants and also have implications when carrying out statistical tests if numerical data are involved. So a select group of measures should be chosen, probably narrowed down from a longer list of potentials, prior to a research study being carried out

4. **Plan for a sufficient sample size**—The ability of a study to find significant results is partly determined by the number of participants included in the study. If the sample is too small, it can look as though there were no significant findings, even if there were (or vice versa). More on choosing the right sample size is provided in Chapter 11. To allow for a sufficient sample size, parallel versions of the intervention may need to be planned, such as back-to-back classes, or more time may be built in for recruitment. Recruitment should not be underestimated in terms of the time it may take nor in terms of the number of dropouts that may occur across the course of a project

5. **Use a computerized online reference manager**—There are a number of software options, both paying and free, available for citing papers including EndNote, RefWorks, and Zotero. These allow readers to capture the details about an article they find online and save it to a database for later use and then allow for the easy citation of papers within documents later. Some even give the option of changing the referencing style with a single click, which can be a helpful way of changing the format of a document to suit the needs of different journals. This automation can save a lot of time formatting references and bibliographies and also will help gather together research articles in a single place for future reading

6. **Collaborate**—Arts in health research often involves multiple different fields, as discussed earlier in this chapter. Science papers are rarely single-authored because of the breadth of expertise required within studies. Arts in health studies should be treated no differently and support should be sought where expertise is not available within the immediate project team. Researchers may be willing to collaborate and help with study design or statistical analysis or other elements of a study or advise on the overall thrust of the research question

7. **Attend conferences**—One of the best ways of keeping up-to-date with new research is to attend conferences, seminars, and other presentations. This too can be a good way of meeting fellow practitioners and researchers with similar interests and discussing research ideas or potential challenges

encountered with others in the field. Some conferences have a specific arts in health focus, whereas others may be broader, for example including more general psychological or social interventions or focusing on specific health conditions. These broader conferences can also be of value as they may reveal specific health challenges where the arts could provide solutions or suggest which measures or research designs are valued most highly within that area of research so you can design future studies in the most effective way. Such events can also be of value in raising the profile of your own work through poster or oral presentations

Recommended journals

Research from the field of arts in health tends to be published across a broad spectrum of academic journals. Often, these are not journals specific to the field, but simply journals that overlap with an element of the research study. For example, a study looking at dance for Parkinson's disease could be published in a neurology journal, a rehabilitation journal, a nursing journal, or an arts journal. Consequently, the only way to identify relevant research is to keep track of publications from a whole host of journals related to your area of interest. Nevertheless, some journals do help to bring together studies relating specifically to arts in health. These include:

- *American Journal of Dance Therapy*
- *Art Therapy*
- *Arts & Health, An International Journal of Research, Policy and Practice*
- *Body, Movement and Dance in Psychotherapy*
- *Canadian Creative Arts in Health, Training and Education Journal*
- *Design for Health*
- *Drama Therapy Review*
- *Dramatherapy*
- *Hektoen International: A Journal of Medical Humanities*
- *International Journal of Art Therapy*
- *International Journal of Arts Medicine*
- *Journal of Applied Arts & Health*
- *Journal of Creativity in Mental Health*
- *Journal of Medical Humanities*
- *Journal of Music Therapy*
- *Journal of Poetry Therapy*

- *Medical Humanities*
- *Music and Medicine*
- *Musicae Scientiae*
- *Psychology of Creativity, Aesthetics and the Arts*
- *Psychology of Music*
- *The Arts in Psychotherapy*
- *The British Journal of Music Therapy*
- *The International Journal of the Creative Arts in Inter-disciplinary Practice*
- *The Journal of the Irish Association of Creative Arts Therapists*
- *Voices: A World Journal for Music Therapy*

Recommended conferences

There are also regular conferences in the field. Many are organized nationally through individual arts or health organizations or universities or a consortium of partners. Others are organized on a larger scale through international associations. A list is provided below of just a few examples of international organizations that organize annual, biennial, or triennial conferences:

- International Music and Medicine Conference organized by the International Association for Music & Medicine
- International Arts Therapies Conference organized by the European Consortium for Arts Therapies Education
- Culture, Health & Wellbeing International Conference organized by Arts and Health South West
- International Health Humanities Conference organized by the International Health Humanities Network
- The Art of Good Health and Wellbeing Conference organized by the Australian Centre for Arts and Health
- The International Symposium on Performance Science organized by the Centre for Performance Science

References

1. **Brown E.** 'Duh' science: Why researchers spend so much time proving the obvious. Los Angeles Times [Internet]. 2011 May 28 [cited 2016 Oct 31]. Available from: http://articles.latimes.com/2011/may/28/science/la-sci-duh-20110529.
2. **Warburton AL, Shepherd JP.** Effectiveness of toughened glassware in terms of reducing injury in bars: a randomised controlled trial. Inj Prev. 2000 Mar 1;6(1):36–40.

3. **Segerstrom SC, Miller GE.** Psychological Stress and the Human Immune System: A Meta-Analytic Study of 30 Years of Inquiry. Psychol Bull. 2004 Jul;130(4):601–30.

4. **Trochim W.** EVALTALK. Archives of EVALTALK@LISTSERV.UA.EDU. 1998.

5. **Coffman J.** Michael Scriven on the Differences Between Evaluation and Social Science Research. Eval Exch Period Emerg Strateg Eval. 2003 Winter/2004;9(4).

6. **Mathison S.** What is the difference between evaluation and research—and why do we care? In: Smith NL, Brandon PR, editors. Fundamental Issues in Evaluation. New York, London: The Guilford Press; 2008. pp. 183–96.

7. **Burgess R.** New Principles of Best Practice in Clinical Audit. London, New York: Radcliffe Publishing; 2011. 215 pp.

8. **White M.** RCTs—The Holy Grail of Arts in Health? [Internet]. Centre for Medical Humanities. 2013 [cited 2016 Oct 31]. Available from: http://centreformedicalhumanities. org/rcts-the-holy-grail-of-arts-in-health/.

9. **Parkinson C.** arts and health blog: Fiction-Non-Fiction (revisited) [Internet]. arts and health blog. 2015 [cited 2016 Oct 31]. Available from: http://artsforhealthmmu. blogspot.com/2015/01/fiction-non-fiction-revisited.html.

10. **Medical Research Council.** A framework for development and evaluation of RCTs for complex interventions to improve health. London: Medical Research Council; 2000 Apr.

11. **Craig P, Dieppe P, Macintyre S, Michie S, Nazareth I, Petticrew M.** Developing and evaluating complex interventions: the new Medical Research Council guidance. BMJ. 2008 Sep 29;337(sep29 1):a1655–a1655.

12. **Craig P, Rahm-Hallberg I, Britten N, Borglin G, Meyer G, Köpke S,** et al. Researching Complex Interventions in Health: The State of the Art. BMC Health Serv Res. 2016;16(1):101.

13. **Rosenfield PL.** The potential of transdisciplinary research for sustaining and extending linkages between the health and social sciences. Soc Sci Med 1992 Dec;35(11):1343–57.

14. **Aboelela SW, Larson E, Bakken S, Carrasquillo O, Formicola A, Glied SA,** et al. Defining Interdisciplinary Research: Conclusions from a Critical Review of the Literature. Health Serv Res. 2007 Feb;42(1 Pt 1):329–46.

Chapter 10

A step-by-step approach to the research process

On the surface, research can appear a mystifying process. Vast numbers of theories, methodologies, designs, and measures are available to researchers, yet the selection of the most appropriate for each individual circumstance can be hard to make. This selection can be confounded by a perceived inherent tension in arts in health research: between the rigour of science and the creativity of arts. Consequently, in 2013, an international working group was formed of leading artists, arts researchers, health researchers, policy-makers, and funders who wished to bring arts in health research more into the research mainstream. The aim was to draw together the needs of health research and arts research and develop a tool that could be a reference point for the field; not a tool that would suggest that arts in health was somehow different or 'exceptional' from other sorts of research (as discussed in Chapter 9) or force either world to compromise, but rather a tool that would enhance collaboration and importantly raise awareness about the range of factors that should be carefully considered when designing an arts in health research project.

The tool developed drew on the UK Medical Research Council's (MRC) guidelines for developing and evaluating complex interventions; interventions that might involve several different components as well as depending on certain environments or other contextual factors to achieve their impact.(1,2) The initial tool was published in 2015 and entitled 'Aesop: A framework for developing and researching arts in health programmes'.(3)

Q More information about the initial project and the framework is published open access in the journal *Arts and Health*.(3)

This chapter takes the original paper published on the framework as its starting point, but moves beyond this, updating some of the scales and steps in the research process, as well as providing detailed explanations about what each step involves to give a bird's eye view of the entire research process, providing an introduction to various decisions that researchers face. Although not explicitly a research methods chapter, it is intended to provide a framework on which more specific knowledge, such as research methods, can be hung. It should be noted that this chapter focuses specifically on researching arts in health *interventions*. For other types of research within arts in health, such as studies profiling arts engagement in different populations, studies looking at the longitudinal impact of the arts engagement on aspects of health, and lab-based mechanistic studies interrogating how and why the arts affect us, aspects of this chapter may still be of interest, but the framework provided here is not intended to cover them.

Broadly speaking, there are four stages to a research project: the development of the initial idea for a research study, the design of the study to explore this idea, the running of the research study, and the outcome of the research study. However, this framework breaks the process down into a number of substages to make it clearer to navigate:

- Developing a research study
  - Identifying the research problem and evidence base
  - Developing research questions
  - Developing a theory
  - Piloting and feasibility
  - Choosing a study team
  - Involving patients and public
- Designing a research study
  - Quantitative strategies
  - Qualitative strategies
  - Mixed methods strategies
  - Economic evaluations
  - Process evaluations
- Running the research study
  - Research implementation
- Outcome of the research study
  - Reporting results
  - Dissemination
  - Further implementation of the intervention

At each stage of a research study, researchers will have to make decisions about their ambitions for a project. Often ambitions are dictated by funding or deadlines: small budgets might mean that a project has to focus its objectives and incorporate a simpler design requiring fewer participants, whereas large budgets and long timescales could support the running of a complex design involving large numbers of participants across multiple sites. Other times, a project simply might not be ready for a more ambitious study: the first time a research study is being undertaken on a specific intervention, it can be sensible to undertake a small pilot study with a focus on exploring potential areas of impact with minimal risk rather than a large-scale, expensive, and time-consuming study. Also, certain research questions do not demand large-scale studies but suit smaller and simpler designs. However, understanding the spectrum of possibilities for each decision within research can help a researcher to make an informed decision about where to situate their study. Consequently, throughout this chapter, the spectrum for each decision is laid out on a scale of 1-5 moving from less comprehensive to more comprehensive. This scale is not intended to imply that levels of 1 or 2 are less valuable than levels 3-5, so studies at the lower end of the scale should not be overlooked but rather appreciated for what they do contribute and how they relate to and inform other studies.

Developing a research study

Identifying the research problem and evidence base

Sometimes, a research project might emerge organically from the development and evaluation of an intervention. For example, a choir set up to support people with lung disease might have such good evaluation results that it is decided that a formal research project to explore these effects in more detail should follow. In this case, the previous consultation work to design the intervention might have involved a thorough search of previous research literature prior to the intervention being run. However, a research project could equally emerge from a research question (such as 'does singing improve lung function in lung disease?') with the plan that an intervention is developed to test this. In this case, a literature search may be undertaken after the initial research idea. Either way, understanding the existing evidence base is a crucial first step in a research project.

At the simplest level, evidence reviews could involve eliciting expert advice from established researchers about what research has been carried out (see Table 10.1, level 1). Such advice is often very helpful in narrowing down the potential area of interest. However, it is not a substitute for exploring the evidence base in more detail. This further exploration can be important both to identify more precisely what questions have been asked and what evidence has been found, and also to find out about interventions that have been explored and how they were designed. Of course, it is possible that the topic may not have been researched at all. In this case, it can be helpful to explore related literature (such as breathing exercises for lung disease) (level 2). With level 3, there is more of an engagement with the literature: previous studies can be reviewed

Table 10.1 The spectrum of options for identifying the evidence base

1	2	3	4	5
Ideas for the research project are formed based on apparent need and expert opinion.	Research in this area may not have been carried out before or may not be suitable. So instead, a review of some similar research projects is undertaken or a detailed explanation of rationale is provided.	A review of some relevant previous studies selected by the researchers is undertaken to show how research in this area has been of benefit before, and a potential gap or research question is identified for this study.	A systematic review is undertaken and detailed conclusions formed about the current evidence base. The research study proposed then forms the next logical step in developing this evidence base.	A systematic review is conducted and a meta-analysis of results is undertaken.

and 'gaps' for further work identified, meaning that the new research project builds on past evidence and takes a logical next step in exploring the topic. In level 4, a systematic review is undertaken. This involves finding every single previous study in the field. It is normally carried out with searches using relevant keywords of online research databases. This ensures that the new research project does not inadvertently duplicate previous work. However, it requires a greater time commitment so is normally reserved for larger research studies. For smaller studies, is it sometimes possible to find systematic reviews that have been published, which could have undertaken much of the work already (although such reviews do date very quickly, so often a manual search for more recent articles is necessary too).

Finally, level 5 involves a systematic review with meta-analysis. A meta-analysis statistically combines the findings from independent studies and looks at the overall aggregated results. So, for example, if a systematic review showed 12 studies about singing and lung function, if the studies had been carried out in similar ways with the similar outcome measures, it might be possible to look statistically at whether all 12 studies together showed evidence that singing helped lung function, providing an overall greater sample size and richer data. However, meta-analyses are often not possible if there are relatively few studies or they have not used comparable interventions.

Q The PRISMA checklist is a 27-item checklist for undertaking systematic reviews and meta analyses, showing what information should be collated and reported. It is available along with further resources at www.prisma-statement.org.

Developing research questions

Based on the evidence base, the next step is then to define some specific research questions. Often research projects have a primary research question that will be the overarching focus of the study and guide its design, and also a set of secondary research questions that will be explored along the way. For example, a primary research question might be 'Does group drumming reduce depression among people with mental health conditions?', and secondary research questions might include 'Does drumming also improve social networks and reduce social isolation?', 'What are the mechanisms by which drumming has these effects?', 'Do

Table 10.2 The spectrum of options for developing research questions relating to health and wellbeing outcomes

1	2	3	4	5
Depth/length				
The study will examine health or wellbeing in a broad way looking for general rather than specific effects with no consideration for how long effects last beyond an intervention.	The study will look at health or wellbeing in more specific terms, perhaps through validated measures or a specific framework	The study will focus on a specific psychological, physiological, or behavioural factor of health and/ or wellbeing through multiple measures or approaches, and may consider how long effects last.	The study will look at multiple psychological and/or physiological and/or behavioural factors, or look in great detail at one aspect of health, and length of effect will be considered.	The study will look comprehensively at the health and wellbeing of participants, using a wide variety of methods. The study will also examine whether changes are long-lasting.
Breadth/reach				
The study will focus exclusively on individuals involved in the intervention.	The study will focus on the core group of participants but will include some additional exploratory research around another group, such as healthcare professionals, relatives, or artists involved.	The study will look in detail at the core group of participants, their close healthcare professionals, and their close relatives/carers.	The study will look at effects on collective groups beyond the main target group such as the healthcare organization and the local community in addition to the target group.	The study will look at the impact of the project on wider communities such as the wider health system and cultural landscape.

these effects last beyond a 6-week project?', 'Is drumming cheaper and more cost-effective than cognitive behavioural therapy?', 'Does the engagement of the mental health patients in drumming also reduce stress among their family or main carers?', or 'Are the participants more skilled musically by the end of the project?'.

Sometimes, depending on the type of research being undertaken, research questions are further shaped into hypotheses (predictions of outcomes), which propose more specifically what it is anticipated will be found. There are many domains across which research questions can sit. These can include health and wellbeing outcomes (Table 10.2), social outcomes (Table 10.3), financial outcomes (Table 10.4), and artistic outcomes (Table 10.5), in relation to the depth and length of impact and the breadth and reach of those affected. Each of these different domains has been set out below. Although not all of the domains may be of interest for a research project, an awareness of them is important, as there are likely to

Table 10.3 The spectrum of options for developing research questions relating to social outcomes

1	2	3	4	5
Depth/length				
The study will not look at social outcomes.	The study will examine social impacts in a broad way looking for general rather than specific trends with no consideration for how long effects last.	The study will examine one or more specific social factors and explore if effects extend beyond the end of the project.	The study will look at multiple social factors and ascertain for how long alteration could last.	The study will look comprehensively at social factors through a wide variety of methods and exploration of longitudinal impact.
Breadth/reach				
The study will focus exclusively on individuals involved in the intervention.	The study will focus on the core group of participants but will include some additional exploratory research around another group, such as healthcare professionals, relatives, or artists involved.	The study will look in detail at the core group of participants, their close healthcare professionals, and their close relatives/carers.	The study will look at effects on collective groups beyond the main target group such as the health or social care organization and the local community in addition to the target group.	The study will look at the impact of the project on wider communities such as the wider health or social care system and cultural landscape.

Table 10.4 The spectrum of options for developing research questions relating to financial outcomes

1	2	3	4	5
Depth/length				
The study will not consider financial outcomes.	The study will catalogue the resources needed to run the intervention and outline the business model.	The study will compare the cost of the intervention to other interventions for the same target group.	The study will look at the financial impact of the project for the health service, focusing on immediate or short-term effects.	The study will look at the long-term financial impact of the project for the health service.
Breadth/reach				
The study will focus exclusively on the costs directly associated with the target health condition	The study will focus on the wider health costs for that individual.	The study will look in detail at the main healthcare organization or system involved and explore implications for close healthcare professionals, carers, or relatives.	The study will additionally look at implications beyond health, such as implications for social care, employment, or housing.	The study will look at the wider implications for society as a whole.

be effects of varying sizes in each domain from an arts intervention, so it may be useful to incorporate ways of capturing these effects in the research design .

Developing a theory

It is also important to consider whether there is a theoretical background to any research being undertaken. Sometimes, theories are developed as hypotheses based on previous research that a new research study seeks to explore. Alternatively, theories can become a lens through which to explore the research question. Other times, theories may emerge from the data. At a basic level, there may be no consideration of theory in a research project (see Table 10.6, level 1). However, many research projects at least reference previous theories as a way of framing the research question being explored (level 2). On a more specific level, a study may be grounded in a number of previous theories and be putting these to test in the research project, either as a way of providing further validation of the initial theories or assessing whether they apply with a new intervention or a new participant group (level 3). As the study becomes more theory-focused, hypotheses may be made up front about what the researchers are expecting to find or a theory may be used as a lens through which to undertake the study,

Table 10.5 The spectrum of options for developing research questions relating to artistic outcomes

1	2	3	4	5
Depth/length				
The research study will not examine artistic outcomes, or artistic outcomes are not applicable.	The study will look at basic artistic outcomes, such as whether participants enjoy the artistic process or learn basic artistic skills.	The study will look at the artistic impact on participants in greater detail, such as whether participants expand their knowledge, appreciation, or experience of an art form.	The study will look in detail at the artistic learning and development including skill acquisition of participants and explore whether there are lasting effects.	The study will examine the artistic effects of the project as a major strand of research, such as whether the intervention leads to participants learning the artistic skills necessary to lead their own projects in the future.
Breadth/reach				
The study will focus exclusively on individuals involved in the intervention.	The study will look at how the artistic experience impacts on the wider life of the individual involved.	As well as focusing on the individual, the study will also look at the possible impacts on the artists/arts leaders involved too.	The study will additionally explore whether those connected to the individual are affected and change their attitude towards or become more engaged with the arts as a result.	The study will look at whether the artistic involvement of the individual (and perhaps the artistic outputs) lead to a shift in public perception towards the target group.

Table 10.6 The spectrum of options for developing a theory

1	2	3	4	5
No use of theory.	There will be some reference to theoretical underpinnings but no application or specific theories to be tested in this study.	There will be comprehensive reference to theoretical underpinnings and their application in selected parts of the research study but no new theories will be tested.	There will be a clear theoretical grounding leading to detailed application of theory within the research study and the development of theory/theories building on these previous ideas to be tested in the study.	There will be a clear theoretical grounding which will be used as a springboard for the exploration and development of a new theory, culminating in a strong new theoretical model.

with the aim of building on this and expanding the theoretical framework at the end of the study (level 4). Finally, a project may set out from the standpoint that there is not a suitable current theory that matches the intervention and participant group, and so attempt to build a new theoretical model or framework (level 5). For this much larger theoretical step to occur, it may be that previous pilot studies have already been undertaken to provide the research team with the confidence that such an ambition is feasible (see 'Piloting and feasibility', next).

Q For more information about theory in research, *Theory and Methods in Social Research* edited by Bridget Somekh and Cathy Lewin (2011) covers a range of theories, including core quantitative and qualitative theories as well as theories that address issues of power such as feminist, race, and queer theory.(4)

Piloting and feasibility

An important step within the development of a research idea is to have a strong intervention that has the best chance of achieving the impacts being explored. This brings into the equation three issues: how well targeted the intervention is to the needs and sensitivities of the participant group, how practical it is to run, and how high the artistic quality is. The first two of these issues were discussed at length in Chapters 5 and 6, and the third was touched on; however, it should not be underestimated. The issue of quality is not to create a false distinction between professional and amateur practice; both have been researched and shown to have benefits for health and wellbeing. Rather it pertains to how well designed the intervention is and how rigorously and creatively the opportunities for maximizing its impact have been explored. For example, consider an intervention in which a dancer teaches a general non-specific dance class to older adults with mobility issues. Then consider an intervention in which a dancer with experience working in healthcare teaches a class to the same older adults incorporating all the recommended physiotherapy exercises into more creative dance steps, using music that the older adults are likely to know and recognize, and providing follow-up resources to encourage practice at home. The difference between these is likely to have a profound effect on the benefits felt by participants, the buy-in of healthcare professionals, and the interest of funders. An intervention of poor quality runs the risk of leading to a research project with no clear or meaningful findings and the concept of 'dance' being good for 'mobility in older adults' being dismissed, when a better-designed dance intervention for the same target group could have found more distinct benefits.

Table 10.7 The spectrum of options for piloting and feasibility

1	2	3	4	5
Feasibility of the arts intervention itself is being/ has been assessed based on expert opinion and information from previous studies.	The arts intervention is being devised in response to patient/ public need. A basic informal consultation is being/has been carried out, involving one or more of the following: service users, staff, health organizations, arts organizations.	A formal consultation process into the need for the arts intervention is being/has been carried out involving an identification of healthcare priorities, research into the psychological/ physical needs and experience of service users, and an assessment of the needs and views of staff/ service users, and a review of similar arts interventions in arts/health settings is undertaken.	In addition to the full formal consultation process, a pilot session(s) of the arts intervention is being/ has been undertaken to assess logistics, costings, and group sizes, and to gain some basic feedback OR the arts intervention is already running successfully.	A full pilot project with preliminary evaluation or previous small research project assessing the intervention is being/has been undertaken to assess fully the strengths and inner workings of the project.

If a research project is following on from the development steps outlined earlier in this book, these issues should have been addressed in previous piloting and feasibility work. But if a research project has arisen more from a specific research question than from an already-existing intervention, piloting and feasibility should be considered. Table 10.7 shows a scale ranging from no piloting but basic feasibility (level 1) to more comprehensive levels of consultation and piloting. Details of how to carry these steps out are covered in Chapters 5 and 6.

Choosing a study team

When developing a research study, selecting the study team is an important consideration. This will draw on decisions about whether multi-disciplinary, inter-disciplinary, or trans-disciplinary working is involved in a project (see Chapter 9). Some studies involve either arts or health specialists, but with no effort to engage the other sector (see Table 10.8, level 1). This strategy runs the risk of important details of research design being overlooked or lower levels of

Table 10.8 The spectrum of options for choosing a study team

1	2	3	4	5
The study team consists of just arts OR just health professionals/ researchers. No significant effort is made to involve people from other quarters in the research study.	The study team consists of professionals in arts OR health, but advice or consultation is sought from other quarters, e.g. artists offering opinions on the arts intervention, or health professionals/ researchers reviewing the study design.	The study team consists of arts OR health professionals, but advisers from other quarters are closely involved in important stages of/decisions in the study and monitor the progress of the project.	The study team contains a mixture of arts and health experts, but there may still be a bias towards arts or health in terms of numbers in the team, or time invested.	The study team involves a combination of both arts and health experts who are fully involved in all stages of the study.

rigour being selected, weakening results from the study. A level up from this involves a core team from one or other sector, but advisers being involved, either offering peer review (level 2) or providing closer advice at important stages of the project (level 3). This can reduce the chance of serious design flaws, but can still mean that opportunities are missed to maximize findings through weaker selection of measures, analysis, or consideration of important artistic or scientific variables. A stronger team would involve both arts and health experts, but perhaps with a bias towards one over the other, or one or the other being phased in and out of the research study as needed (level 4). However, the strongest team should involve a combination of arts and health professionals staying closely involved throughout (level 5). Often decisions about the size of a study team depend on organizational partnerships and the level of research funding available. Nevertheless, the decision not to involve equal input from arts and health experts has to be consciously and carefully made so that appropriate safeguards can be put in place to avoid jeopardizing the research (for more on safeguarding, see Chapter 8).

Patient and public involvement

A related topic is how to engage patients and the public in the research plans. Some research projects do not include PPI (patient and public involvement) at all (see Table 10.9, level 1). However, there is increasingly a requirement from ethics committees to include PPI to demonstrate that the intervention is suitable

Table 10.9 The spectrum of options for patient and public involvement

1	2	3	4	5
No involvement of patients or public beyond participation in the intervention.	Limited patient or public involvement in one part of the study (e.g. setting research priorities or helping to publicize results).	Patients and public are involved in multiple stages of the research study.	Patients and public are involved in all stages of the project, but perhaps in an advisory capacity rather than as active partners.	Patients and public are systematically involved as active partners in every stage of the research project and their views have a direct impact on the study.

for participants, recruitment is being planned appropriately to reach the target group, the research documents are understandable and clearly written, likely questions participants might have are answered, the research techniques are not too onerous, and the data will be disseminated to people for whom the outcomes will be relevant. Limited PPI (level 2) might involve seeking advice on basic elements of the research, such as support in deciding on the initial research questions. However, better PPI uses patient and public advice at multiple stages (level 3) or all stages (level 4) of a research project, including proof-reading of study documentation, practice runs of data collection, overviewing of research management, and the dissemination of results. For the highest level of PPI, patients and the public will be active partners in the research project, such as chairing a research governance group or working as members of the research team. PPI can be particularly helpful for studies in identifying potential problems in advance to avoid these later down the line.

> Q In the UK, the resource INVOLVE from the National Institute of Health Research provides briefing notes on how to undertake PPI within healthcare, as well as helpful resources, case studies of successful PPI, and training opportunities: www.invo.org.uk.

Designing a research study

Once a research question and intervention have been developed, a study can be more officially designed. Broadly, there are three strategies of enquiry that can be taken in research, with different designs and methods depending on the strategy: quantitative strategies (which employ surveys or experiments and collect data on numerical instruments that are analysed statistically), qualitative strategies (which employ strategies based on words and collect open-ended, emerging data from which themes develop), and mixed methods strategies (which involve different types of data being collected and analysed either simultaneously or sequentially). Which strategy is used will depend on the research question being asked and the anticipated audience for the research.

Quantitative strategies

Study designs

Within a quantitative strategy of enquiry, there are three broad types of design that can be employed: 'pre-experimental', 'quasi-experimental', and 'true experimental'. However, for the purposes of illustrating these three types in more detail, they have been split into five levels (see Table 10.10).

Pre-experimental designs are often the easiest study design to run, as they are resource-light and do not involve putting participants through any intervention other than the main arts activity. However, they can leave key questions unanswered, such as how involvement in an intervention might compare either with no intervention (a control group) or involvement in a different kind of intervention (a comparison group). If control or comparison groups

Table 10.10 The spectrum of options for quantitative study designs

1	2	3	4	5
Pre-experimental or non-experimental design—a study that assesses an individual or single group of participants. No measures are taken at the start of the project, but participants are assessed either during the intervention or at the end. No controls are used.	Pre-experimental design—a study that compares participants before and after the project, but does not include controls OR a project that includes a control but only takes measurements at the project end.	Quasi-experimental design—involves pre- and post-testing and includes a control group but generally does not involve randomization or follow-up OR the effect of the project on a single group is studied longitudinally with repeated measurements collected both when participants are and are not involved in the intervention.	True experimental design—the study is controlled and randomized.	True experimental study including some additional element such as blinding, a comparison activity, a comparison with a medical intervention or some form of follow-up after the intervention finishes.

are involved, it is important that they are comparable demographically to the intervention group. Although this similarity gets left partly to chance in quasi-experimental studies (although careful and balanced recruitment strategies can reduce the chance of imbalance between groups occurring), randomization in true-experimental studies can greatly reduce this chance. Randomization can involve simple coin tosses to determine to which group people are allocated or more sophisticated techniques including stratification (whereby people are split into different demographic groups and randomized in a way that creates balance between these groups in the different experimental conditions) to try and ensure that groups are similar on demographic factors.

As explained at the start of this chapter, quasi- and true-experimental designs are not necessarily 'better' than pre-experimental designs. Rather it is about selecting the most suitable design to help answer the research questions. For example, if the research question is 'does pottery lead to reduced anxiety in new mothers?', a pre-experimental design could be used initially to assess whether there are indications of change (and whether it is worth embarking on a larger study or developing an intervention further). A quasi- or true-experimental study could then be potentially carried out to ascertain whether this reduction is greater than if people do not engage in pottery, or than if they engage in a separate activity. Also, as discussed in Chapter 9, different types of research questions require different designs. Consequently, a level 5 study is not necessarily more valuable or important than a level 1 study: it is more about the context and aims of the research questions.

Q For more information on different study designs, John W. Creswell provides a clear introduction to many of the most common designs in *Research Design: Qualitative, Quantitative, and Mixed Methods Approaches* (2013).(5)

Research methods

With regards to quantitative research methods, there are a range of options. Some studies may not involve any quantitative techniques (see Table 10.11, level 1) or may involve quite basic gathering of numerical data (level 2). For example, feedback forms could ask participants to self-report whether clay modelling has reduced their anxiety over the past 6 weeks. Figures from this may be presented in descriptive statistics (which describe the data) such as percentages, but no further analysis will be undertaken. However, there are also more robust quantitative techniques that can be employed in research. Quantitative data could be analysed using inferential statistical techniques (which make inferences or predictions about the population based on the data). This will normally require

Table 10.11 The spectrum of options for quantitative research methods

1	2	3	4	5
No quantitative study undertaken.	A survey or numerical questionnaire that assesses the number and demographics of participants involved and their personal reactions to a project (in numerical terms), but does not involve statistical testing.	A survey or numerical questionnaire that is then analysed statistically.	Validated quantitative methods, such as psychological scales or physiological tests that are analysed statistically.	Multiple quantitative methods employed simultaneously using more advanced statistical techniques.

the use of a computer-based statistical programme. Depending on the study design that has been selected, this may involve comparisons of pre-test and post-test results, comparisons between experimental and control groups, or analyses of effects for different subgroups of participants. A further level of rigour (level 4) could include use of validated quantitative methods, such as psychological scales testing particular constructs such as anxiety. Validated scales (described further in Chapter 6) have been designed and tested to confirm that their psychometric properties are reliable. Alternatively, studies could involve physiological measures such as heart rate or stress hormones. Finally, level 5 could involve the use of multiple quantitative techniques to compare findings from different measures, as well as more advanced statistical techniques such as regression analyses to look at predictors of change.

> Q John Field provides a very accessible introduction to statistical techniques and some of the major software packages used in research in his *Discovering Statistics* books (2013).(6,7)

Qualitative strategies

Study approaches

Within qualitative strategies, establishing sliding scales of options is more challenging, perhaps because qualitative research does not rely on numbers but also because the qualitative research process is often emergent rather than tightly prescribed. Nevertheless, there are a range of possibilities for qualitative study approaches, of which those in the list below are some of the most common:

- Case studies involve in-depth exploration of the effects of an intervention on one or more individuals

- Narrative research involves the study of an individual's involvement in an intervention, with the information then retold in a narrative chronology
- Phenomenological research involves identifying common patterns in participants' subjective experiences of an intervention to develop patterns of meaning
- Grounded theory involves building a theoretical model around an intervention grounded in the views of participants involved
- Ethnography involves studying participants in an intervention in relation to data gathered about the setting and other individuals
- Related to qualitative strategies, arts-based research involves art forms being used either as types of data themselves or as ways of analysing or interpreting data to convey meaning about an experience

Q For more on arts-based methods specifically, Patricia Leavy considers how narrative, poetry, music, dance, visual arts, theatre, drama, and film can be used in research in her book *Method Meets Art*.(8)

As with quantitative research, the qualitative approach is usually selected based on the research question being asked. Overall, qualitative research can help to establish how participants personally experience an intervention and the meaning it has for them.

Research methods

Qualitative research can involve a broad range of types of data. These can include observations of interventions, interviews, focus groups, feedback forms, documents such as diary entries or letters, and audio-visual material such as photographs, video diaries, and film. Often, qualitative research draws on multiple sources of data, with information then pooled to make sense of the bigger picture.

There are also specific analytical techniques that can be used depending on the study approach. Many techniques use thematic analysis, in which patterns or 'themes' that emerge from the data are identified. Sometimes, these themes are allowed to emerge organically from the data, whereas other times searches are made for specific themes. For example, if a study is looking to see whether participation in an intervention leads to specific outcomes such as enhanced wellbeing, a wellbeing model such as the PERMA model (which looks at five indicators of wellbeing: positive emotion, engagement, positive relationships, meaning, and accomplishments (9)) may be applied to see whether there is evidence that any of these specific indicators are affected. However, as well as thematic analysis, each different qualitative approach outlined above also has its own set of analytical techniques. For example, in case studies and ethnographies, detailed descriptions of the setting or individuals are often presented, followed by discussions around these descriptions. In narrative research, structural devices such as plots are constructed to tell the story. In phenomenological research, significant statements are coded into units of meaning. And in grounded theory, information is coded and positioned within a theoretical model. Where data are coded or themes identified, more than one researcher may be involved so that codes can be cross-checked.

As qualitative data can be time-consuming to collect and also yield a rich body of data, often not all participants involved in an intervention are involved in qualitative research, but instead just a sample are selected. This selection or sampling can either be representative (i.e. it aims to reflect a larger entity, such as the overall demographics of the intervention group) or non-representative. Representative samples can either be random (where participants have an equal chance of being selected to be interviewed or be involved in observation) or stratified (in which researchers split participants into different demographic groups such as ages or ethnicities and then sample randomly from within these groups). Non-representative samples can involve quota sampling (similar to stratified sampling but with participants volunteering rather than being randomly selected from within different demographic groups), purposive sampling (whereby specific participants are invited who have a particular relevance for the research question), or convenience sampling (where participants are asked to volunteer to be involved).

Q For a clear and readable introduction to qualitative research approaches and methods, *Qualitative Research* edited by David Silverman (2016) gives an overview, providing a useful framework for more in-depth reading.(10)

Mixed-methods strategies

In Chapter 9, we discussed some of the challenges around conducting RCTs in arts in health research, yet RCTs remain one of the most respected types of study within healthcare. Mixed-methods strategies can be very powerful for arts in health as they offer the opportunity for both experimental and alternative research designs to be used to explore an intervention.

There are three main considerations that determine how mixed-methods strategies are employed. First, researchers have to decide on the timing of the selection of different types of data: sometimes different types of data are collected sequentially through different phases; sometimes they are collected concurrently. Sequential designs mean that two separate studies can be set up: one using a quantitative research design and one using a qualitative approach. Concurrent designs often mean that there is an over-riding quantitative research design (such as an RCT), but nested within this is a qualitative study, for example focusing just on the group of participants involved in an intervention. Often this decision between sequential and concurrent is made based on funding or logistics. However, it can also be strategic to allow the data from one to feed into another: for example if quantitative methods are used first, qualitative methods could then be selected to elucidate more of the quantitative findings, such as understanding more about the characteristics or mechanisms of quantitative changes found. Alternatively, qualitative methods could be used first to guide the selection of quantitative methods, which can then be used to explore the qualitative results in more detail.

A second consideration relates to the weighting of different methods. In some studies there may be an equal weighting planned, whereas in others one type of data may be privileged above the other, because of the nature of the research question, the expertise of the researchers involved, or the audience for which the research is intended. Related to this, a third consideration is how different methods are mixed. In some studies, different methods are simply connected, such as two different phases exploring different aspects of an overarching research question or topic. In other studies, different types of data may be compared or 'triangulated' to see if they show complementary aspects of the same phenomenon (such as whether participants have demonstrated both decreases in depression on a validated scale and spoken about experiencing improvements in their mental health), or, if they diverge, where this divergence occurs and why. Finally, data can be embedded, by which one form of data is selected to provide supportive information for the other. For example, qualitative methods could be used to explore outliers from quantitative analyses to see why the experiences of some participants diverged from others.

Q For more information on mixed-methods strategies, Creswell and Clark cover aspects of choosing mixed–methods designs and collecting, analysing, and writing up data.(11)

Economic evaluations

While qualitative and quantitative strategies can be used to assess health, well-being, social, and artistic outcomes of arts interventions, different strategies are required to assess the financial outcomes. Often in arts in health research, no financial considerations are involved in research (see Table 10.12, level 1),

Table 10.12 The spectrum of options for undertaking economic evaluations

1	2	3	4	5
No consideration of cost will be undertaken.	The cost of the project will be assessed and cost-per-heads calculated, potential funding sources identified, and a case created for the financial sustainability of the project.	A study of the cost-effectiveness of the project for the healthcare service will be undertaken.	A study of the cost-utility of the project for the health service (including measures such as quality-adjusted life years) will be undertaken.	An economic evaluation of the project from a societal perspective, such as the cost for society (including the health service, welfare, and employers) will be undertaken, OR a full cost-benefit analysis converting impacts into monetary values will be undertaken.

either because the intervention is deemed too early in its design to be evaluated on an economic basis, or because the true cost is not felt to be reliably determinable, perhaps because the intervention is being run for relatively small numbers, compared with the larger service delivery that would be envisaged. However, basic costs of an intervention can be calculated, such as the cost-per-head for individuals involved in the intervention (level 2). This may support the development of the intervention by providing a stronger financial case for the project's sustainability beyond the end of the research. A further level of rigour (level 3) involves undertaking a cost-effectiveness analysis. This compares the relative costs and outcomes of the intervention compared with the alternative process (such as patients not having access to the intervention, or having access to a different intervention, such as the current gold-standard intervention available). As a level up from this, a cost-utility analysis may be taken. Although this term is sometimes used in conjunction with cost-effectiveness, it more specifically relies on the estimation of the ratio between the cost of the intervention and the benefits yielded, so it goes hand-in-hand with the qualitative and (more often) quantitative findings from the research. Finally at level 5, a cost-benefit analysis may be undertaken, in which a monetary value is assigned to the measure of effect to balance the benefits versus the drawbacks of investing in an intervention, or an economic evaluation may be designed taking a wider societal perspective (such as considering the effects of the intervention on sectors outside healthcare, e.g. employment in days of sick leave for example, or welfare in the amount of disability benefits claimed). The more rigorous analyses of levels 3-5 often require specialist input from economists, but are ultimately required if there are plans for an intervention to receive core healthcare funding or long-term investment.

 Health Economics: An Introduction for Health Professionals by Ceri J. Phillips (2008) provides a simple introduction to the field.(12)

Process evaluations

In addition to outcome research (as outlined above with both quantitative and qualitative techniques), there is increasing emphasis within healthcare on evaluating the process involved in an intervention. Process evaluations assess the resources required to deliver the intervention, the practical problems encountered, and the ways such problems are resolved. Process evaluations seek to answer questions such as 'has the intervention reached the target group?', 'are participants and stakeholders satisfied with the intervention?', 'has the intervention been implemented as intended?', and 'what changes are required to improve the intervention?'. Many of these questions may have been explored in the development of the intervention. Indeed, an entire process evaluation may have already taken place at an earlier stage of the intervention's lifespan as part of its evaluation (as discussed in Chapter 6). However, as part of a research project, a process evaluation may be conducted in more detail to inform the findings from the quantitative and qualitative methods involved.

At a basic level (see Table 10.13, level 1), a process evaluation consists of a rich description of the intervention, such as 'manualizing' it as discussed in

Table 10.13 The spectrum of options for undertaking process evaluations

1	2	3	4	5
An overview of the process involved in the project is given to help guide future groups who may want to repeat the project.	The intervention is fully documented and data to assess the implementation of the project (such as the fidelity of the intervention and the 'dosage' received by individuals) are explored.	A wide range of methods is used to assess both the implementation and the context within which the intervention was delivered, exploring how contextual factors may have influenced potential effects.	The intervention is fully described and comprehensive details relating to its implementation, context, and its potential mechanisms of effect are analysed.	In addition to level 4, a full ethnographic study of the process is undertaken.

Chapter 6. This provides the information needed to replicate the intervention (so should be the minimum level provided in research write-ups), but does not go into detail about the effectiveness of the process or what could have been improved. A step up from this (level 2) involves exploring the implementation of the project in more detail (such as how well the intervention adhered to its original plans). Level 3 involves also considering the context in which the intervention is delivered, while level 4 explores the potential mechanisms by which the intervention has an effect. Finally, process evaluations can be made even more detailed through ethnographic methods (the in-depth recording and analysis of, in this case, an intervention based usually on richly detailed observation). Although ethnography has not developed specifically for process evaluation, it provides a powerful tool for understanding the complex dynamics underlying the process of implementing an intervention. This technique is by far the most time-consuming and essentially adds another wave of research to the outcome research, but does provide rich data on how the intervention aligns to its environment. Across a process evaluation, methods such as interviews, focus groups and surveys with participants, stakeholders, and staff as well as analysis of diaries of those involved or case studies can help to build up a three-dimensional view of how the intervention works in its environment. Such information can be valuable in helping future teams assess whether they could take the intervention forwards. It can also help to contextualize the outcomes from a research study and make them more comprehensible.

Q The *BMJ* has published guidelines on how to undertake a process evaluation of a complex intervention.(13) In addition, an article published in *BMC Health Services Research* by Bunce et al. (2014) provides an overview and case study of ethnographic process evaluations in a healthcare setting.(14)

Running the research study

Research implementation

Once a research study has been designed and received funding and ethical approval (see Chapter 12), it can be carried out. Ideally, the project will run as anticipated (see Table 10.14, level 5). Issues around the process may be identified during the process evaluation, which could be improved in future iterations, but for this 'level' participants will pass through the intervention smoothly and data will be collected as planned. However, even with careful planning, research projects can hit problems. Some of these problems may be easily assimilated into the research analysis (level 4). For example, a project that was intended to recruit adults aged 18-50 but recruited only adults aged 30-50

Table 10.14 The spectrum of options for how a research study runs

1	2	3	4	5
A number of conflicting factors have occurred which mean the research project has had to take a different turn and is not able to test the research question as originally intended.	The research has been carried out to completion. However some variables or external events are anticipated to have significantly affected results.	The research has been successfully carried out, although some minor variables or external events may have affected results. These are described alongside findings.	The research has been successfully carried out and, although additional variables or unexpected events are noted, they are all believed to have been factored into the testing of results so that their influence is minimized or removed.	The research has been carried out exactly to plan and no unforeseen circumstances or unmeasured variables are thought to have occurred that might interfere with the validity of results.

could still provide valuable data for this more limited demographic, but the demographic must be discussed in the research limitations and the results may not be as generalizable as hoped. However, sometimes it may not be possible to control for such unexpected events in analysis, such as higher levels of drop-outs from the study than anticipated. This could affect analysis, limiting the opportunity for the study to obtain strong findings (level 3). At the least, these should be discussed in research write-ups as limitations, but they are also likely to feature strongly in the process evaluation. If the effects of this are great, it will reduce the effective running score for the study to level 2 and may compromise the validity of the study altogether. Such an outcome is what happens in level 1, in which conflicting events mean that the research project is entirely unable to answer the original research question. This could include major changes to a patient process meaning that patients are involved in a conflicting intervention alongside the intervention in this research study, biasing all the data. Or funding may run out before the study can be completed. It is important that this is carefully documented, partly so that biased data are not released.

Outcome of the research study

Reporting results

If a research study has been well planned up front, with specific research questions and hypotheses, reporting the outcomes of the study should be relatively simple. In general, results are best mapped against the original questions. However, to support this, 5-point scales have been proposed below to assess

Table 10.15 The spectrum of options for health and wellbeing research outcomes

1	2	3	4	5
Depth/length				
The study has not found significant changes or has found significant changes that do not support the hypotheses.	The study has found significant changes in a broad sense, but the specifics of these effects and length of the effect remain unknown.	The study has found significant changes in factors of health and wellbeing and there may be preliminary indications that these extend beyond the end of the sessions.	The study has found significant changes in multiple factors of health and wellbeing and data suggest that these changes will have an effect beyond the end of the study.	The study has found a comprehensive effect on health and wellbeing with lasting impact.
Breadth/reach				
The study may or may not have found changes for the target participants, but either way has found no evidence of change for other people immediately involved, such as artists or healthcare professionals.	The study has found significant changes for target participants but no evidence of change in close family, carers, or staff who did not participate in the intervention.	The study has found significant changes for people immediately involved and those close to them but no evidence of change at an organizational or community level.	The study has found significant changes at organizational or community levels.	The study has found benefits extending to society more generally, reaching large numbers of people as a result of the project.

how well results have met the initial hypotheses and contextualize the strength of these findings (see Tables 10.15-10.18). For example, a small-scale study may have shown strong findings immediately after the intervention for participants involved in the project, but the 5-point scales help to show that these findings are still relatively limited if we do not know how long they lasted for, who else might have been affected, or whether there were any lasting financial benefits, etc. As always, the aim is not to judge studies for not being more ambitious or not asking more questions, but rather to appreciate their findings in proportion to what they have shown. While 'significant' is a term typically used to describe quantitative findings that are 'statistically significant' (meaning that

Table 10.16 The spectrum of options for social research outcomes

1	2	3	4	5
Depth/length				
The study has not found significant changes or has found significant changes that do not support the hypotheses.	The study has found significant changes in social factors in a broad sense, but the specifics of these effects and length of the effect remain unknown.	The study has found significant changes in social factors and there may be preliminary indications that this may extend beyond the end of the sessions.	The study has found significant changes in multiple social factors and there are data suggesting that these changes will have an effect beyond the end of the study.	The study has found a comprehensive effect on social factors with lasting impact.
Breadth/reach				
The study may or may not have found changes for the target participants, but either way has found no evidence of change for other people immediately involved, such as artists or social or healthcare professionals.	The study has found significant changes for target participants, those immediately involved, but no evidence of change in close family, carers, or staff who did not participate in the intervention.	The study has found significant changes for people immediately involved and those close to them but no evidence of change at an organizational or community level.	The study has found significant changes at organizational or community levels.	The study has found benefits extending to society more generally, reaching large numbers of people as a result of the project.

the probability of the effect being found if in fact there is no effect is small), it is also used here in relation to meaningful qualitative findings.

Dissemination

There are various ways in which the results of research studies can be disseminated (see Table 10.19). A level 1 of dissemination, involving very restricted (or no) dissemination of results, is rarely advised. Even if a study does not result in significant or meaningful findings, there are still a number of reasons why it is ethical to make these results available. This is covered more in Chapter 12. The

Table 10.17 The spectrum of options for financial research outcomes

1	2	3	4	5
Depth/length				
The study has not considered financial outcomes or has found financial losses from the project.	The study has demonstrated a sustainable use of resources and a reliable business model to run the arts intervention.	The study has demonstrated that the intervention is more cost-effective than similar interventions for the same target group.	The study has demonstrated financial benefits for the wider health service, focusing on immediate or short-term effects.	The study has demonstrated long-term financial benefits from the intervention for the health service.
Breadth/reach				
The study did not find any financial benefits focusing on the costs directly associated with the target health condition.	The study has demonstrated financial benefits in relation to the individual's wider health costs.	The study has demonstrated financial benefits for the main healthcare system in relation to individuals involved in the intervention and healthcare professionals, carers, or relatives.	The study has demonstrated financial benefits of the intervention extending beyond health, such as in social care, employment, or housing.	The study has demonstrated financial benefits for society as a whole.

exception to this might be if conflicting events seriously impact on the study meaning that data are unreliable, but in this case a detailed process evaluation may be publishable. Level 2 involves some research dissemination, but with only a local reach, such as a report going to stakeholders involved in the study. Stronger dissemination (level 3) involves publicizing findings in academic and public arenas, across both the arts sector and health sector so that patients, arts practitioners, and researchers become aware of the outcomes. This could include public-facing reports, magazine articles, conference presentations, or videos summarizing results. Level 4 involves more detailed reporting. This level of dissemination should involve peer-review journal publication of findings and may be accompanied by more public messaging, such as social media to further the reach outside academia. Finally, a high level of dissemination could, in addition, involve a distinct strategy to engage healthcare professionals and provide training related to the findings, such as programmes to teach arts practitioners how to lead a similar intervention themselves. Dissemination could in

Table 10.18 The spectrum of options for artistic research outcomes

1	2	3	4	5
Depth/length				
The research study did not examine artistic outcomes, or there was evidence of poor artistic outcomes for individuals involved.	The study has demonstrated basic artistic outcomes, such as enjoyment from participants in the artistic process or the acquisition of basic artistic skills.	The study has demonstrated the artistic impact on participants in greater detail, such as showing that participants have expanded their knowledge, appreciation, or experience of an art form.	The study has demonstrated artistic learning and development including skill acquisition for participants and shown indications of lasting effects.	The study has demonstrated meaningful improvements in the acquisition of artistic skills among participants, meaning they could lead their own projects in the future.
Breadth/reach				
The study found no evidence of effects on the individual involved in the intervention.	The study found evidence that the artistic experience impacted on the wider life of the individual involved, outside the intervention.	The study found evidence of impact on the artists involved too.	The study additionally found that those connected to the individual were affected and changed their attitude towards or became more engaged with the arts as a result of the intervention.	The study found that the artistic involvement of the individual (and perhaps the artistic outputs) led to a shift in public perception towards the target group.

Table 10.19 The spectrum of options for disseminating research findings

1	2	3	4	5
Basic or restricted dissemination of results is attempted.	Some dissemination of results and publicity about the project is undertaken but it is informal and predominantly local.	Good reports of results take place across arts and health sectors, across both academic and public arenas, with some national reach.	Full reporting takes place through academic streams (adhering to reporting guidelines on good practice) and public streams (perhaps with multi-media links or public performances) with national reach.	The project dissemination has a distinct strategy with a goal of engaging public and professionals, promoting learning, and possibly offering training/capacity-building at national and international level.

turn lead to increased chances of the intervention being taken forwards in the future, leading into the next point: implementation.

Q Guidelines exist to support thorough reporting of studies, such as the TREND statement, which provides a checklist for reporting controlled studies in sufficient detail (www.cdc.gov/trendstatement), or the CONSORT statement for randomized controlled studies (www.consort-statement.org).

Further implementation of the intervention

Depending on the level of rigour involved in the study and the strength of the findings, it may be possible to turn the data into a strategy for further implementation of the intervention. In some cases, this may be premature (see Table 10.20, level 1) either because findings were not convincing enough or because the study was relatively small-scale with a simple study design, so the next step would involve undertaking a larger-scale, more rigorous design to ascertain more about the effects or mechanisms. The next level up (level 2) could involve recommendations for future practice, but no practical steps being taken immediately. A preferable scenario is often that findings lead to the intervention being continued or recommissioned in the site at which the research took place (level 3) or even being spread to more sites (level 4), with the strongest outcome being that an intervention is rolled out nationally or even further afield (level 5). Such large-scale roll-outs often require very strong evidence, including rich process evaluations and clear financial benefits. However, if an intervention has undergone multiple phases of research, this may be the ultimate aim and this has certainly happened with some past arts in health interventions. Yet even

Table 10.20 The spectrum of options for further implementation of the intervention

1	2	3	4	5
Implementation is not possible or not appropriate at this stage.	The project demonstrates how findings could be translated into routine practice or policy, although no steps are currently being taken.	The project is being commissioned again for the same (or similar) groups of participants.	The project is being commissioned and spread to more centres, perhaps being adopted regionally or through one particular health programme.	The project is being rolled out nationally, with potential to support its development abroad in the future.

then, this final stage of the research process may lead to the recommencing of the cycle outlined in this chapter once again to interrogate the effects and mechanisms yet further.

Summary

This chapter has outlined many of the different stages involved in undertaking an arts in health research project and hopefully demystified the component parts involved. As is clear from the 5-point scales provided for each step, it is possible for research to be undertaken by arts experts or health experts on their own with relatively low levels of resources, rather like a heightened form of evaluation. Indeed, these low-resource research projects have enormous value, for example as proof-of-concept projects to provide preliminary data to secure buy-in from stakeholders or funding. However, the decision to undertake research this way should be made with a full awareness that such research is likely to provide less robust data, and have smaller implications for the intervention's future. Larger-scale, truly collaborative efforts may be a larger time and resource commitment to undertake but they have the potential to lead to important outcomes both for the intervention being researched and for the field more broadly. In Chapter 11, we will explore how to turn the decisions made about researching an intervention using the step-by-step guide here into a comprehensive research protocol, providing all the necessary details to carry out a research study.

References

1. **Craig P, Dieppe P, Macintyre S, Michie S, Nazareth I, Petticrew M.** Developing and evaluating complex interventions: the new Medical Research Council guidance. BMJ. 2008 Sep 29;**337**(sep29 1):a1655–a1655.

2. **Medical Research Council.** A framework for development and evaluation of RCTs for complex interventions to improve health. London: Medical Research Council; 2000 Apr.

3. **Fancourt D, Joss T.** Aesop: A framework for developing and researching arts in health programmes. Arts Health. 2015 Jan 2;7(1):1–13.

4. **Somekh B, Lewin C, editors.** Theory and Methods in Social Research. 2nd ed. edition. Los Angeles ; London: SAGE Publications Ltd; 2011. 368 pp.

5. **Creswell JW.** Research Design: Qualitative, Quantitative, and Mixed Methods Approaches. SAGE Publications; 2013. 305 pp.

6. **Field A.** Discovering Statistics Using IBM SPSS Statistics, 4th Edition. 4th edition. SAGE Publications Ltd; 2013. 915 pp.

7. **Field A, Miles J, Field Z.** Discovering Statistics Using R. SAGE; 2012. 994 pp.

8. **Leavy P.** Method Meets Art: Arts-Based Research Practice. 2 edition. New York ; London: Guilford Press; 2015. 334 pp.

9. **Seligman MEP.** Flourish: A Visionary New Understanding of Happiness and Well-being. New York: Simon and Schuster; 2012. 370 pp.

10. **Silverman D.** Qualitative Research. SAGE; 2016. 670 pp.

11. **Creswell JW, Clark VLP.** Designing and Conducting Mixed Methods Research. SAGE; 2011. 489 pp.

12. **Phillips CJ.** Health Economics: An Introduction for Health Professionals. John Wiley & Sons; 2008. 161 pp.

13. **Moore GF, Audrey S, Barker M, Bond L, Bonell C, Hardeman W**, et al. Process evaluation of complex interventions: Medical Research Council guidance. BMJ. 2015 Mar 19;**350**:h1258.

14. **Bunce AE, Gold R, Davis JV, McMullen CK, Jaworski V, Mercer M**, et al. Ethnographic process evaluation in primary care: explaining the complexity of implementation. BMC Health Serv Res. 2014;**14**:607.

Chapter 11

Writing a research protocol

An introduction to protocols

Within the world of screen, 'show bibles' are created for each production; full reference documents detailing the film or TV series' characters, settings, backstories, and major plotlines. As series continue or more films are made, show bibles are updated to include important details, such as a character's mother's name, or his/her favourite food, ensuring that all future plotlines are accurate and have internal consistency. Show bibles have several aims, including:

1. Explaining the rationale for the production: who it is targeted at, what it will achieve, why there is a gap in the market for it, and what its impact might be

2. Explaining how the production will unfold: where the story will take place, what the plot lines will be, who the characters are, and how they interact with one another

3. Discussing the feasibility of the production: how long the series will be, over what timescale it will be set and filmed, how many characters are involved, and which actors might play the parts

The information in the show bible is important both to the production team members, ensuring that the relevant details have been worked out in advance of the filming commencing to ensure it runs smoothly, and to any partners, funders, and stakeholders, showing what the production actually entails and aims to achieve.

Much like the world of screen, the world of research also has its own 'show bibles': research protocols. Protocols share similar aims to show bibles:

1. The rationale: a research protocol is an opportunity to present a strong and convincing rationale for a study, showing where the key gaps lie in the current literature, demonstrating that there is a need for research that fills these gaps, showing that the research question can be researched, detailing precisely what the aims and objectives are, and explaining what the implications of this will be for future research and practice

2. The methods: the protocol should demonstrate how the study will go about answering the research questions: which design and methods will be used, why these are appropriate, how these will prevent issues of bias, how these fit in with legal and ethical regulations, and whether results will be generalizable or applicable beyond the immediate research setting

3. The feasibility: the protocol should explain how the study will be carried out, what the timescale is, where the responsibilities lie, what resources are needed, how and at what rate participants will be recruited, whether the team have the appropriate experience to carry out the study, and the benefits and risks of participation for individuals

As with show bibles, protocols have multiple audiences. They are important internal documents for those involved in the study, mapping out the responsibilities and activities required; they can seek to convince stakeholders and possible funders of the value and integrity of a study; and they form the core document underpinning all ethical approval applications (see Chapter 12). Protocols often undergo multiple iterations, and it is possible too that they change once a project is under way. However, once a study has ethical approval, changes may require resubmitting for approval, so protocols are often very detailed and well-worked through to avoid the delays that this resubmission causes. For studies involving arts interventions, it may not appear on the surface that research protocols are necessary: participants are engaging in enjoyable arts-based activities with no evident risks. However, as Chapter 12 will discuss, even arts-based interventions can involve significant ethical risks. Furthermore, the principles of clearly explaining the rationale and carefully mapping the logistics of a study both for internal and external records remain, just as in other non-arts studies. So even if an organization does not officially require a protocol, it is recommended that one be created for these reasons.

Different organizations have different templates for research protocols that vary in exact format depending on the nature of the study. For example, studies involving vulnerable populations have to include large sections on participant safeguarding; studies involving observational research but no active intervention may be much shorter; and studies involving identifiable patient records may need to demonstrate clearly their modes of data protection and confidentiality. However, the broad headings and sections of research protocols generally remain the same. Consequently, this chapter provides a template protocol suitable for a range of research projects, whether a small pilot or a large-scale randomized controlled trial. The key headings found in research protocols are outlined and for each section a description is given of what it normally entails. It is up to each individual study and the organizations involved to determine which sections require the most attention, or which sections may not be required.

To facilitate the use of this template, the following symbols are used throughout the chapter:

✍ **Sample text** that could be included in a protocol if it is appropriate for the study

❷ **Explanations** of terms that may be unfamiliar

Writing a protocol

Covering page

Research protocols generally start with a covering page containing logos of key organizations involved alongside the essential information, including the title, ethics reference, date and version number, a list of investigators, funders and sponsors, and important statements on confidentiality and conflict of interest:

Full study title

The full study title should be descriptive rather than creative. The UK research ethics service recommends the IPOC rule for choosing a study title: Intervention, Population, Outcome, Comparator (if there is one). This often leads to a dense title, such as 'The impact of recorded music vs. benzodiazepine in reducing pre-surgical anxiety among adults undergoing elective gastrointestinal surgery'.

Internal reference number/short title

The short title for a research study is typically no more than 20 characters and is a recognizable simple reference to the project, such as an acronym or the key words.

Ethics reference

If the study requires ethical approval, the ethics reference number is often stated right at the start. Prior to ethical approval being granted, this section is often left blank, with the number added once ethical approval is received. Once the study has ethical approval, it is not normally possible for changes to the protocol to be made without additional correspondence with the ethics committee.

Date and version number

Protocols are normally dated and given 'version' numbers. This is a way of ensuring that the most current protocol is in circulation and any changes made are transparent.

Investigators

There are three main types of investigators in research studies. The 'chief investigator' is the person in charge of the whole project who is ultimately responsible for its design and running. If the study has multiple locations, there may also be 'principal investigators' who take local responsibility and report back to the chief investigator (although sometimes 'chief' and 'principal' investigator are used interchangeably). Other people involved in the study in positions of responsibility are called 'co-investigators'. There may also be research assistants, project managers, consultants, healthcare professionals and students involved.

Sponsor

The sponsor is the individual or organization taking ultimate responsibility for the whole project, including initiating, managing, and financing it (or sourcing the funding). This may well be the research and development department within a hospital or other institution, or the employer of the chief investigator or an educational institution or the funder themselves. Sometimes there may be more than one sponsor, but in this case a 'lead sponsor' should be nominated.

Funder

The funder is the individual or organization providing the money for the research project. They should be listed on the protocol to make it clear if there are any competing interests. Any grant reference numbers are normally included on protocols.

Conflict of interest statement

All the investigators named in this initial section of the protocol should declare if they have any affiliations or involvement with any organization with any financial interests or non-financial interests in the research, for example if a researcher has shares in the organization funding the research, or if there are any professional or personal relationships with the sponsor or funder. They will not necessarily cause any problems with the project, but ethics boards and other people involved in the project have a right to know. If there is no known conflict of interest, you may write:

✍ *The investigators declare no known conflict of interest*

Confidentiality statement

Many research protocols also contain a confidentiality statement. This makes it clear to anybody who might be reading the protocol that it is not for public discussion or dissemination or that it may include sensitive information. This can help to protect protocols in their early stages of development from being copied by other people. Confidentiality statements may take a form similar to this:

✍ *This document contains confidential information that must not be disclosed to anyone other than the sponsor, the investigator team, host organization, and members of the Research Ethics Committee, unless authorized to do so*

Chief investigator signature

Once the protocol has been approved by those involved, the chief investigator should sign it and date it as confirmation of its high-level approval.

Format

In addition to specific sections, the formatting of protocols is fairly standardized. Protocols often have headers reiterating the version number and date, and footers giving the short title of the protocol and providing a confidentiality statement.

Table of contents

Following the covering page, protocols often have a table of contents outlining the main sections. These often include the following, each of which will be discussed individually:

- Summary information
- Background and rationale
- Objectives and outcomes
- Study design
- Participant identification
- Study procedures
- Intervention
- Analysis
- Data management
- Ethical and regulatory considerations
- Finance and insurance
- Publication policy
- References

Summary information

Synopsis

Following the table of contents, it is common to see study synopses. These set out the basic information about the study, partly as an aide-memoire, and partly so that the reader can instantly get an idea of the aim and design of the study. Synopses are normally directly copied from text later in the protocol, so are often the last thing to be completed to ensure they most accurately reflect the rest of the document. Synopses typically include the study title, study design, study participants, planned sample size, planned study period, and primary objectives and endpoints, all of which are discussed in more detail below.

Abbreviations

Protocols also often have an abbreviations list. This can reduce the text needed later in the protocol, making it more concise to read. Abbreviations may include common terms relating to the healthcare service or organizations involved, technical terms routinely involved in research studies, or short-hand for the intervention or project partners. Table 11.1 shows some examples of some of the standard terms included in research protocols and their definitions. In general, all abbreviations are written out in full the first time, with the abbreviation in brackets, before the abbreviation is used on its own in future references.

Background and rationale

The background and rationale is one of the most important parts of the protocol. It clarifies what the research problem is and how it is being tackled, so has a significant amount of weight with an ethics committee and also often forms the initial information needed for the introduction section for papers or research reports. Specifically the background/rational should include:

◆ A broad overview of the field being researched

◆ A more specific focus on research projects that have been undertaken related to the one proposed. This often takes the form of a condensed version of an in-depth literature search showing a clear awareness of what has previously been found and what questions remain to be answered

◆ A traceable path between past projects and the project being proposed so it is clear how this study builds on previous knowledge and is a logical 'next step'

◆ A brief summary of what the intervention entails (this will be expanded later in the protocol)

◆ An explanation of what this study will add to the literature and to practice. Studies with a clear implication, either for future research or practice, have a higher likelihood of receiving funding and ethical approval as their purpose is more tangible and the consequent need for the study to be carried out can be perceived as greater

Table 11.1 A glossary of common terms found in research and ethics

Acronym	Definition
CI	Chief investigator or coordinating investigator
AIHW	Australian Institute of Health and Welfare
CNIH	Canadian National Institute of Health
CRF	Case report form (the name of the form on which the study data for each patient is reported each time it is collected)
CTMS	Clinical trial management system
EHR/EMR	Electronic health record/electronic medical record
GP	General practitioner (doctor)
GCP	Good Clinical Practice (an international quality standard for undertaking trials with online and face-to-face training available for researchers)
IRAS	Integrated Research Application System (UK) (the online system used to make and manage ethics applications)
CF/ICF	Informed consent form (the form that patients will sign to agree to take part in the study (see Chapter 12))
NHS	National Health Service (UK)
NIH	National Institute of Health (US)
NIHR	National Institute of Health Research (UK)
NRES	National Research Ethics Service (UK)
PIS/PIL	Participant/patient information sheet/leaflet (the document that informs participants of what is involved in a study (see Chapter 12))
PI	Principal investigator
PPI	Patient-public involvement (the involvement of patients and the public in research (see Chapter 10))
R&D	Research and development
EC/REC/ REB	Research ethics committee/board (the committee who will decide if a study is ethical and can go ahead)
RCT	Randomized controlled trial (see Chapter 9)
(S)AE	(Serious) adverse event (a serious unforeseen medical event that occurs during the research but not necessarily causally related to the research)
(S)AR	(Serious) adverse reaction (a serious unforeseen medical event that occurs as a result of the research or intervention)
SIF	Site investigator file (the file that contains the core study documents specific to each site)
SLA	Service level agreement (a contract between service providers (such as arts organizations or artists) and the recipients (such as health organizations) that specifically define what work will be undertaken and its terms)
SOP	Standard operating procedure (the normal process a patient will follow in the course of their visit or treatment)
TMF	Trial master file (the overall file containing core documents for the study)
WHO	World Health Organization

Objectives and outcomes

Primary objective

Research studies often have multiple objectives. The primary objective is the main outcome that is being measured in the study and normally equates to the main research question. Objectives are often expressed as purposes, for example, 'To assess whether an iPad app used for 30 minutes pre surgery can reduce stress levels by 20% in children undergoing anaesthesia'. Chapter 6 included details about SMART objectives, which can be helpful in defining research objectives. The primary objective is copied into the summary table at the start of the protocol.

As well as setting out the objective, it is also necessary to explain how it will be measured: its outcome measure or endpoint. This should include information on the measurement tool. Sometimes, outcome measures are left broad, especially when it is a preliminary study. However, studies often also specify what level of improvement will be considered a result, for example 'a decrease of 20% in blood pressure from before to after the intervention using a wrist blood pressure monitor'. If the objective is being measured in more than one way, this can be listed here.

Secondary objective(s)

Secondary objectives are other constructs being tested by the study that could clarify findings from the primary objective or show potential additional effects. Although multiple secondary objectives and outcome measures are common in studies, caution should be applied as using too many measures can overburden research participants and complicate later analysis, so each measure being included should be carefully considered.

Tertiary objective(s)

Tertiary objectives are those that are not part of the core study plans and not crucial to the study but might occur simultaneously and be of broader interest. For example, a study might have the primary objective of exploring whether crafts activities improve social resilience among dementia patients, and secondary objectives focusing on mood. A tertiary objective might be that the crafts also improve social resilience among staff.

Study design

The study design section explains how the study will be conducted. Often study designs can be summarized in a few words, but this section of the protocol is intended to expand on this and explain the procedure. For example, a study might be summarized as a 'three-arm randomized controlled trial' with further elaborations as to the activity involved in each 'arm' (or 'branch') of the trial outlined (prior to being described fully later), and what participants will be required to do, where, when, and for how long. Study design sections often contain a procedure diagram in the form of a flowchart, showing what will happen to participants. The flowchart should give the reader a quick and thorough overview of the study process. A sample flow chart is given in Figure 11.1.

Participant identification

Study participants

Study participants should be clearly defined to focus the study and avoid biased recruitment. Even if participant groups are very broad, defining features such as location, gender, age range, etc., should be included. For example, 'people aged 18 or over living within the borough of Camden in London' or more specifically 'women aged 18-30 with moderate depression (defined as a score of 11-15 on

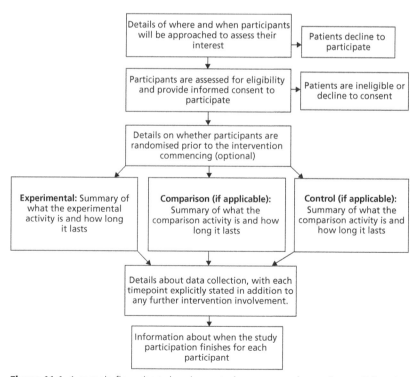

Figure 11.1 A sample flow chart showing a study process and mapping participant involvement.

the Hospital Anxiety and Depression Scale)'. For some arts interventions, it may be considered unethical to exclude some people from taking part in an activity because they do not fit the inclusion criteria for a study. However, it may be possible to allow a broader range of people to take part in an activity, perhaps including friends or carers of participants, but with the research only involving those who fit the specific criteria for the study. Alternatively, it may be possible to offer delayed joining options for participants, meaning that the initial few months will be for research participants only, but thereafter the intervention will become freely available to others.

Inclusion criteria

Inclusion criteria narrow down specifically which participants will be targeted. One essential criterion is:

✎ *Participant is willing and able to give informed consent for participation in the study*

In addition, there may be others, such as:

◆ Either male or female, aged 18 years or above
◆ In the community clinic awaiting a routine dental check-up

Exclusion criteria

Exclusion criteria ensure that people with conflicting health conditions or other issues do not enter the study. This section should start with the following statement:

✎ *The participant may not enter the study if ANY of the* following *apply:*

This should then be followed by a list of criteria, such as:

◆ A language barrier or dementia that prevents participants from being able to provide informed consent
◆ Severely impaired sight or hearing (to the level that would affect their ability to participate in the intervention)
◆ Attendance in other activities that might compromise the research (e.g. if the intervention involves participation in a weekly choir, participants who are already members of weekly choirs may be excluded)
◆ Other participant demographics, medications, or activities that may conflict with the research study

It is important when controlling essential variables within the study to strike a balance between being robust and being overly exclusive to the point that not enough participants will be eligible to take part.

Study procedures

Screening and eligibility assessment

Screening and eligibility involves checking whether potential participants meet the inclusion and exclusion criteria set out earlier. Criteria will need to be checked with participants before they are officially enrolled on the study. Sometimes this occurs before informed consent, and sometimes afterwards depending on the study design. Eligibility assessments can either be done with a tick list that participants complete to confirm that they do not meet any of these criteria, or the criteria may be checked by a researcher by talking with the participant. The process planned for a study should be outlined in this section.

Sometimes screening involves accessing patient medical records to identify potentially eligible participants and invite them to take part. If patient medical records are being accessed, details of who will access them (whether somebody within or outside the care team), how patients' confidential data will be protected, and whether patients will be informed that they are being screened should be carefully outlined.

> Q There are different ways of selecting or 'sampling' the participants to be involved in a study. Some of these are outlined in Chapter 10. For a comprehensive overview of different sampling strategies, *Sampling Essentials* by Johnnie Daniel is recommended.(1)

Recruitment

It is important to be clear about when and where patients will be recruited for the study. The first thing to clarify is how participants will find out about a study, for example 'posters will be placed in oncology clinics at the County Hospital' or 'patients attending the art therapy group will be handed leaflets at the end of their weekly sessions'. Then it is important to plan who will approach potential participants and when, for example 'patients will be approached by a member of the study team at the weekly art therapy group 1 week after receiving the leaflet'.

The recruitment plan should explain when eligibility will be assessed and information provided, and how long participants will have to consider if they would like to be involved (e.g. 'participants will have up to 2 weeks to consider whether they would like to be involved'; or if the intervention has fixed dates, 'participants will be able to sign up until 1 week prior to the intervention commencing'). If a standard information and consent process is being followed, the sentence below may be included:

✍ *The researcher will check the participant's eligibility criteria and explain the study, as well as providing the participant information sheet, before taking informed consent*

Informed consent

❷ *The process of informed consent means telling the participant enough about the study so that they can make an informed decision about whether or not they want to take part. Generally, a participant information sheet is used to provide the necessary information. Once a participant has agreed to take part, they will be asked to sign a consent form. This is discussed further in* Chapter 12.

Because informed consent is a standard process for participants, often important routine information about the process is included. This is modulated based on the study protocol, but may follow a format similar to the following:

✍ *Participants will personally sign and date* the *informed consent form, co-signed by a member of the research team, before any study-specific procedures are performed. Written and verbal versions of the participant information and informed consent will be presented to the participants detailing the exact nature of the study and what it will involve for the participant. It will be clearly stated that the participant is free to withdraw from the study at any time for any reason without prejudice to future care, and with no obligation to give the reason for withdrawal. A copy of the signed informed consent will be given to the participant. The original signed form will be retained at the study site. The participant will have the opportunity to question a member of the research team to decide whether or not to participate in the study*

Potential risks and benefits

Many arts interventions may not have specific risks, and it is not necessary to over-analyse any risks that might occur. For example, when leading a singing group, there is always a chance that somebody may trip over a chair or a cable when they are in the room. However, this risk would exist even if they were not part of a research study. It is important to identify any such risks in a risk assessment (see Chapter 8), but the more important risks for this protocol are the study-specific ones. For example, if a study involves providing confidential medical data, it may be necessary to explain how it will be stored so participants are not concerned about private information being made public. There may also be other disadvantages to involvement, for example providing a blood sample may be painful or the study may involve repeat trips to a clinic, which could involve people's time and perhaps money for travel. If any aspect of the research could cause distress, such as the posing of sensitive questions, this needs to be clearly outlined too. If there is any chance that the study could find clinically relevant data, such as a study involving heart rate monitoring showing that a participant has a heart murmur, the plans for how the participant or their healthcare professional are to be notified should be outlined. If there are no obvious risks, then this should be stated, identifying whether aspects of a study are non-invasive and pain-free.

Benefits should also be stated to demonstrate why participants may want to take part. Benefits could include participation in free arts workshops or participants being provided with some of their study data, such as copies of their own brain scans. In line with potential hypotheses in the study, benefits could also be experienced through participation in the intervention. Another benefit could be that taking part in a study might lead to improved experience for future patients at a clinic. Although not directly relevant to the participant, they may feel encouraged to know that their participation could have a positive effect longer term.

Randomization, blinding, and code-breaking

❷ *Randomization involves allocating patients to either an experimental group, where they will receive the arts intervention being tested, or a control or comparison group who are not receiving that intervention*

Randomizing aims to reduce the bias of allocation, so neither participants nor researchers can select in which group they are included. There are various methods of randomization, ranging from a coin toss with a 50:50 probability of being allocated to either group, to more complex statistical methods involving weighting the probability in favour of different outcomes, or stratifying patients to ensure that there are equal balances of sex/age/health conditions, for example, in each group.

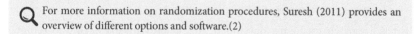

Q For more information on randomization procedures, Suresh (2011) provides an overview of different options and software.(2)

❷ *Blinding involves either not telling a participant whether they are in the experimental group or the control/comparison group, or not telling a researcher collecting or analysing which group a participant is in. It is intended to add another level of rigour to a research design and minimize bias*

Blinding can be difficult as participants may realize that they are receiving music, for example, and know they are in the experimental group. However, sometimes it is still possible. For example, if you are testing whether singing is more effective than listening to singing for improving depression in older adults, it may be possible to recruit people to a study looking at the effects of 'music' on depression and then randomize people to the singing or listening group. Both groups will receive music so will think they are receiving an active intervention, but in fact the singing will be the experimental group and the listening a comparison group. Blinding can also refer to the experimenters. For example, if a study involves assessing whether magic tricks can improve the hand function of children with paralysis, the occupational therapist may not be told whether the child being assessed has yet been exposed to the magic trick therapy, to reduce bias in the data being collected. In addition to these types of blinding, sometimes study designs involve 'deception', where participants are told the focus of the study is one thing to distract their attention away from the true focus; in other words, they are blind to the true aim of the study. For example, if a public dance performance aims to reduce the perceived time of waiting in a clinic, if patients know that 'reducing perceived time of waiting' is the primary objective of the study, they may keep an eye on the clock. So instead, participants may be told that the aim is to assess the general experience of a waiting area. The questionnaire they complete will then ask about other variables such as mood alongside perceived waiting time to hide the real aim of the study. However, designs involving deception have to be carefully worked out to ensure that they are still ethical, and participants are not duped into providing information they may not want to provide.

> Q Mike Cardwell and Cara Flanagan include an accesible section on deception in research in their companion guide for students *Psychology AS* (2005).(3)

❷ *Code-breaking or 'unblinding' involves either telling participants who were previously 'blinded' whether they are in the experimental or control group, or telling the researcher collecting or analysing the data which group a participant is in or possibly even the identity of a participant*

If it is a participant being 'unblinded', this usually means having to remove them from the study as knowing which group they are in may bias results. Unblinding is most commonly found in drugs studies in which, if patients start having unusual symptoms, it may be necessary to tell them whether they were taking an active drug or a placebo so they know whether their symptoms are side effects. However, it may also be necessary to unblind a researcher collecting or analysing the data, such as if a questionnaire response indicates that a participant is feeling suicidal, and it is necessary to identify who the participant is to provide support to them. The ethical implications of this are discussed in Chapter 12.

If randomization, blinding, or code-breaking are involved in a study, details must be provided to help the ethics committee decide whether the plans are ethical. For example, a protocol may explain which software is used to create a randomization sequence, the type of randomization used, the blinding strategy, and how blinding will be tested (such as with a questionnaire to ascertain whether participants thought they were in the experimental or control group). The strategy for unblinding studies should also be mapped out. This may involve one member of the study team having access to a database explaining which intervention each participant is part of, or a locked database that links anonymous ID codes with names.

Baseline assessments

Baseline assessments are the pieces of data collected at the very start of the study before any intervention takes place. It should be clear when baseline assessments are going to take place, for example 'following consent but prior to randomization'. Bullet points of the types of assessment should be given in this section of the protocol, such as:

1. 'Complete an anonymous questionnaire assessing demographic data'

2. 'Take part in a 30-minute focus group with other participants'

3. 'Provide a 1mL saliva sample through a straw into a 2mL tube'

Often, data collection measures such as questionnaires are provided as appendices to the protocol.

Subsequent assessments

Subsequent assessments are the pieces of data collected at any other timepoint of the study. If there are multiple different timepoints, this section should state exactly which data are being collected at each timepoint, when timepoints occur, and when the study will finish. If assessment plans are relatively complex in design, tables or Gantt charts (a type of chart used for mapping workplans discussed in Chapter 5) may help to clarify when and how data will be collected.

Discontinuation/withdrawal of participants from study

In most research studies, participants are free to withdraw at any point in a study, and if this is the case, it should be stated. If it is not the case, for example if it is anticipated that a participant will lose the capability to consent or withdraw during the course of the study such as in a longitudinal study involving dementia patients, the plans for how this will be handled should be outlined carefully. It is also advisable to explain the circumstances in which a participant might be terminated from a study early at the investigator's instigation. Suggested reasons for discontinuation may include the following along with the associated text:

✍ *Each participant has the right to withdraw from the study at any time. In addition, the investigator may discontinue a participant from the study at any time if the investigator considers it necessary for any reason including:*

✍ *Ineligibility (either arising during the study or retrospectively having been overlooked at screening)*

✍ *Significant protocol deviation*

✍ *Significant non-compliance with study requirements*

Other reasons for discontinuation could include a change in a participant's status that makes it impractical to continue having them in the study, for example if their doctor changes the hospital at which a participant is being treated, they may not be able to continue receiving music therapy at the original site. Sometimes, attempts are made to retain participants for data collection, even if they can no longer take part in the intervention. This is sometimes called an 'intention-to-treat' analysis and can give a helpful picture of what proportion of people do complete the intervention and how their results differ from the results of those who do not complete the intervention. This can be useful in estimating true intervention effectiveness by replicating what happens in the 'real world' (e.g. people do move away or lose interest in interventions).

Information should also be given on what will happen to a participant's data if they do withdraw. Data are either destroyed or kept in the study but no further data taken. A sample paragraph is:

✍ *If a participant withdraws from the study, data already collected with consent will be retained and used in the study. But no further data will be collected or any other research procedures carried out on or in relation to the participant. The reason for withdrawal will be recorded*

Definition of end of study

The end of the study is when the last piece of data has been collected, both for each participant and for the study as a whole. For participants, this might coincide with the end of an intervention or the last piece of data collection. The end of study as a whole might be when the recruitment target is hit, or the end of a period of funding (often stated as 'whichever comes sooner' to prevent studies from carrying on for too long if recruitment is clearly not on target.) Both are often stated in protocols.

Intervention

A crucial part of the protocol is describing the intervention. Depending on who is reading the protocol, different levels of detail will be required for this section. For ethics applications, often just the key pieces of information will be required, such as where the intervention will take place/who will lead it/ how many participants will take part/how long for/what the principal activity will be. However, for funders, stakeholders, and team members, a more comprehensive description may be required. In addition to the main intervention being described, any comparison or control group activities should also be outlined. (More on describing interventions is provided in Chapter 6 in relation to the TIDieR checklist.)

Analysis

Description of analytical methods

The description of the analytical methods often starts with identifying any software packages to be used. Following this, explanations should be given of the processes planned, such as the statistical tests for quantitative data or the theoretical frameworks and plans for data analysis or coding for qualitative data. Ethics boards are often in favour of comprehensive detail at this stage to prevent 'cherry-picking' later, by which different tests or methods are used to increase the likelihood of finding something significant. Of course, for exploratory studies, it may be that multiple tests and methods are planned to gain as much insight as possible into the data. However, even in this case, there are certain aspects that can be planned, such as the types of tests or methods and, importantly for quantitative research, the statistical level that will be required to say that a result was significant (see Chapter 10).

Q There are a range of software programs that can support data analysis. IBM SPSS, Stata, and R are examples of statistical packages used in analysis of quantitative data, while Nvivo and ATLAS.ti are packages for analysing qualitative data. More information can be found on the websites for these packages.

Sample size

Protocols require the study team to justify the number of participants involved in the study. The number of participants may be decided by logistics. For example, if a study is assessing the response of A&E nurses in one hospital to recorded music, there may only be 15 nurses who can take part in the study. Alternatively, it may be that a sample size calculation can be performed before the study commences. Sample sizes should account for dropouts and be realistic within the planned timeframe.

❓ *Sample size calculations are a statistical test used to determine how many people are needed in a study to have a good chance of achieving statistical significance in tests, based on the anticipated size of effect the intervention. If a study is underpowered, it may not achieve significance even though the effect being examined may be occurring (also known as type II error), leaving results ambiguous or even meaning that the intervention is dismissed as not effective.*

Sample size calculations can be performed using statistical programs such as G*Power or on paper using graphs called nomograms

 For more information on sample sizes, Andy Field provides good introductions in his statistics books.(4,5)

Data management

Access to data

In addition to planning the study and analysis, protocols also explain how the data will be safeguarded. In general, data should be kept secure and confidential, for example only visible to the immediate study team. But it may be necessary to grant access to the data to other people more broadly involved in the study. Often protocols contain a paragraph like the one below:

✍ *Data will be accessible only to the immediate study team. However, direct access will be granted to authorized representatives from the sponsor or host institution for monitoring and/or audit of the study to ensure compliance with regulations*

Data recording and record keeping

All study data should be carefully stored, for example data may be stored on secure computers at a single site to minimize the chance of data being leaked. Protocols often contain information about the programs that will be used to host data, such as Microsoft Excel, and propose systems such as password-protection or encryption of documents to ensure they are secure. Where data are being gathered anonymously, this should be stated in this section as a mitigation of risk. This section should also outline what will happen to the data after the end of the study. Universities and hospitals may have a set period of months or years for which data should be kept. Alternatively, the study team may decide to destroy all identifiable data, such as participants' contact details, shortly after the study and then either upload the anonymous data to a public repository or destroy it after a certain number of years.

Quality assurance procedures

For studies taking place within healthcare institutions, there will often be standard quality assurance procedures to follow. In this case, these regulations can be briefly explained followed by a statement confirming accordance with them, such as:

✍ *The study may be monitored, or audited in accordance with the current approved protocol, relevant regulations, and standard operating procedures*

For studies outside specific institutions, details of how the study team will monitor quality assurance should be set out, such as through audits or following the procedure of the university or host organization. It may be necessary to provide some of these documents as appendices.

Ethical and regulatory considerations

Declaration of Helsinki

❷ The Declaration of Helsinki *is a set of ethical principles set out for health research studies by the World Medical Association for studies involving human subjects. It consists of a set of general principles, including acknowledging that the health and safety of participants comes above the research, recognizing the particular need for protection of vulnerable groups, and upholding the value of research protocols*

If this is being observed, the sample sentence below is often included here. If any aspect of the declaration is not being followed, strong justifications for this will be required.

✍ *The investigator will ensure that this study is conducted in accordance with the principles of the Declaration of Helsinki*

In addition, some protocols may require descriptions of other regulations that will be followed, such as the ICH Guidelines for Good Clinical Practice (CPMP/ICH/135/95) July 1996; an international set of standards for clinical trials.

Approvals

The plan for gaining ethical approval also should be mapped out in the protocol. This may involve a national ethics committee or university or organizational approval. It should be listed which documents (e.g. participant information sheet, protocol, and consent form) will be submitted for review.

Reporting

At the end of a study, two forms are often produced: one to close the study, reporting final participant figures and any deviations from the planned protocol; and an end of study report of the findings, which may instead take the form of research papers. This section usually outlines which documents are planned and confirms which bodies, such as ethics committees, will see them, for example:

✍ *An 'end of study' notification and final report will be submitted to all parties involved*

Participant confidentiality

Participant confidentiality is important for the process of recruiting people to the study. Wherever possible, studies should be carried out anonymously and medical records should not be accessed. In addition, participants should be assigned identification numbers rather than their names being used. A common way this is conducted is through linked-anonymized data, whereby participants are assigned identification codes which are used for all their data provided during the study and a separate database exists linking their name to their identification code. If the link needs to be broken and participants need to be informed about results, this can be done. This, and other methods for protecting participant confidentiality are discussed further in Chapter 12. These processes should be explained in this section, including who will have access to the linking database, in what circumstances the links will be broken, and when this database will be destroyed after the study. Documents should be stored securely and these secure processes (such as locked cabinets, password-protected computers, and authorized personnel only) should be outlined. If the study requires participants' medical records or involves sensitive information, safeguards for these data should be carefully explained, and this information should be clearly stated to participants before they give consent to take part.

Finance and insurance

Funding

Details should be given of who is funding the study and the reference numbers for any grants.

Insurance

If the study is taking place within a healthcare institution or other company, there may be local or national insurance and indemnity that will apply in the case of any participants making a claim against the design, conduct, or management of the research study. Of course, the risks of this are much less than for drugs studies where the drugs may have serious consequences for participants. Nevertheless, there are many occasions where accidents could occur or data could still be mishandled. If organizational or institutional insurance and indemnity is not available, other options may include insurance being available through the funder or sponsor, if they are willing to take on this responsibility, or private insurance being taken out directly for the study. Accompanying proof of this insurance is often required with protocols, especially for ethics applications.

Publication policy

The plans for publication should be set out here; specifically who will be responsible for articles. Often, this takes the following form:

✍ *The investigators will be involved in reviewing drafts of the manuscripts, abstracts, press releases, and any other publications arising from the study. The chief investigator will have final approval of manuscripts*

Authorship should also be planned in advance. The standard practice is to follow the guidelines such as the Vancouver Protocol from the International Committee of Medical Journal Editors. This sets out regulations about what level of involvement is necessary to constitute an author and is discussed further in Chapter 12. The recommended paragraph is:

✍ *Authorship will be determined in accordance with the Vancouver protocol and other contributors will be acknowledged*

Acknowledgement is normally made at the end of research publications, thanking other people who have been involved but who have not made a contribution significant to constitute an author. Funders are usually recognized in acknowledgement sections too.

🔍 Further information about authorship, editorship, peer review, and conflicts of interest, including the Vancouver protocol, is available on the website for the International Committee of Medical Journal Editors www.icmje.org.

References

Finally, any references given in the protocol should be provided here in full reference format.

Summary

This chapter has set out a template format for a research protocol, breaking each section down and outlining what it involves and what decisions must be made prior to a research study going ahead. Many of the considerations in this chapter build on the step-by-step guide to research in Chapter 10, with a research protocol essentially tying together many of the decisions that have to be made in designing a research study. However, a research protocol also brings to the fore important questions around research ethics. Chapter 12 will consider ethics in more detail.

References

1. **Daniel J.** Sampling Essentials: Practical Guidelines for Making Sampling Choices. Los Angeles, London, New Delhi: SAGE; 2011. 321 pp.
2. **Suresh K.** An overview of randomization techniques: An unbiased assessment of outcome in clinical research. J Hum Reprod Sci. 2011;4(1):8–11.

3. **Cardwell M, Flanagan C. Psychology AS.** Hadenham: Nelson Thornes; 2005. 246 pp.

4. **Field A, Miles J, Field Z.** Discovering Statistics Using R. London: SAGE; 2012. 994 pp.

5. **Field A.** Discovering Statistics Using IBM SPSS Statistics, 4th Edition. 4th edition. London: SAGE Publications Ltd; 2013. 915 pp.

Chapter 12

Research ethics

Arts in health interventions often have a clear positive aim: to provide support and enjoyment to an individual or group, by improving experience and/or improving outcomes. Consequently, it is easy to see why people might ask are there any real ethical implications for arts in health interventions? Are ethics anything more than a tick-box exercise to allow a project to move forwards? How can a consideration of ethics add any value to a project?

In 2000, medical sociologist Professor Dame Sally Macintyre and her colleague Mark Petticrew wrote an article in the *Journal of Epidemiology and Community Health* entitled 'Good intentions and received wisdom are not enough.'(1) In this editorial, Macintyre and Petticrew discussed the relevance of ethics through some examples of projects that, like many arts in health interventions, had only good intentions. For example:

1. Implementing school-based bicycle safety education programmes ('Bike Ed') to reduce the risk of bicycle injury in children

2. Organizing visits to prison for juvenile delinquents so that adult inmates could discourage them from getting involved in criminal activity

3. Lying babies on their fronts to reduce the risk of inhaling vomit or choking

4. Prescribing vitamin E supplements to smokers to reduce the incidence of cancer

However, these projects are in fact examples of the dangers of assuming that good intentions are enough, as these studies actually had rather alarming results:

1. A case-control study involving 278 children aged 9-14 found that 'Bike Ed' encouraged more risk-taking behaviours and led to twice as many accidents for boys (2)

2. A systematic review of 'Scared Straight' programmes showed that meeting inmates normalized prison to juvenile delinquents, leading to an increase in delinquency rates (3)

3. Lying babies on their fronts led to a 4.6-fold increase in SIDS (sudden infant death syndrome) deaths, and for babies who were unaccustomed to sleeping on their fronts, the death rate was nearly 20 times higher (4)

4. A meta-analysis of 11 RCTs showed that vitamin E supplementation was associated with an increase in all-cause mortality (5)

Consequently, far from being ethically risk-free, these studies are pertinent examples of precisely why ethical considerations are so important: not only did a good intention not have any positive benefit, but it actually led to dangerous results. Arts in health interventions may set out with only good intentions, but it is still possible that they lead to unanticipated negative outcomes.

Ethics are typically brought to the fore of any intervention or research at the point that ethical approval needs to be secured for the project to move ahead. However, ethical considerations should pervade any research project, from its inception through to its conclusion. In this chapter, we will consider both general ethics of conduct when working in arts in health as well as returning to the research journey mapped out in Chapter 10 and considering the importance of ethics across the lifespan of a research project.

General ethics of conduct

A broad range of organizations consider ethics in a way that is relevant to arts in health. Examples include medical associations in different countries, such as the British Medical Association, American Medical Association, and World Health Organization, and different research bodies internationally, such as the American Sociological Association and British Psychological Association. Although there may be individual distinctions between different bodies, many of these ethical guidelines share concerns around the same topics. These can be broadly split into general ethics of conduct and specific ethics of practice.

Regarding general ethics of conduct, all people involved in arts in health interventions, whether arts professionals, health professionals, arts managers researchers, or volunteers (referred to here under the umbrella of 'professionals') should ensure that they follow important ethical standards in their research and practice. The British Psychological Association proposes four: respect, competence, responsibility, and integrity.

1. Respect

Respect involves valuing the dignity and worth of patients, staff, and members of the public involved in projects. Respect can include:

- General respect, including respecting individual, cultural, and role differences; respecting people's knowledge, insight, experience, and expertise; avoiding practices that might be seen as unfair or prejudiced; and being willing to explain the bases for their ethical decision-making

- Privacy and confidentiality, including keeping appropriate records; avoiding inadvertent disclosure of confidential information and obtaining consent for any planned disclosure; ensuring participants are aware of when information may be passed back to other parties including families and healthcare professionals; ensuring permissions are granted for any audio, video, or photographic recordings and only using these in ways approved by participants; and reporting breaches of confidentiality

- Informed consent, including ensuring participants understand what the intervention involves; recording and storing consents appropriately; identifying participants who may not be able to provide informed consent and working with carers or relatives to ensure activities are carried out in the participant's best interests; and withholding information about an intervention or intentionally deceiving participants only when it is essential for the preservation of participant welfare, the efficacy of professional services, or the integrity of evaluation or research activities (see Chapter 11 for more on deception in research studies)

- Self-determination, including supporting participants to make their own decisions about involvement; ensuring participants know they have the right to withdraw; and supporting participants who do withdraw, such as destroying personal records unless permission has been granted for these to be maintained

2. **Competence**

Professionals involved in interventions also have a responsibility to ensure the development and maintenance of high standards in their own professional abilities, especially in the following four areas:

- Professional ethics, including maintaining an awareness of current ethical principles and relevant ethical codes and integrating these into their professional practice

- Ethical decision-making, including recognizing ethical dilemmas when they arise; taking responsibility for attempting to resolve these; being able to justify their actions on ethical grounds; and taking particular care where legal obligations may intersect with or contradict ethical principles, working to ensure a path is chosen that is both legal and adheres as much as possible to ethics

- Recognizing limits of competence, including practising within the boundaries of one's competence; making sure one has the appropriate training to undertake an activity; engaging in continued professional development; keeping up-to-date with developments in the field; and seeking support and advice where circumstances begin to challenge one's expertise

◆ Recognizing impairments, including monitoring one's own lifestyle to recognize signs of impairment; seeking professional support or advice if health or other personal problems arise that may impair professional competence; refraining from practice when competence is seriously impaired; and providing appropriate support for colleagues to include informing appropriate bodies if a colleague appears unable to recognize their own impairment to protect staff, participants, and the public

3. **Responsibility**

Professionals also have responsibilities towards participants, the general public, and colleagues. Broadly, these fall into two areas:

◆ General responsibility, including avoiding deliberate harm; avoiding personal or professional misconduct; remaining aware of the activities of colleagues in particular employees, assistants, supervizees, and students; and being mindful of the potential risks to oneself

◆ Termination and continuity of care, including making clear to colleagues and participants the conditions under which one will terminate professional activities; terminating activities where participants do not appear to be deriving benefit and are unlikely to do so; and referring participants to alternative sources of assistance if projects are terminated to ensure continued support

4. **Integrity**

Professionals should also ensure honesty, accuracy, clarity, and fairness in their interactions with colleagues, participants, and members of the public. These activities fall under four headings:

◆ Honesty and accuracy, including presenting professional affiliations, qualifications, training, knowledge, and skills accurately; ensuring these are not misrepresented by others either; being honest in conveying professional conclusions and opinions as well as contractual obligations and financial matters; ensuring participants are aware upfront about any costs or obligations of participation; claiming appropriate ownership or credit for work or writings and acknowledging others' contributions in collaborative work; and not encouraging unrealistic expectations of the outcomes of work

◆ Avoiding exploitation and conflicts of interest, including avoiding forming relationships that may impair professional objectivity; handling existing relationships sensitively; clarifying for colleagues and participants any conflicts of interest that might potentially arise; refraining from abusing professional relationships to advance interests; and recognizing that conflicts of interest may apply even after professional relationships are formally terminated

◆ Maintaining personal boundaries, including refraining from inappropriate relationships with participants for whom there is a duty of care; recognizing and avoiding harassment of any sort and ensuring employees, students, supervizees, and trainees understand appropriate behaviours; and cultivating an awareness of tensions within groups or teams and dealing with them appropriately

◆ Addressing ethical misconduct, including challenging colleagues who appear to have engaged in ethical misconduct and/or bringing it to the attention of those responsible; avoiding allegations that involve malice or breaches of confidentiality other than those absolutely necessary; and assisting enquiries if allegations are made against oneself

> Q The British Psychological Society provides further details about these values and potential challenges that may arise in their Code of Ethics and Conduct, which can be downloaded from www.bps.org.uk.

Developing a research study

There are further specific guidelines that affect different stages of the lifecycle of a research project. For this reason, ethics should be considered from the initial conception of the research questions. Ethical research questions will focus on problems that have the potential to benefit the participants being studied. For some studies, this benefit may be clearly identifiable, such as studies examining the effectiveness of an intervention for a target patient group, where, if benefits are found, there may be a rationale for scaling up the intervention to reach more people. However, for other studies the benefit may not be as immediate. For example, a research study looking at how different parameters of music affect heart rate variability will not immediately lead to patient or public benefit, but the information derived from that study could have a significant effect in the future, such as in the choice of music to help patients relax in stressful situations like hospital waiting areas. Therefore, both basic and applied research can have potential benefits, and identifying what these benefits might be and when they are likely to occur is an important part of deciding whether a research question is ethical. However, if there is no clear impact from undertaking a research study, for example because the question is too obscure or specific and thus not likely to have any real-world implications, it may be questioned whether it is ethical to spend money on the study or to put participants through involvement in the research.

Related to this selection of an ethical research question is a consideration of any potential conflicts of interest. A research study naturally combines the individual agendas of researchers, who have areas of research in which they want to develop and become known; funders, who have strategic priorities for how their money is spent; and sponsors, who want to prioritize support for studies which are in line with their own strategies. Balancing these different agendas is important to ensure a study remains ethical. If any one of these three parties becomes too dominant, a study could be at risk of bias. For example, if a funder wants to test whether their new music software is capable of reducing stress hormones in people with anxiety disorder, it is important for the researcher to be allowed enough autonomy to design an objective research study, as well as to analyse the data appropriately, avoiding misleading presentation of results. It is also important that participants are aware of the individual interest of the funder in the study. As another example, it is important to ensure that the arts intervention being proposed for a research project is truly suitable for the target participant group, rather than merely being the one promoted by the arts organization involved. Preliminary evaluations, focus groups, and pilot projects undertaken as part of consultancy processes (outlined in Chapters 5 and 6) can be of help in confirming that the intervention is suitable for those involved. Although many of these issues will arise at later stages of the project, being aware of the potential for conflicts of interest is important at the start of a study so that appropriate agreements can be drawn up regarding the roles of the different parties.

Q The American Medical Association discusses potential conflicts of interest and ways to minimize and mitigate them as part of its Code of Medical Ethics available at www.ama-assn.org.

Finally, ownership of data and any potential intellectual property arising from a project should be clarified at the outset of a study. Personal agreements, such as Brunswick Agreements, can be developed between institutions to ensure that all parties are in agreement about arrangements once data are collected.

Q Brunswick Agreements were developed by the Brunswick Group to facilitate collaborative research between two universities or similar not-for-profit organizations. More information can be found on the Association of Research Managers and Administrators website www.arma.ac.uk.

Designing a research study

When designing a research study, it should be carefully considered whether there is a risk that participants can come to any harm. Harm could include (1) physical harm, such as older adults in a dance class getting injured; (2) psychological harm, such as participants becoming distressed by sensitive questions in an interview; (3) social harm, for example HIV patients' diagnosis becoming public knowledge through participation in a project; (4) economic harm, such as participants having to spend excess money travelling or paying for carers while involved in the project; or (5) legal harm, such as participation in the study leading to complications with rights to healthcare insurance. Harm can also extend to researchers, healthcare professionals, and artists involved in a project. Consequently, care should be taken at the design stage to consider how and when harm might occur and what steps can be taken to mitigate this. Safeguarding procedures such as risk assessments and confirmation of insurance and indemnity for the host organization should be undertaken prior to any study activity taking place (see Chapter 8).

It is also important that there is a careful consideration of how to ensure participant confidentiality. This extends to how and when participants are given anonymized participant codes, where any databases linking identifiable information with participant data are kept and who will have access to them, and under what circumstances the codes will be 'broken' (meaning data are linked back to the individuals who provided them). For example, if a psychological questionnaire reveals that a participant is contemplating self-harm, there may need to be a system in place to allow the data to be de-anonymized and the healthcare professional responsible for that participant to be notified so that they can be provided with support. Details such as how data will be kept anonymous and when codes will be broken need to be planned in advance and communicated to potential participants to ensure they are happy with how their data will be handled (see Chapter 8 for more on confidentiality).

Q The British Medical Association has developed a toolkit entitled 'Confidentiality and the Disclosure of Health Information' available as part of its 'Ethics: A to Z' on its website www.bma.org.uk.

Care also should be taken to make sure data collection measures are appropriate to the participant group. Here, patient and public involvement (PPI), which was discussed in Chapter 10, is especially important, as people from the target participant group can be asked in advance to check through questionnaires or interview schedules to confirm that questions are appropriate and not likely to cause undue distress. Where participants are to be drawn from a vulnerable group, the support of parents or carers may be crucial to the project being ethical, so their role and how they will be involved needs to be identified early on.

There are also ethical issues in recruitment. Some eligible participants may be easy to reach, such as through newspaper advertisements and online public advertisements. However, other participants may be harder to reach who do not access these channels. It is important to ensure that a wide range of people who are eligible are given the chance to participate to ensure that opportunities are not biased towards subsets of participant populations. Recruitment strategies, and in particular who will make the first approach to potential participants, should be mapped out in advance.

Running the research study

Once a study commences, participants will usually need to undergo informed consent. This was referenced in Chapter 11 and is outlined later in the chapter along with a consideration of the key documents involved in this process. However, broadly, this involves making sure that participants fully understand what the study is exploring, what their participation will involve, any risks and benefits, and that they have the right to withdraw whenever they like. Crucially, participants should not be coerced into participating but rather given plenty of time to consider whether they would like to take part, discuss the project with friends or family, and ask any questions they may have.

> Q Good Clinical Practice (GCP) is an international quality standard developed by the International Council for Harmonisation of Technical Requirements for Pharmaceuticals for Human Use (ICH). There are both face-to-face and online GCP courses offered internationally which provide further training on key aspects of running a research study including informed consent in both adults and children. Some ethics review boards require investigators involved in a research study to be GCP trained prior to the study starting.

Participants need to be treated with respect throughout the study, avoiding any imbalances of power between researcher and participant that could lead to participants feeling like 'guinea-pigs' in the project. If there are sensitivities around participants' health conditions, researchers need to be trained or have experience in how to deal with these sensitivities, especially how to handle any difficult situations that may arise. Safeguarding of participants is paramount, so processes need to be in place for researchers should unplanned information arise during the course of the study, such as a participant disclosing abuse or plans to harm somebody. Similarly, if mistakes occur on the part of the research team during a research study, such as the divulging of personal participant data, plans need to be in place for how to deal with this in an open and transparent way, both ensuring that participants are subsequently safeguarded and that appropriate action is taken to prevent similar mistakes occurring again. An important part of this is confirming responsibility and accountability prior to a study starting (see Chapter 8).

Finally, the study should be monitored to ensure that it does not inadvertently cause distress or harm to participants, with appropriate steps taken if there are signs of this occurring and, most crucially, careful decisions made about whether a study should be discontinued if there are concerns about the effect it might be having. The World Medical Association Declaration of Helsinki states 'in medical research involving human subjects, the wellbeing of the individual research subject must take precedence over all other interests'.(6) This should be true too of arts in health research, even if it is to the detriment of the research data.

Outcome of the research study

Once data have been gathered, there are two broad areas in which ethical considerations must be taken into account:

Data analysis

It is paramount in research that the anonymity of participants, where this has been guaranteed, is preserved. Data must be stored correctly, and only made accessible to those who are involved in the project. Any identifiable information should be disassociated from responses during data analysis. Data also should be preserved for a suitable number of years (often organizations have their own local rules), before being discarded to allow the verification of analyses. Where there are plans to make data publicly available, such as through the publication of anonymized datasets, this should be carried out carefully and with appropriate checks in place so that no participants' details are compromised. If audio recordings are being made as any part of data collection, these should be destroyed once they have been analysed, unless express permission is sought to keep them (see Chapter 8 for more details about permissions relating to recordings, photographs, and filming).

Another ethical issue in data analysis pertains to how the data are actually analysed. For quantitative analysis, appropriate statistical tests should be carried out that avoid bias towards positive results. Statistical techniques should be comprehensively reported in any journal articles to ensure that they can be replicated. Some journals now stipulate that data need to be made publicly available to allow other researchers to check results. However, this should always be done in line with the protocol and the consent of participants. For qualitative research, analyses should be cross-checked by a second person, where possible, to avoid researcher bias, and again full details about how the data have been analysed and who has checked this should be reported to ensure transparency.

Dissemination

When looking to publish data, reports should be written in a way that is sensitive to the participant group involved. Language should be unbiased, not allowing gender or racial stereotypes without qualification. Labels should be carefully applied, such as in linking different ethnic groups together. The authorship of studies is also an ethical issue, and should not merely be attributed as personal favours or in the hope of eliciting authorship on other studies in return. The Vancouver Protocol was developed by a group of medical journal editors in Vancouver, British Columbia in 1978 to set out uniform requirements for manuscripts submitted for journal publication, including setting out guidelines for who should be named as an author on research. According to the protocol, authorship should be based only on substantial contributions to:

1. Conception and design OR analysis and interpretation of data

2. AND drafting the article or revizing it critically for important intellectual content

3. AND on final approval of the version to be published

To be named as authors, those involved must satisfy all three conditions. Notably, involvement in acquisition of funding or collection of data on its own does not justify authorship, nor does general supervision of the research group undertaking the research. People who do not fulfil the three criteria but who have contributed to the project should instead be 'acknowledged', which is often through a separate section on a research paper.

Another ethical issue pertains to which data are reported and how. Problems that can arise within science include the falsifying of data, suppressing negative or insignificant results, and even inventing data to support specific conclusions. At best, these practices lead to wasted money and ineffectual treatments. At worst, they can lead to participants being harmed. Given the large amounts of data that are collected in research studies, it is common for not all of them to be reported. However, certain principles can guide whether reporting is ethical or not. Suggestions for these include:

♦ Demographic data should be provided with enough detail that it is clear who is represented by the study results. If participants in a study are all musically trained, this is an important point for inclusion in a study about a music intervention as it could imply that the intervention only has effects on people with musical backgrounds. However, other pieces of demographic data that may have been collected, such as what city people live in, may not be as important if this is not part of the study hypotheses and if the defining features of their city living (such as socioeconomic status) are already being reported

- Non-results should be acknowledged. If there are some findings alongside other null findings, it is encouraged that both types are reported. If the entire study finds no significant results, it can be a challenge to find a journal that will publish it. However, there are now a wide range of science and arts journals that publish results from well-designed studies, regardless of the outcome. And it is also possible to publish study reports on project websites so that people can be aware of null findings

- Limitations should be outlined. All studies have limitations, whether a weakness in the study design, a limited number of participants, or questions that could not be answered yet are still relevant to the topic. These should be honestly stated so that readers can judge for themselves how much store to place on findings and can develop follow-up research

Q The topic of publication in research was made famous by doctor Ben Goldacre, who for more than a decade wrote a column in the *Times* entitled 'Bad Science', as well as producing best-selling books *Bad Science* (2009) and *Bad Pharma* (2013).(7,8)

Finally, when publishing results, the opportunity for repercussions based on these results should be considered: comprehensive limitations sections can help to reduce sweeping generalizations; press releases that accompany results should be carefully worded to ensure they do not mispresent results to a non-scientific reader; and if there are contentious issues brought to light by data, these should be discussed within the 'discussion' section of a research paper, in particular with any caveats to interpreting the data carefully outlined.

Obtaining ethical approvals

This chapter has so far demonstrated how ethics should be embedded in every aspect of a project, rather than focusing on the point at which ethical approval from a committee is required. However, the specific process of obtaining a research ethics committee approval can be complex. Each country has its own research ethics approvals in place, either operating at a national or institutional level. Depending on whether a study specifically involves patients or members of the public, ethical approval may be sought directly through the healthcare system or healthcare institution, or it may be sought through a university affiliated with the research. Each research ethics committee will have different requirements. However, there are certain aspects that remain fairly constant between institutions and countries. In general, there are three particularly important documents required by ethics committees:

- Research protocol
- Participant information sheet
- Consent form

Research protocol

In Chapter 11 we looked at what a research protocol is and which different sections are normally included. The research protocol is a crucial element of ethics approval as it shows exactly what is involved at each stage of the project and how participants will be safeguarded. Some committees expect to see the protocol as its own document. Others have their own ethics forms. However, the sections of ethics forms are often identical or very similar to sections of the research protocol, so it is still advisable to put together the protocol while the study is being designed to ensure all avenues of ethics have been considered and facilitate the submission of the ethics form later. If there is no obvious ethical challenge posed by the project, ethics committees may have a system for fast-tracking proposals for expedited review. If there is an ethical challenge, the study may require a more comprehensive review. This normally involves peer review by a combination of researchers, healthcare professionals, and members of the public.

Participant information sheet

The second document that forms a fundamental part of ethics committee decisions is the participant information sheet (PIS). This is designed to help people make informed decisions about whether or not to take part in research. This PIS has to be carefully targeted at the participant group and written in easily comprehensible language while containing enough detail to allow participants to balance the different options. However, depending on the participant group, the level of detail may vary. For example, a study aimed at recruiting children may have two participant information sheets: a full one for parents or guardians that contains more detailed information, and a simplified age-appropriate one for the children explaining the important details, perhaps aided by pictures. If a study involves recruiting adults who cannot consent for themselves, for example people with advanced dementia, it may be that a PIS is directed entirely to relatives or legal representatives.

A PIS draws heavily on information provided within the research protocol. Indeed, there must not be discrepancies between these documents, or this could lead to inconsistencies in running the study or ethical issues. There is no single fixed template for a PIS, but they often contain specific sections to ensure that participants have been given enough information. These sections are outlined below along with details about what they usually contain and some suggested text. This section is best read in conjunction with Chapter 11. As in Chapter 11, to facilitate the use of this template, the following symbol is used:

✍ *Sample text that could be included in an information sheet or consent form if it is appropriate for the study*

Invitation to participate

A PIS normally starts with the study title (taken from the research protocol) and an introductory paragraph that explains the purpose of the PIS document so that participants understand why they are reading it. For example:

✍ *You are being invited to take part in a research study. The information below is intended to help you understand why the research is being done and what it will involve so you can decide whether or not you would like to take part. Please take time to read the following information carefully and discuss it with others if you wish. You will have the opportunity to ask any questions or request further information. Thank you for reading this*

What is the purpose of the project?

This section gives a quick overview of why the project is important and what it is being undertaken to test. If there is a clear impact that the research could have or if it could lead to important new information, this is often outlined to demonstrate the value of the project. This section is often drawn heavily from the research protocol, but sometimes simplified and shortened to adjust it to a public audience rather than research or ethics board.

Why have I been chosen to take part?

Participants need to understand why they have been selected, for example 'you are being asked to take part because you are an adult attending an out-patient appointment in the eye clinic during March'. Sometimes details such as planned sample size are given here too.

Do I have to take part?

To allow informed consent, potential participants should understand that their participation is entirely voluntary and, importantly, that not taking part will not have any negative impact on their care. If participants are allowed to withdraw, this should also be stated. This paragraph may take the following form:

✍ *It is up to you to decide whether or not to take part. If you refuse to take part, you will not receive any penalty and it will not affect your routine care. If you do decide to take part, you will be given this information sheet to keep and be asked to sign a consent form. However, you are still free to withdraw at any time without giving a reason*

What will taking part involve?

Participants should understand completely the steps that will be involved in participating so that they can decide whether they have enough time available and if they are happy to take part. This section should outline the requirements of both participating in any active component (such as attending workshops, including details about what the workshops will involve, how many people will be taking part together, and when and where they take place) and providing research data (such as completing questionnaires or providing samples, etc.). This will draw on the flow diagram given in the research protocol in Chapter 11 (Figure 11.1), but again full details may be simplified to suit the audience reading the PIS. If participants underestimate how much time participating will take, it could lead to high levels of dropouts from studies, which will have a detrimental effect. It should be clear which elements of participating are simply part of participants' standard care (e.g. if a blood test is required but this can be carried out at the same time as a routine blood test that will be required for treatment or monitoring purposes anyway), and which will involve additional time. If the study involves travelling for additional appointments where a cost might be incurred, it should be stated whether these costs will be covered by the study or not. If data will be accessed from participants' medical records, it should be discussed what will be accessed and by whom so participants understand what details will be visible to the study team.

If there are options available for people other than taking part in the study, this should also be explained. For example, if the study is exploring whether community arts workshops could support mental health in people with mild depression, participants should understand that this is not the only option available, and that if they decline to participate they can still explore other options for supporting their depression with their doctor. Similarly, if a study involves randomization into different conditions, participants (where possible) should be informed about what each condition involves so they are prepared for all options and understand how the randomization process will work (a notable exception to this is if the study is 'blinded'; see Chapter 10).

This section of the PIS often also discusses 'pre' aspects of the study, such as how participants' eligibility for the study will be checked, and 'post' aspects, such as if the study involves a therapeutic intervention, what provision will be available for participants to continue receiving support once the study formally stops.

What are the disadvantages and benefits of taking part?

Chapter 11 explored disadvantages and benefits of taking part for participants and how these are catalogued in a research protocol. These will need to be outlined clearly and honestly for participants in the PIS so they are aware of what participating could mean for them.

Will my data be kept confidential?

Details about how participants' anonymity will be protected should be clearly stated, including whether data will be stored anonymously, where data will be stored, who will have access to the data, whether participants will be identifiable from any research papers, and how and when data will be destroyed following the end of the study. Again, these details should be drawn from the research protocol.

What will happen to the results of the research project?

If there are plans for results to be published in peer-reviewed journals, presented at conferences, or made publicly available, these should be outlined. Participants may wish to see copies of their individual data, so it should be made clear whether this is possible or not. If there are plans for the data to be kept for future analysis as part of another project, this should also be explained.

Who has reviewed the project?

Participants should be told who has provided ethical review, and also whether any patients or members of the public were involved in design of the study or if they will be involved in its management and dissemination.

Who is organizing and funding the study?

Listing funders and partners can help participants to make a decision about whether they want to be involved, based on whether there appear to be any conflicts of interest. If there is a clear conflict, this may need to be explained.

Further information

A PIS often contains details of somebody who can be contacted for further information about the study, as well as somebody who is not formally involved in the research but who can provide more balanced advice about participation. There is often also a section providing details about who to contact if somebody is unhappy or has a complaint to make.

In addition to the sections outlined above, a PIS may contain other details tailored to the project. Patient and public involvement (PPI) can be of enormous support in selecting which information is most important to include, in high-lighting if there are any questions that remain unanswered once the PIS has been read, and in checking that the PIS is comprehensible even to somebody not involved in the arts, healthcare, or medicine.

The exact length of PIS and the amount of detail needed will vary depending on the study. Repetition should be avoided between sections to minimize length and documents should be well formatted to make them easily readable. A PIS should also always be version-controlled, so there is a date and version number on it. This will ensure that the version that has received ethical approval is the one in circulation.

> Q The UK's Health Research Authority provides some excellent online guidance on writing a PIS, including advice on how to phrase responses to common questions, details on how to adapt a PIS to different reading levels (such as children versus adults) and checklists of what participants should be informed about: www.hra-decisiontools. org.uk/consent/content-sheet-support.html.

Participant consent form

The third fundamental document involved in ethical review is the consent form (CF). Once participants have read the PIS and had a chance to ask any questions, if they decide to take part they will need to sign a CF, which is the record of their agreement to take part in the study. For studies involving participants being present in person, the CF is normally signed in person and countersigned by a member of the research team. However, if the study is carried out remotely, such as an online arts intervention involving online data collection, the CF can simply be presented as a series of tick boxes as part of the online process often, with a much shorter PIS prior to consent being given.

As with a PIS, the CF starts with the study title and is version-controlled to ensure the same copy approved by an ethics board is the copy that remains in use. There may also be spaces for the participant's ID, so that if data are anonymous, it is still possible to confirm that the participant has provided consent.

Depending on the participant group, the CF will contain varying levels of detail and styles of language. For children under the age of 16, it is common for a parent or guardian to sign an official CF but for the child to provide 'assent', either verbally or in writing to confirm they are happy to take part. For adults lacking the capacity to consent, the CF may be entirely directed at a relative or legal representative, who may also be required to sign a declaration form outlining their rights to sign on behalf of the participant.

Consent statements

CFs normally contain the following statements (or variations on them), each followed by a box for participants to initial:

✍ *I confirm that I have read and understand the information sheet dated [insert date on PIS] for the above study and have had the opportunity to ask questions and receive satisfactory answers*

✍ *I understand that my participation is voluntary and that I am free to withdraw at any time without giving any reason, and without my medical or legal rights being affected*

✍ *I agree to take part in this study*

In addition to these core statements, there are a number of additional statements that are not essential but are often included depending on the design of the study:

- If data are anonymous, some studies choose to highlight this in the CF, such as:

  ✍ *I understand that my responses will be anonymized before analysis. I give permission for members of the research team to have access to my anonymized responses. I understand that all personal data about me will be kept confidential*

- If the research may be audited by an external body, it is necessary to inform participants that their data may be seen by those outside the study team:

  ✍ *I understand that relevant sections of my medical notes and data collected during the study, may be looked at by individuals from [sponsor name], from regulatory authorities or from the [healthcare system], where it is relevant to my taking part in this research. I give permission for these individuals to have access to my records*

- If data from the study may be accessed in future studies, either participants' details must be kept on file so they can be contacted and consented for the future analysis or participants need to give explicit permission for future use of their data here, such as:

  ✍ *I understand that the information collected about me will be used to support other research in the future, and may be shared anonymously with other researchers*

- If participants' doctors are being informed about their participation, or if there is a safety system in place so that any abnormal data or safeguarding concerns are reported to a doctor, this is often also explicitly stated:

  ✍ *I agree to my general practitioner/doctor being informed of my participation in the study and consent to them being informed about any unusual results identified during the course of the study*

The CF is also an opportunity to confirm participation in any additional, non-compulsory elements of the study. For example, if participants are given the option of taking part in any additional invasive tests, if they are also involved in subgroup focus interviews, if permission is being sought for photographs or verbatim quotations, or if participants are happy to be contacted for follow-up data collection additional to the main study design, these can be added as optional consent boxes on the form.

Participants are often provided with a copy of the CF and PIS to take away with them as confirmation of their involvement. In addition copies are often added as appendices to medical notes as well as being kept by the research team.

Summary

This chapter has explored some important issues relating to research ethics, including at what stages of research ethics should be considered, some of the common ethical issues that arise, some potential solutions to these issues, and some of the key processes that may be involved in obtaining ethical approval. It has also provided templates for creating the other two documents that, along with a research protocol, form the core documents that are often submitted for ethical review. However, what this chapter has also highlighted is that ethics are not just of relevance to research but also overlap with practice. As such, this chapter follows on from Chapter 8 in discussing some of the complexities and sensitivities around delivering arts interventions in healthcare.

> Q For more information about the history and development of research ethics, Tsiris, Farrand, and Pavlicevic (2014) provide an overview at the start of their *Guide to Research Ethics for Arts Therapists and Arts & Health Practitioners*. The book also contains guidance on UK research ethics processes, although it must be noted that some of the processes described have changed since the book was published.(9)

In the final part of this book, we move from a consideration of research practice to research findings. Chapter 2 explored some of the biopsychosocial impacts of the arts for health, citing key research from the last few decades. In the fact file in Part IV, we will explore further how the arts have been found to support specific health conditions, with reference to inspiring case studies, more resources, and a bank of ideas for new projects.

References

1. Macintyre S, Petticrew M. Good intentions and received wisdom are not enough. J Epidemiol Community Health. 2000 Nov 1;54(11):802–3.

2. **Carlin JB, Taylor P, Nolan T.** School based bicycle safety education and bicycle injuries in children: a case-control study. Inj Prev. 1998 Mar 1;**4**(1):22–7.

3. **Petrosino A, Buehler J, Turpin-Petrosino C, Petrosino A, Buehler J, Turpin-Petrosino C.** Scared Straight and Other Juvenile Awareness Programs for Preventing Juvenile Delinquency: A Systematic Review. Campbell Syst Rev [Internet]. 2013 May 2 [cited 2016 Jul 8];9(5). Available from: http://campbellcollaboration.org/lib/project/3/

4. **Mitchell EA, Thach BT, Thompson JD, Williams S, for the New Zealand Cot Death Study.** Changing infants' sleep position increases risk of sudden infant death syndrome. Arch Pediatr Adolesc Med. 1999 Nov 1;**153**(11):1136–41.

5. **Miller I, Edgar R, Pastor-Barriuso R, Dalal D, Riemersma RA, Appel LJ, Guallar E.** Meta-Analysis: High-Dosage Vitamin E Supplementation May Increase All-Cause Mortality. Ann Intern Med. 2005 Jan 4;**142**(1):37–46.

6. **World Medical Association.** Declaration of Helsinki—Ethical Principles for Medical Research Involving Human Subjects [Internet]. Fortaleza, Brazil: World Medical Association; 2013 Oct [cited 2016 Nov 1]. Available from: http://www.wma.net/en/30publications/10policies/b3/.

7. **Goldacre B.** Bad Science. London: Fourth Estate; 2009. 288 pp.

8. **Goldacre B.** Bad Pharma: How Drug Companies Mislead Doctors and Harm Patients. Reprint edition. New York: Farrar, Straus and Giroux; 2013. 448 pp.

9. **Tsiris G, Farrant C, Pavlicevic M.** A Guide to Research Ethics for Arts Therapists and Arts & Health Practitioners. London: Jessica Kingsley Publishers; 2014. 162 pp.

Part IV

Fact file of arts in health research and practice

Introduction

In this book, we have moved from a consideration of the broad historical, theoretical, political, and global context for arts in health through to the specifics of individual case studies in different countries around the world. We have followed the path of an arts in health intervention from its initial inception through to its implementation and roll-out. We have undertaken a journey through the lifecycle of a research project. And we have considered the many moral, ethical, practical, and personal challenges of undertaking work in this field. As has been demonstrated, this is a field of enormous variety with the potential to support health in a vast number of ways. However, the seemingly limitless potential of arts in health can also make it daunting. Even if the steps suggested in this book are followed when designing an intervention, for example, it is also necessary to use imagination: have a vision for what the arts could achieve and a determination to identify how this vision could be realized.

Consequently, this final part comprises a fact file of arts in health research and practice designed to stimulate ideas. Thirteen major areas of health and medicine have been selected and are presented. For each area, the following sections are provided:

♦ Overview—a summary of what each area entails with common technical terms explained

♦ Key research findings—five engaging findings demonstrating how the arts can support each area

♦ Project ideas—a sample of project ideas related to each area. Some of these ideas are already under way in pilot or larger-scale projects in different countries, others may provide inspiration for future research or practice

♦ Further reading and resources—suggested resources for each area, including books, research articles, websites, and case study projects

Naturally, many of the ideas and research findings presented in each area are also applicable to other areas. For example, arts interventions relating to brain trauma in children could be relevant to both 'paediatrics' and 'neurology'. However, given the large number of research studies and resources that are available, no single item is entered twice, providing a total of 65 research findings, over 100 research articles, 40 project ideas, and over 80 resources. Consequently, for projects that involve more than one area of health or medicine, it is advised that all the sections that could be of relevance are consulted.

The aim of this fact file is to provide inspiration, serving as a reference guide for people working in the field. For healthcare professionals, this could highlight some of the ways that the arts could support a particular area of work. For artists and arts organizations, it could provide guidance on how the arts could be applied in different settings and what outcomes they could help to support. And for researchers, this resource file could help to identify what work has already been carried out in a specific area, and consequently where the gaps are for future studies.

Fact file 1: Critical care and emergency medicine

Overview

Emergency medicine involves the care of patients who require immediate medical attention. The specialty encompasses a broad range of medical disciplines, including anaesthesia, cardiology (a field related to the heart), neurology (a field related to the brain), plastic surgery, orthopaedic surgery (surgery relating to the bones or muscles), and cardiothoracic surgery (surgery relating to the heart, chest, or lungs). There are also a number of subspecialties including extreme environment medicine, disaster medicine and sports medicine. Related to emergency medicine is the specialty of critical care medicine, which is concerned with the care of patients with life-threatening conditions often treated in intensive care settings.

Key research findings

1. Arts- and design-enhanced accident and emergency departments can lead to a reduction in threatening body language and aggressive behaviour from patients (1)
2. Recorded music in intensive care can reduce the quantity of sedative drugs needed, decrease stress hormones, blood pressure, and inflammation, and increase growth hormones (2)
3. Diaries written by staff and families for patients in intensive care can reduce symptoms of post-traumatic stress (3,4)
4. Music during interventional radiology procedures, colonoscopies, spinal anaesthesia, and in intensive care can reduce doses of sedative and analgesia (5–7)
5. Music can reduce anxiety among parents of children in emergency department waiting rooms (8)

Project ideas

- Could the arts be used to provide emotional support for relatives of emergency or critical care patients?

- How could emergency vehicles be designed to maximize patient comfort and reduce distress without distracting from their function?
- Could arts-based awareness campaigns be used to educate the public on how to provide first aid support and manage emergency situations?

Q The Design Council's 'A&E Design Challenge' in the UK aimed to reduce the number of physical assaults in English NHS hospitals through the use of design. Their website www.designcouncil.org.uk outlines the problem, consultation plan, intervention, and evaluation, following some of the steps outlined in Chapters 5 and 6. For a case study of how an emergency department can be redesigned to maximize patient experience, Chelsea and Westminster Hospital has integrated visual and digital arts across the different areas of the department. Details are available on the website of the hospital's charity: www.cwplus.org.uk.

The Centre for Arts in Medicine at the University of Florida has delivered a vast number of performances in critical care settings, including at the UF Health Shands Hospital Adult Emergency and Trauma Centre, where over 5,000 musical interactions with patients have been recorded. Based on this work, the centre has developed an online resource website providing recommendations for practice for artists working in emergency and trauma care: www.arts.ufl.edu/academics/center-for-arts-in-medicine/research.

The value of the arts in creating a healing environment in intensive care units is also discussed in some nursing textbooks. For example, chapter 3 of *Critical Care Nursing: Synergy for Optimal Outcomes* by Roberta Kaplow and Sonya R. Hardin (2007) explores the impact of various sensory experiences including design, music, lighting, and smell on psychological and physiological measures and makes recommendations for creating a healing environment.(9)

References

1. **Design Council**. Reducing violence and aggression in A&E: Through a better experience [Internet]. London: Design Council; 2013 [cited 2015 Nov 16]. Available from: http://www.designcouncil.org.uk/what-we-do/ae-design-challenge.
2. **Conrad C, Niess H, Jauch K-W, Bruns CJ, Hartl W, Welker L**. Overture for growth hormone: requiem for interleukin-6? Crit Care Med. 2007 Dec;35(12):2709–13.
3. **Garrouste-Orgeas M, Coquet I, Périer A, Timsit J-F, Pochard F, Lancrin F**, et al. Impact of an intensive care unit diary on psychological distress in patients and relatives. Crit Care Med. 2012 Jul;40(7):2033–40.
4. **Jones C, Backman C, Griffiths RD**. Intensive Care Diaries and Relatives' Symptoms of Posttraumatic Stress Disorder After Critical Illness: A Pilot Study. Am J Crit Care. 2012 May 1;21(3):172–6.
5. **Kulkarni S, Johnson PCD, Kettles S, Kasthuri RS**. Music during interventional radiological procedures, effect on sedation, pain and anxiety: a randomised controlled trial. Br J Radiol. 2012 Aug;85(1016):1059–63.

6. **Koch ME, Kain ZN, Ayoub C, Rosenbaum SH.** The sedative and analgesic sparing effect of music. Anesthesiology. 1998 Aug;89(2):300–6.

7. **Lepage C, Drolet P, Girard M, Grenier Y, DeGagné R.** Music decreases sedative requirements during spinal anesthesia. Anesth Analg. 2001 Oct;93(4):912–6.

8. **Holm L, Fitzmaurice L.** Emergency department waiting room stress: can music or aromatherapy improve anxiety scores? Pediatr Emerg Care. 2008 Dec;24(12):836–8.

9. **Kaplow R.** Critical Care Nursing: Synergy for Optimal Outcomes. Jones & Bartlett Learning; 2007. 810 pp.

Fact file 2: Dentistry

Overview

Dentistry involves the study, diagnosis, prevention, and/or treatment of diseases, disorders, and conditions of the oral cavity, including the teeth, gums, and tissues. Dentistry is thought to be one of the first areas of specialization to emerge from medicine, with evidence of drilled teeth dating back 9,000 years. The most common conditions treated within dentistry involve tooth decay (dental caries) and gum disease (periodontal disease), with common dental procedures including x-rays, restorative treatments (such as fillings, crowns, and bridges), prosthetics (dentures), orthodontics (such as teeth braces), tooth extraction and endodontic (root canal) therapy. Dentistry also involves public health work such as the encouragement of oral disease prevention through dental hygiene and check-ups.

Key research findings

1. A singing toothbrush guiding blind children in how to brush their teeth has been shown to reduce plaque and bacteria over 6 weeks (1)
2. Video eye-glasses can support good behaviour in children undergoing dental examination (2)
3. Relaxing music during dental treatment has been shown to reduce stress hormones and increase levels of the immune-optimizing protein salivary immunoglobulin A (3,4)
4. Ten-minute cartoon animations on dental care have been shown to reduce plaque and improve dental health awareness (5)
5. Lavender smells can reduce anxiety in patients in a dental waiting room and orange smells can increase happiness (6,7)

Project ideas

- Could an arts-based app be used to help people check their oral health?
- Can the digital arts be used to broadcast a public health message about dental hygiene to families in low-income countries?

♦ How could the dentist chair be redesigned to maximize comfort and reduce anxiety in patients?

Q For a comprehensive overview of popular and advanced cosmetic procedures, George A. Freedman's *Contemporary Esthetic Dentistry* is highly recommended. It provides over 2,400 full-colour photographs of procedures and outcomes, playing close attention to the 'artistic' side of dentistry, including manipulations of colour, shade, texture, and polish.(8)

The arts have also been discussed for their relevance to dental aesthetics. An article by TS Valo in *Current Opinion in Cosmetic Dentistry* (1995) entitled 'Anterior esthetics and the visual arts: beauty, elements of composition, and their clinical application to dentistry' discusses how the nature of beauty explored in the visual arts can enhance the work of cosmetic dentists, while I Ahmad's article 'Geometric considerations in anterior dental aesthetics: restorative principles' in *Practical Periodontics and Aesthetic Dentistry* (1998) discusses how geometrical principles including the Golden Ratio can enhance aesthetics.(9,10)

There are also several universities that now incorporate the arts into training for dentistry students. For example, the Melbourne Dental School uses visual arts in training its students to support their work in Special Needs Dentistry. The programme is discussed in *Creative Arts in Humane Medicine* edited by Cheryl McLean (2014): a collection of essays that explores how the arts can facilitate self-care and awareness among healthcare professionals and improve patient care.(11) Similarly, Boston University Henry M. Goldman School of Dental Medicine teaches dental students art appreciation through visiting the Isabella Stewart Gardner Museum to improve patient care. A talk entitled 'Why Art is Important to Dentists: Dr. Neal Fleisher Explains' available on the Boston University website by Dr Neal Fleischer, Clinical Associate Professor in the department, describes the programme in more detail: www.bu.edu.

The link between visual art and dentistry has also resulted in a special art gallery in Georgia Regents University in the USA that contains over 175 pieces of art by dentists. A news item on the programme entitled 'Double Dip: Dentistry meets visual artistry in Georgia Regents University dental school gallery' is available through www.ada.org.

References

1. **Shetty V, Hegde A, Varghese E, Shetty** V. A Novel Music based Tooth Brushing System for Blind Children. J Clin Pediatr Dent. 2013 Apr 1;**37**(3):251–6.

2. **Ram D, Shapira J, Holan G, Magora F, Cohen S, Davidovich** E. Audiovisual video eyeglass distraction during dental treatment in children. Quintessence Int Berl Ger 1985. 2010 Sep;**41**(8):673–9.

3. **Oyama T, Hatano K, Sato Y, Kudo M, Spintge R, Droh** R. Endocrine Effect of Anxiolytic Music in Dental Patients. In: Spintge D med R, Droh D med R, editors. Musik in der Medizin/Music in Medicine [Internet]. Springer Berlin Heidelberg; 1987 [cited 2015 Nov 9]. pp. 223–6. Available from: http://link.springer.com/chapter/10.1007/978-3-642-71697-3_20.

4. **Goff LC, Rebollo Pratt R, Madriga JL.** Music listening and S-IgA levels in patients undergoing a dental procedure. Int J Arts Med. 1997;5:22–6.

5. **Ness A.** The Effects of the Preventive Dentistry Audio-Visual Instructional Program on the Knowledge, Attitude and behavior of Elementary School Aged Children in Romania. University of Wisconsin-Stout; 2010.

6. **Lehrner J, Marwinski G, Lehr S, Johren P, Deecke L.** Ambient odors of orange and lavender reduce anxiety and improve mood in a dental office. Physiol Behav. 2005 Sep 15;86(1–2):92–5.

7. **Kritsidima M, Newton T, Asimakopoulou K.** The effects of lavender scent on dental patient anxiety levels: a cluster randomised-controlled trial. Community Dent Oral Epidemiol. 2010 Feb;38(1):83–7.

8. **Freedman GA.** Contemporary Esthetic Dentistry, 1e. 1 Har/Psc edition. St. Louis, Mo: Mosby; 2012. 832 pp.

9. **Valo TS.** Anterior esthetics and the visual arts: beauty, elements of composition, and their clinical application to dentistry. Curr Opin Cosmet Dent. 1995;24–32.

10. **Ahmad I.** Geometric considerations in anterior dental aesthetics: restorative principles. Pract Periodontics Aesthetic Dent PPAD. 1998 Sep;10(7):813–822; quiz 824.

11. McLean CL, editor. Creative Arts in Humane Medicine. 1 edition. Brush Education; 2014. 240 pp.

Fact file 3: Geriatric medicine

Overview

From the Greek 'γέρων' (geron) meaning old man, and 'ιατρός' (iatros) meaning doctor or healer, geriatric medicine focuses on the health of elderly people. Geriatric medicine includes preventing and treating impairments, such as impaired vision, hearing, memory or intellect, immobility and incontinence, and dealing with increasing health complexities such as multiple health conditions and multi-medication usage. One of the main areas of attention is around dementias including Alzheimer's disease. The field also encompasses practical and ethical issues around supporting independence, daily functioning. and self-care in elderly people as well as attention on wellbeing and quality of life.

Key research findings

1. Dance and movement workshops can improve gait and lead to a reduction in falls among older adults (1,2)

2. Background music can decrease aggression and agitation in dementia patients during bathing and mealtimes (3,4)

3. Reminiscence workshops can reduce withdrawal from daily life and improve cognitive function in patients with Alzheimer's disease (5,6)

4. Design elements such as lighting, noise level, and use of contrasting colours have been found to improve behaviour, cognition, wellbeing, and orientation in people with dementia (7)

5. Singing has been shown to improve quality of life and reduce anxiety and depression in older adults (8)

Project ideas

◆ How could the arts be used to reduce delirium and confusion in elderly people in hospital or a nursing home?

◆ How could the arts be used to help dementia patients remember who their family members are?

◆ Could arts-based technologies be harnessed to connect elderly people and help them to feel less lonely?

◆ How could the arts be used to educate elderly people about the importance of staying active?

Q There are a number of online resources relating to geriatric medicine. For more information about dementia, 'Barbara's story' is a short film about the experiences of a patient with dementia in hospital aimed at educating viewers on the challenges faced by dementia patients, available through the website of Guy's and St Thomas' Hospital in London: www.guysandstthomas.nhs.uk.

For environmental design, the King's Fund ran a multi-year project entitled 'Enhancing the Healing Environment', focusing on how to design hospital and care home environments to support elderly people. Their 'Dementia Assessment Tool' helps to assess whether an environment is supportive of elderly people, and their resources page on their website www.kingsfund.org.uk includes case studies from NHS acute, community, and mental health hospitals in the UK showing how the arts were used to provide practical and cost-effective improvements.

There are several films that demonstrate the impact of the arts in dementia care. 'Alive Inside' is a documentary about an elderly man called Henry Dryer showing the effects that music can have in supporting memory www.youtube.com/watch?v=XBuG8xwIvYY. And the UK charity Wishing Well has also produced a video about the effects of live music on dementia patients www.wishingwellmusic.org.uk/film. 'I remember better when I paint' is a documentary about the impact of creative arts on dementia: www. iremembetterwhenipaint.com. The accompanying book edited by Berna F Huebner provides scientific insight into Alzheimer's disease and how the arts can have an impact, as well as containing case studies from artists about their experience working with patients with the condition.(9)

There are also many practical guides to running arts workshops with older adults, such as *Connecting Through Music with People with Dementia* by Robin Rio (2009), *Art Therapy and Creative Coping Techniques for Older Adults* by Susan I. Buchalter (2011), and *Music Therapy and Geriatric Populations* by Melita Belgrave, Alice-Ann Darrow, Darvy Walworth, and Natalie Wlodarczyk (2011).

Two reports from the Baring Foundation map out suggestions for engagement of older adults in the arts: 'Creative Homes, How the Arts' can contribute to quality of life in residential care explores case studies of impact in care homes, including top tips for care home managers and arts practitioners. And 'Ageing Artfully: Older People and Professional Participatory Arts in the UK' examines the personal and societal benefits from arts organizations working with older people both within and outside the UK. They are both available on the website www.baringfoundation.org.uk.

For case studies of practice, there are a vast number of organizations delivering projects across the world, including 'Singing for the Brain' from the Alzheimer's Society UK www.alzheimers.org.uk, the US charity Music and Memory who use digital technology to connect older adults with the arts www.musicandmemory.org, and 'Come Dance with Me' delivered by Alzheimer's Australia https://qld.fightdementia.org.au.

References

1. Shigematsu R, Chang M, Yabushita N, Sakai T, Nakagaichi M, Nho H, Tanaka K. Dance-based aerobic exercise may improve indices of falling risk in older women. Age Ageing 2002;31(4):261–262.

2. Wittwer JE, Webster KE, Hill K. Music and metronome cues produce different effects on gait spatiotemporal measures but not gait variability in healthy older adults. Gait Posture. 2013 Feb;37(2):219–22.

3. Goddaer J, Abraham IL. Effects of relaxing music on agitation during meals among nursing home residents with severe cognitive impairment. Arch Psychiatr Nurs. 1994 Jun;8(3):150–8.

4. Thomas DW, Heitman RJ, Alexander T. The Effects of Music on Bathing Cooperation for Residents with Dementia. J Music Ther. 1997 Dec 21;34(4):246–59.

5. Ashida S. The effect of reminiscence music therapy sessions on changes in depressive symptoms in elderly persons with dementia. J Music Ther. 2000;37(3):170–82.

6. Tadaka E, Kanagawa K. Effects of reminiscence group in elderly people with Alzheimer disease and vascular dementia in a community setting. Geriatr Gerontol Int. 2007 Jun 1;7(2):167–73.

7. Marquardt G, Bueter K, Motzek T. Impact of the Design of the Built Environment on People with Dementia: An Evidence-Based Review. HERD Health Environ Res Des J. 2014 Oct 1;8(1):127–57.

8. Coulton S, Clift S, Skingley A, Rodriguez J. Effectiveness and cost-effectiveness of community singing on mental health-related quality of life of older people: randomised controlled trial. Br J Psychiatry J Ment Sci. 2015 Sep;207(3):250–5.

9. Huebner BG, Butler RN, Cohen GD, Noronha A, Lazarus LW, Sheppard JG, et al. I Remember Better When I Paint: Art and Alzheimer's: Opening Doors, Making Connections. Glen Echo, MD: Bethesda Communications Group; 2012. 138 pp.

Fact file 4: Healthcare staff

Overview

The field of medicine involves a wide range of jobs including doctors/physicians, dentists, nurses, midwives, radiologists, dieticians, physiotherapists, occupational therapists, psychologists, psychiatrists, porters, healthcare managers, data analysts, healthcare assistants, support workers, technicians, and many others. Recent reviews have highlighted the effects of demanding healthcare jobs and shift work on the functioning and wellbeing of staff, with particular focus on negative working conditions such as long hours and short-staffing leading to staff burnout. Consequently, many countries are now placing an emphasis on providing additional support for staff to improve retention rates and optimize the level of care provided for patients.

Key research findings

1. Doctors' surgeries with enhanced design can reduce patient anxiety, increased satisfaction with patient-doctor communication, and improved staff satisfaction (1)

2. Art therapy can reduce stress and burnout among nurses, help the processing of grief, and build team morale (2,3)

3. Visual arts can be used to enhance the visual diagnostic skills of trainee doctors (4,5)

4. Staff witnessing music therapy sessions for patients have been shown to experience greater self-awareness, improved mood, better teamwork, and perceived improvement in their patient care (6)

5. Arts and design-enhanced hospitals can improve the mood of hospital staff, influence their decision to apply for a job and affect their decision to remain in their current job (7)

Project ideas

- Could arts interventions be designed to help staff unwind and switch off from work at the end of hospital shifts?
- How could the arts be used in training programmes to improve staff communication?

◆ Could arts-based technologies be used to connect healthcare staff to improve peer support?

Q Carnegie Hall's Weill Music Institute commissioned a paper by WolfBrown in 2011 that included a review of how music can support healthcare staff. The review entitled 'Music and HealthCare' summarizing a range of studies exploring this topic is available at www.wolfbrown.com/images/books_reports/documents/Music_and_Health_Care.pdf.

There are also a range of music ensembles for healthcare staff in different countries. For example, in the UK, York Hospital have their own staff choir who have featured on BBC radio, while Lewisham and Greenwich NHS Trust have appeared on television in a work choir competition and were the Christmas #1 in 2015.

For more information about arts in medical training, CLOD Ensemble in the UK feature a number of resources on their website www.clodensemble.com. And *Creative Arts in Humane Medicine* edited by Cheryl McLean (2014) contains a series of chapters discussing how the arts including role-play, fabric art, drama, and the visual arts can support the education and personal development of healthcare professionals.(8) Further resources relating to healthcare staff are discussed in Chapter 5.

References

1. **Rice G, Ingram J, Mizan J.** Enhancing a primary care environment: a case study of effects on patients and staff in a single general practice. Br J Gen Pr. 2008 Jul 1;**58**(552):e1–8.

2. **Nainis NA.** Art Therapy with an Oncology Care Team. Art Ther. 2005 Jan 1;**22**(3):150–4.

3. **Repar PA, Patton D.** Stress reduction for nurses through Arts-in-Medicine at the University of New Mexico Hospitals. Holist Nurs Pr. 2007 Jul;**21**(4):182–6.

4. **Dolev JC, Friedlaender LK, Braverman IM.** Use of fine art to enhance visual diagnostic skills. JAMA. 2001 Sep 5;**286**(9):1020–1.

5. **Naghshineh S, Hafler JP, Miller AR, Blanco MA, Lipsitz SR, Dubroff RP,** et al. Formal art observation training improves medical students' visual diagnostic skills. J Gen Intern Med. 2008 Jul;**23**(7):991–7.

6. **O'Callaghan C, Magill L.** Effect of music therapy on oncologic staff bystanders: a substantive grounded theory. Palliat Support Care. 2009 Jun;**7**(2):219–28.

7. **Staricoff RL, Duncan J, Wright M, Loppert S, Scott J.** A study of the effects of visual and performing arts in health care. London: Chelsea and Westminster Hospital; 2002.

8. McLean CL, editor. Creative Arts in Humane Medicine. 1 edition. Brush Education; 2014. 240 pp.

Fact file 5: Neurology

Overview

Neurology focuses on diagnosing and treating conditions affecting the nervous system, which encompasses the brain and peripheral nervous system (involving the nerves and nerve cell clusters that connect the brain to the limbs and organs) and the muscular system. Some neurological conditions are present from birth, such as cerebral palsy; while some develop during childhood, such as Duchenne muscular dystrophy; and others typically affect older people, such as Alzheimer's and Parkinson's diseases. Neurology also deals with acquired brain injuries, strokes, and cancers affecting the brain and spine.

Key research findings

1. Listening to music after a stroke can enhance the recovery of early sensory processing and support better cortical connectivity and enhanced cognitive recovery (1–3)
2. Music-based movement therapy can improve walking speed, stride length, and gait symmetry in patients with acquired brain injury (4)
3. Music can improve social responsiveness in children with autistic spectrum disorders (5–7)
4. Museum object handling and art viewing can improve wellbeing, confidence, and optimism in people with Alzheimer's disease and their caregivers (8)
5. Clay manipulation can reduce emotional and somatic symptoms in patients with Parkinson's disease (9)

Project ideas

- Could the arts be used in occupational therapy to help neurology patients with daily tasks such as making a cup of tea?
- Could arts interventions be designed to support speech and language therapy?
- How could patients with brain injury use the arts to express to family or friends the lived experience of their condition?

Q For an engaging introduction to how music can help a range of neurological conditions, Oliver Sach's best-selling *Musicophilia: Tales of Music and the Brain* (2011) provides an accessible insight. For further research insight into the impact that music can have, the Music Therapy Centre of California has produced fact sheets for how music therapy can support a whole range of neurological conditions including cerebral palsy, autism, Parkinson's disease, and Rett syndrome: www.themusictherapycenter.com. And Cerebrum online journal has published a summary of research in the field through an article from 24 March 2010 entitled 'How music helps to heal the injured brain': www.dana.org. Music therapists may also be interested in Michael H. Thaut and Volker Hoemberg's *Handbook of Neurologic Music Therapy* (2014), which provides a comprehensive overview of different techniques and models.

For more information about other arts therapies, *Arts Therapies and Progressive Illness: Nameless Dread* edited by Diane Waller (2002) considers interventions from therapeutic dance circles to art therapy for different neurological conditions, while *Art therapy for Neurological Conditions* edited by Sally Weston and Marian Liebmann (2015) focuses specifically on art therapy for both acquired and hereditary conditions.(10,11)

There are a number of lectures online that provide further information, including a lecture by Frederike van Wijk, Professor in Neurological Rehabilitation at Glasgow Caledonian University on how music can improve life after stroke given on 16 November 2015 available via the Live Music Now website www.livemusicnow.org.uk, and a lecture by Dr Christina Devereaux, Associate Professor in Dance Movement Therapy at Antioch University New England on dance and movement therapy in autism: www.youtube.com/watch?v=65DLHYrHIlM.

There are a large number of charities and organizations supporting people with neurological conditions through the arts. Dance for Parkinson's works in partnership with organizations including English National Ballet; Music for Autism operates in the UK and US; and The Amber Trust, a charity supporting blind and partially sighted children across the UK, includes a significant amount of work with autism. For more on music and autism, *In the Key of Genius* by Adam Ockelford explores the life of Derek Paravicine, a musical prodigy with autism and *Comparing Notes* builds theoretically on musical work with autistic children to consider how we make sense of music.(12,13)

A large number of organizations globally deliver projects for people with neurological conditions. For example, the Aphasia Community Chorus in Michigan, USA is a social singing group for people with aphasia or other communication disorders www.aphasia-centermi.org/chorus.html. Painting with Parkinson's is an art therapy programme delivered in Australia www.paintingwithparkinsons.org.au, and the Amy Winehouse Music Therapy Programme delivers workshops for children with cerebral palsy, with details available at www.cplondon.org.uk.

References

1. Särkämö T, Tervaniemi M, Laitinen S, Forsblom A, Soinila S, Mikkonen M, et al. Music listening enhances cognitive recovery and mood after middle cerebral artery stroke. Brain. 2008 Mar 1;131(3):866–76.

2. Särkämö T, Pihko E, Laitinen S, Forsblom A, Soinila S, Mikkonen M, et al. Music and Speech Listening Enhance the Recovery of Early Sensory Processing after Stroke. J Cogn Neurosci. 2009 Nov 19;**22**(12):2716–27.

3. Altenmüller E, Marco-Pallares J, Münte TF, Schneider S. Neural Reorganization Underlies Improvement in Stroke-induced Motor Dysfunction by Music-supported Therapy. Ann N Y Acad Sci. 2009 Jul 1;**1169**(1):395–405.

4. Bradt J, Magee WL, Dileo C, Wheeler BL, McGilloway E. Music therapy for acquired brain injury. In: Cochrane Database of Systematic Reviews [Internet]. John Wiley & Sons, Ltd; 2010 [cited 2015 Nov 16]. Available from: http://onlinelibrary.wiley.com/doi/10.1002/14651858.CD006787.pub2/abstract.

5. Whipple J. Music in Intervention for Children and Adolescents with Autism: A Meta-Analysis. J Music Ther. 2004 Jun 20;**41**(2):90–106.

6. LaGasse AB, Thaut MH. Music and rehabilitation: neurological approaches. In: MacDonald RAR, Kreutz G, Mitchell L, editors. Music, health, and wellbeing. Oxford: Oxford University Press; 2012. pp. 153–63.

7. Finnigan E, Starr E. Increasing social responsiveness in a child with autism A comparison of music and non-music interventions. Autism. 2010 Jul 1;**14**(4):321–48.

8. Johnson J, Culverwell A, Hulbert S, Robertson M, Camic PM. Museum activities in dementia care: Using visual analog scales to measure subjective wellbeing. Dement Lond Engl. 2015 Oct 13;

9. Elkis-Abuhoff DL, Goldblatt RB, Gaydos M, Corrato S. Effects of Clay Manipulation on Somatic Dysfunction and Emotional Distress in Patients With Parkinson's Disease. Art Ther. 2008 Jan 1;**25**(3):122–8.

10. Higgins R. Arts Therapies and Progressive Illness: Nameless Dread. 1 edition. Waller D, editor. Hove, East Sussex ; New York, NY: Routledge; 2002. 206 pp.

11. Ashley J, Michaels D, Bell S, Hyde IVS, Connelly C, Knight A, et al. Art Therapy with Neurological Conditions. 1 edition. Liebmann M, Weston S, editors. London: Jessica Kingsley Publishers; 2015. 368 pp.

12. Ockelford A. In The Key of Genius: The Extraordinary Life of Derek Paravicini. London: Cornerstone Digital; 2009. 298 pp.

13. Ockelford A. Comparing Notes: How We Make Sense of Music. Main edition. Profile Books; 2017. 352 pp.

Fact file 6: Obstetrics, gynaecology, and neonatology

Overview

Obstetrics (a branch of medicine focusing on childbirth and midwifery), gynaecology (a field of medicine specific to women and girls with a particular focus on the reproductive system), and neonatology (a subspecialty of paediatrics focused on the care of newborn infants, especially those who are premature) cover the whole span of pre-conception, pregnancy, childbirth, and the postpartum period for both mothers and babies. The topics covered by these disciplines include family planning, reproductive medicine, menopausal and geriatric (older adult) gynaecology, maternal medicine, and female urology. Because of the breadth of these disciplines, care teams involve hospital clinicians, surgeons, family doctors, nurses, midwives, doulas, and health visitors, among others.

Key research findings

1. Hip-hop videos have been used with African-American teenagers to improve awareness about HIV prevention, condom use, and protective sexual behaviours among teenage girls (1,2)

2. Babies can recognize sounds heard as early as 20 weeks into pregnancy and remember them after birth (3,4)

3. Playing lullabies to premature infants can stabilize physiological measures, increase oxygen saturation, and shorten their hospital stay (5–7)

4. Musical reinforcement can be used to increase babies' feeding ability and weight (8,9)

5. Creative arts therapy provides social support and increased self-esteem and confidence in mothers with postnatal depression (10)

Project ideas

- Could arts-based apps be developed to support the physical health or mental wellbeing of new mothers?

- How could the arts be integrated into hospitals to improve women's experiences of labour?
- Could an arts programme be developed to support the bereaved parents of newborn infants?

Q There are a number of pregnancy and labour guides that reference the value of the arts. *The Pregnancy Journal and Coloring Book* by Lisa Greenhut (2016) encourages colouring and journaling to deal with pregnancy-related stress and mental preparation for motherhood.(11) *Easing Labor Pain: The Complete Guide to a More Comfortable and Rewarding Birth* by Adrienne B. Lieberman and Dan Rosenberg contains a chapter entitled 'Charms to Soothe: Music', which gives guidance on how to use music to best effect during the birth.(12) There are many projects internationally applying the arts in this field, such as 'The Birthing Sanctuary' in southern India, which uses art and dance therapy for birth preparation or postnatal debriefing: www.birthingsanctuary.com/wellness-center.

For working with neonates, *Music Therapy and Parent Infant Bonding* edited by Jane Edwards (2011) offers an in-depth insight into different types of music interventions with specific populations including mothers who experienced abuse, families with new babies affected by cancer, and mothers in marginalized communities.(13) *Music Therapy with Premature Infants: Research and Interventions* by Jayne M. Standley and Darcy Walworth (2010) explores how music can be of support both in neonatal intensive care units and when families transition back to their own homes.(14)

There are also a range of resources for working in bereavement. The Yinstill Reproductive Loss and Art Therapy programme gives practical guidance for art therapists working with women who have experienced a miscarriage or miscarriage http://www.yinstill.com/reproductive-loss-and-art-therapy-program. Laura Seftel's book *Grief Unseen: Healing Pregnancy Loss Through the Arts* (2005) is a personal account of how art supported the author through miscarriage including a step-by-step guide to supportive arts practices.(15)

As an example of a wider arts project, *The Art for Baby* series in support of NSPCC (the National Society for the Prevention of Cruelty to Children) is a wonderful case study of how the arts can be used to fundraise for research and support for mother and babies.(16) Each book brings together leading global artists including Julian Opie, Takashi Murakami, Damien Hirst, and Gary Hume to create new pieces of art designed to be appropriate for new babies through high-contrast colours and bold shapes, with a portion of the proceeds going to charity.

References

1. **Stokes CE, Gant LM**. Turning the tables on the HIV/AIDS epidemic: hip hop as a tool for reaching African-American adolescent girls. Afr Am Res Perspect. 2002;**8**(2):71–81.
2. **Lemieux AF, Fisher JD, Pratto** F. A music-based HIV prevention intervention for urban adolescents. Health Psychol. 2008;**27**(3):349–57.

3. **Shahidullah S, Hepper PG.** The developmental origins of fetal responsiveness to an acoustic stimulus. J Reprod Infant Psychol. 1993 Jul 1;**11**(3):135–42.

4. **Partanen E, Kujala T, Tervaniemi M, Huotilainen M.** Prenatal Music Exposure Induces Long-Term Neural Effects. PLoS One. 2013 Oct 30;**8**(10):e78946.

5. **Cassidy JW, Standley JM.** The Effect of Music Listening on Physiological Responses of Premature Infants in the NICU. J Music Ther. 1995 Dec 21;**32**(4):208–27.

6. **Lorch CA, Lorch V, Diefendorf AO, Earl PW.** Effect of Stimulative and Sedative Music on Systolic Blood Pressure, Heart Rate, and Respiratory Rate in Premature Infants. J Music Ther. 1994 Jun 20;**31**(2):105–18.

7. **Caine J.** The effects of music on the selected stress behaviors, weight, caloric and formula intake, and length of hospital stay of premature and low birth weight neonates in a newborn intensive care unit. J Music Ther. 1991 Winter;**28**(4):180–92.

8. **Standley JM.** The effect of music-reinforced nonnutritive sucking on feeding rate of premature infants. J Pediatr Nurs. 2003 Jun;**18**(3):169–73.

9. **Standley JM.** The Role of Music in Pacification/Stimulation of Premature Infants with Low Birthweights. Music Ther Perspect. 1991 Jan 1;**9**(1):19–25.

10. **Perry C, Thurston M, Osborn T.** Time for Me: The arts as therapy in postnatal depression. Complement Ther Clin Pract. 2008 Feb;**14**(1):38–45.

11. **Greenhut L.** Pregnancy Journal and Coloring Book. 1 edition. Turtle Moon Press; 2016. 178 pp.

12. **Lieberman A.** Easing Labor Pain: The Complete Guide to a More Comfortable and Rewarding Birth. Revised edition. Boston, Mass.: Lanham, Md: Harvard Common Press; 1992. 288 pp.

13. **Edwards J.** Music Therapy and parent infant bonding. 2 edition. Oxford ; New York: Oxford University Press; 2011. 240 pp.

14. **Standley JM, Walworth D.** Music Therapy with Premature Infants: Research and Developmental Interventions. American Music Therapy Association; 2010. 248 pp.

15. **Seftel L.** Grief Unseen: Healing Pregnancy Loss Through the Arts. London ; Philadelphia: Jessica Kingsley Pub; 2006. 191 pp.

16. **NSPCC.** Art for Baby. 01 edition. Dorking: Templar Publishing; 2008.

Fact file 7: Oncology

Overview

Oncology is a branch of medicine focusing on the prevention, diagnosis, and treatment of cancers; one of the leading causes of death in the world. Early records of cancer have been found in fossils from mummies in ancient Egypt and are discussed in some ancient manuscripts, attesting to the long history of the condition. Oncology teams often encompass medical oncologists (who can specialize in chemotherapy, immunotherapy, hormonal therapy, and targeted therapy), surgical oncologists, radiation oncologists, and doctors with specialities in the organs affected.

Key research findings

1. Virtual windows (artistic films of the outside world) can reduce anxiety and improve treatment experience in cancer patients undergoing stem cell transplantation (1)

2. Video games explaining cancer treatments to children can increase medication adherence and promote healthy behaviours (2)

3. Art therapy improves collaborative behaviour and coping in children with leukaemia in hospital undergoing painful procedures (3)

4. Singing for 1 hour reduces stress hormones and increases proteins of the immune system in cancer patients, carers, and the people who have been bereaved (4)

5. Dance has been shown to improve physical functioning, body strength, quality of life, and depressive symptoms in women in remission from breast cancer (5,6)

Project ideas

- How could chemotherapy wards be redesigned to maximize comfort and minimize distress during treatment?

- Could the arts be used as part of a public health campaign to encourage people to reduce behaviours known to increase the risk of cancer?

- How could the arts provide psychological support for patients transitioning from treatment to remission?

Q There are a large number of inspiring programmes using the arts to support people affected by cancer such as The Ernest H. Rosenbaum MD Art for Recovery programme and the Art for Cancer Foundation in the US, which use creative arts to help adults express feelings arising from their experience of cancer including a Breast Cancer Quilt Project, and a Healing Through Writing programme: www.cancer.ucsf.edu/support/afr. Welsh charity Tenovus Cancer Care have established over 20 choirs for people affected by cancer, including patients, carers, and people who have been bereaved www.tenovuscancercare.org.uk/singwithus. There are also a number of charities such as Art V Cancer, which use the arts to raise money for cancer research www.artvcancer.com.

The benefit of the arts for cancer care is evidently being recognized: the UK National Health Service has developed a toolkit for allied healthcare professionals on how to improve healthcare and save money, which includes descriptions of the impact of music and in particular art therapy on improving cancer outcomes and the economic rationale for its integration into care. Entitled 'How AHPs improve patient care and save the NHS money', it can be found at www.networks.nhs.uk.

The arts have also been discussed as complementary treatments for cancer in a number of books, including those related to cancer treatments such as *Cancer and Cancer Care* edited by Debby Wyatt and Nicholas Hulbert-Williams (2015), complementary medicine books such as *Enhancing Cancer Care: Complementary Therapy and Support* edited by Jennifer Barraclough (2007), and in relation to survivorship, as in *Survivorship: Living Well During and After Cancer* by Barrie R. Cassileth (2014).(7–9) There are also some texts on specific arts interventions, such as *Art Therapy and Cancer Care* edited by Diane Waller and Caryl Sibbett (2005).(10)

References

1. McCabe C, Roche D, Hegarty F, McCann S. 'Open Window': a randomized trial of the effect of new media art using a virtual window on quality of life in patients' experiencing stem cell transplantation. Psychooncology. 2013 Feb 1;22(2):330–7.

2. Kato PM, Cole SW, Bradlyn AS, Pollock BH. A video game improves behavioral outcomes in adolescents and young adults with cancer: a randomized trial. Pediatrics. 2008 Aug;122(2):e305-17.

3. Favara-Scacco C, Smirne G, Schilirò G, Di Cataldo A. Art therapy as support for children with leukemia during painful procedures. Med Pediatr Oncol. 2001 Apr 1;36(4):474–80.

4. Fancourt D, Williamon A, Carvalho LA, Steptoe A, Dow R, Lewis I. Singing modulates mood, stress, cortisol, cytokine and neuropeptide activity in cancer patients and carers. ecancermedicalscience [Internet]. 2016 Apr 4 [cited 2016 Oct 18];10. Available from: http://www.ecancer.org/journal/10/631-singing-modulates-mood-stress-cortisol-cytokine-and-neuropeptide-activity-in-cancer-patients-and-carers.php.

5. **Kaltsatou A, Mameletzi D, Douka S.** Physical and psychological benefits of a 24-week traditional dance program in breast cancer survivors. J Bodyw Mov Ther. 2011 Apr;**15**(2):162–7.

6. **Sandel SL, Judge JO, Landry N, Faria L, Ouellette R, Majczak M.** Dance and movement program improves quality-of-life measures in breast cancer survivors. Cancer Nurs. 2005 Aug;**28**(4):301–9.

7. **Wyatt D, Hulbert-Williams N.** Cancer and Cancer Care. 1st ed. Los Angeles: SAGE Publications Ltd; 2015. 640 pp.

8. Barraclough J, editor. Enhancing Cancer Care: Complementary Therapy and Support. 1 edition. Oxford ; New York: Oxford University Press; 2007. 224 pp.

9. **Cassileth B.** Survivorship: Living Well During and After Cancer. 1 edition. Ann Arbor, MI: Spry Publishing LLC; 2014. 216 pp.

10. **Waller D, Sibbett C.** Art Therapy and Cancer Care. 1 edition. Maidenhead, England ; New York: Open University Press; 2005. 288 pp.

Fact file 8: Paediatrics

Overview

Paediatrics focuses on the medical care of infants, children, and adolescents. The term derives from the Greek 'παῖς' meaning child and 'ἰατρός' meaning doctor or healer. While adult medicine is split into different subfields (such as neurology, oncology, cardiology, etc.), paediatrics encompasses all of these sub-fields, making it a vast field of medicine. Medical conditions in children often present differently to medical conditions in adults, partly due to the physiological differences in the bodies of a child and an adult. Furthermore, paediatrics can be an ethically and legally complex field as it requires adults to give consent on behalf of children, meaning that the entire family unit can be involved in medical decisions.

Key research findings

1. Music can significantly improve the experience and enjoyment of chest physiotherapy among infants and young children with cystic fibrosis and their families (1)

2. Art therapy among children with leukaemia can reduce resistance and anxiety and improve collaborative behaviour during painful procedures and improve parents' coping abilities (2)

3. Dance/movement therapy can improve mood in adolescents in psychiatric hospitals (3)

4. Theatre has been shown to engage families in dialogue about adolescent sexual health (4)

5. Dance interventions can be more effective than regular physical activity in reducing BMI and heart rate as well as reducing unhealthy behaviours in adolescents (5,6)

Project ideas

- Could X-ray machines and scanners be redesigned by artists to make them more fun and less daunting to young children?
- Could the arts be used to educate children on what 'being in hospital' involves to reduce anxiety during visits?

♦ Could arts-based games be used to educate teenagers about which procedures to follow during emergency situations and how to administer first aid?

Q There are a wealth of practical projects for children and the arts. Some focus on supporting play and healthy development in infants and young children, such as Jo Jingles in the UK and Australia www.jojingles.com and Kindermusik in the USA www.kindermusik.com. Others have a special focus on children with health conditions. Chickenshed is an inclusive theatre company that brings together children from different social backgrounds and both with and without different mental and physical health conditions. Over the past 30 years, the organization has delivered theatre workshops in communities, schools, and hospitals in the UK and Russia www.chickenshed.org.uk.

In particular, there are very varied arts programmes across children's hospitals worldwide, with notable examples being the Go Create programme at Great Ormond Street Children's Hospital in London www.gosh.nhs.uk/about-us/our-priorities/go-create-arts-programme, the Creative Arts Programme at Boston Children's Hospital www.childrenshospital.org/patient-resources/family-resources/creative-arts-program, and the Royal Children's Hospital in Australia http://www.rch.org.au/arch/. All show videos of their work, examples of projects and evaluations on their websites.

For more information on how arts therapy can be applied in paediatrics, *Clinical Applications of Music Therapy in Developmental Disability, Paediatrics and Neurology* edited by Tony Wigram and Jos De Backer (1999) provides some insightful case studies and *Art Therapy in the Early Years* edited by Julia Meyerowitz-Katz and Dean Reddick (2016) discusses approaches for individual work, family and dyad work, and group work.(7,8) There is also specialist guidance for the use of the arts in more specific situations, such as *Creative Arts Therapies Approaches in Adoption and Foster Care: contemporary strategies for working with individuals and families* edited by Donna J Betts (2003) and *Adopted and Wondering: Drawing Out Feelings* by Marge Eaton Heegaard (2007), which both explore how the arts can support children coming to terms with adoption.(9,10)

References

1. Grasso MC, Button BM, Allison DJ, Sawyer SM. Benefits of music therapy as an adjunct to chest physiotherapy in infants and toddlers with cystic fibrosis. Pediatr Pulmonol. 2000 May 1;29(5):371–81.

2. Favara-Scacco C, Smirne G, Schilirò G, Di Cataldo A. Art therapy as support for children with leukemia during painful procedures. Med Pediatr Oncol. 2001 Apr 1;36(4):474–80.

3. Anderson AN, Kennedy H, DeWitt P, Anderson E, Wamboldt MZ. Dance/movement therapy impacts mood states of adolescents in a psychiatric hospital. Arts Psychother. 2014 Jul;41(3):257–62.

4. Causey K, Zuniga M, Bailer B, Ring L, Gil-Trejo L. Using Theater Arts to Engage Latino Families in Dialogue about Adolescent Sexual Health: The PATH -AT Program. J Health Care Poor Underserved. 2012 Feb 26;23(1):347–57.

5. **Robinson TN, Killen JD, Kraemer HC, Wilson DM, Matheson DM, Haskell WL,** et al. Dance and reducing television viewing to prevent weight gain in African-American girls: the Stanford GEMS pilot study. Ethn Dis. 2003;13(1 Suppl 1):S65-77.

6. **Flores R.** Dance for health: improving fitness in African American and Hispanic adolescents. Public Health Rep. 1995;110(2):189–93.

7. **Backer JD.** Clinical Applications of Music Therapy in Developmental Disability, Paediatrics and Neurology. 1 edition. Wigram T, editor. London ; Philadelphia: Jessica Kingsley; 1999. 316 pp.

8. Meyerowitz-Katz J, Reddick D, editors. Art Therapy in the Early Years: Therapeutic interventions with infants, toddlers and their families. Reprint edition. Abingdon, Oxon ; New York, NY: Routledge; 2016. 216 pp.

9. **Betts DJ.** Creative Arts Therapies Approaches in Adoption and Foster Care: Contemporary Strategies for Working With Individuals and Families. 1 edition. Springfield, Ill., USA: Charles C Thomas Pub Ltd; 2003. 342 pp.

10. **Heegaard ME.** Adopted and Wondering: Drawing Out Feelings. Fairview Press; 2007. 40 pp.

Fact file 9: Palliative care

Overview

Palliative care is support for seriously ill patients and their families. The aim of palliative care is to minimize pain and discomfort as much as possible and provide psychological, social, and spiritual support. An important part of palliative care is end-of-life care, which aims to improve quality of life as much as possible while patients are alive and then help them to die with dignity.

Key research findings

1. Storytelling can help families to make sense of illness and death in palliative care and bereavement (1–3)

2. Participation in creative arts can provide a sense of purpose, permanence, and hope for patients in hospices (4)

3. Music therapy has been shown to improve quality of life in terminally ill patients (5)

4. Collaborative arts projects between school children and terminally ill patients have been shown to promote healthier attitudes towards death and dying and support coping with loss (6)

5. Music therapy and song-writing can improve behaviour and grief in bereaved children (7,8)

Project ideas

◆ Could an arts intervention be designed to help patients to say goodbye to friends and relatives and give them the opportunity to leave something permanent behind?

◆ Could the arts be used to bring together people who have been bereaved to enhance their social support networks?

◆ Could the arts be used to educate friends and relatives on how to provide effective emotional support to patients with terminal conditions?

Q For further general reading, *The Creative Arts in Palliative Care* edited by Nigel Hartley and Malcolm Payne (2008) explores how to develop arts interventions for palliative care and contains case studies of experiences working with a broad range of art forms from pottery to digital arts to crafts.(9) In addition, *Creative Engagement in Palliative Care* edited by Lucinda Jarrett (2007) offers an extensive range of ideas and practical advice on developing service users' creativity including song making, drama, dance, creative writing, music, video, and visual arts.(10) For further project ideas, *Dying, Bereavement and the Healing Arts* edited by Gillie Bolton (2007) describes a range of successful arts programmes by artists, writers, nurses, musicians, therapists, social workers, and chaplains in palliative care settings.(11)

For a powerful insight into the world of palliative care, UK charity Rosetta Life has developed a series of documentaries: www.rosettalife.org. The organization aims to use performance, film, and writing projects to allow people with life-limiting conditions to contribute to cultural life and have their voices heard.

There are also a range of inspiring programmes in palliative care settings. For example, Marie Curie hospices in the UK offer arts therapy and have hosted exhibitions of artwork with the Royal Academy Schools using art to give a glimpse of life for people with serious and terminal illness: www.mariecurie.org.uk/help/hospice-care/hospices/hampstead/about/art-exhibition.

Bespoke training courses exist for working with the arts in palliative care, such as the Expressive Arts and Palliative Care course offered by Fleming College in Canada: www.flemingcollege.ca/continuing-education/courses/expressive-arts-in-palliative-care. The National Hospice and Palliative Care Organization in the USA even hosts a Creative Arts Contest each year, with brochures of past shortlisted projects and winners available on their website www.nhpco.org/creative-arts-contest-winners.

References

1. **Noble A, Jones C**. Benefits of narrative therapy: holistic interventions at the end of life. Br J Nurs Mark Allen Publ. 2005 Apr 24;**14**(6):330–3.

2. **Frank AW**. Just listening: Narrative and deep illness. Fam Syst Health. 1998;**16**(3):197–212.

3. **Romanoff BD, Thompson BE**. Meaning Construction in Palliative Care: The Use of Narrative, Ritual, and the Expressive Arts. Am J Hosp Palliat Med. 2006 Aug 1;**23**(4):309–16.

4. **Kennett CE**. Participation in a creative arts project can foster hope in a hospice day centre. Palliat Med. 2000 Sep;**14**(5):419–25.

5. **Hilliard RE**. The effects of music therapy on the quality and length of life of people diagnosed with terminal cancer. J Music Ther. 2003 Summer;**40**(2):113–37.

6. **Tsiris G, Tasker M, Lawson V, Prince G, Dives T, Sands M**, et al. Music and arts in health promotion and death education: the St Christopher's schools project. Music Arts Action. 2011 Apr 11;**3**(2):95–119.

7. **Hilliard RE**. The effects of music therapy-based bereavement groups on mood and behavior of grieving children: a pilot study. J Music Ther. 2001;**38**(4):291–306.

8. **Dalton TA, Krout RE**. The Grief Song-Writing Process with Bereaved Adolescents: An Integrated Grief Model and Music Therapy Protocol. Music Ther Perspect. 2006 Jan 1;**24**(2):94–107.

9. Hartley N, Payne N eds. The Creative Arts in Palliative Care. 1 edition. London, Philadelphia: Jessica Kingsley Publishers; 2008. 206 pp.

10. **Jarrett L.** Creative Engagement in Palliative Care: New Perspectives on User Involvement. 1 edition. Oxford; New York: CRC Press; 2007. 248 pp.

11. Bolton G, ed. Dying, Bereavement, and Healing Arts. 1 edition. London, Philadelphia: Jessica Kingsley Publishers Ltd; 2007. 216 pp.

Fact file 10: Public health

Overview

Public health is defined by the World Health Organisation as 'the science and art of preventing disease, prolonging life and promoting health through organised efforts of society'.(1) Public health looks at populations, from small communities through to entire continents, identifying factors that cause and exacerbate physical and mental health problems, and promoting healthy behaviours. Public health is an inter-disciplinary field that incorporates epidemiology, healthcare services, behavioural health, health economics, and public policy, among others.

Key research findings

1. Attending cultural events is linked with better perceived health (2)
2. Stimulating leisure activities, including reading, painting, and attending cultural events may protect against dementia in later life (3)
3. Arts participation among both teenagers and adult men is associated with reduced obesity (4,5)
4. Arts and cultural engagement is associated with reduced mortality risk (6,7)
5. Mother-infant singing is associated with enhanced wellbeing, self-esteem, and mother-infant bond, as well as fewer symptoms of postnatal depression (8)

Project ideas

- Could the digital arts be used to enhance awareness of key public health messages around healthy eating and exercise and reward healthy lifestyles?
- Could arts-based campaigns be used to enhance public understanding and reduce stigma around certain health conditions?
- How could the arts be used to help educate women in developing countries about the benefits of breastfeeding?

Q For a comprehensive book on the arts and public health, the *Oxford Textbook of Creative Arts, Health and Wellbeing* edited by Stephen Clift and Paul M. Camic (2015) explores what public health is and how it is researched as well as charting research findings from across the lifespan and giving case studies of practice from countries across the world.(9)

For examples of practice, one of the most widespread initiatives globally is the El Sistema. Founded in 1975 in Venezuela, it aims to use music to support personal and social development among young people http://fundamusical.org.ve/el-sistema-2/. Since its beginnings, the El Sistema model has spread to other countries, where it continues its aim to create social change among deprived communities. Videos and research from the programme are available at the websites for different countries, including Sistema Scotland www.makeabignoise.org.uk, Saint James Music Academy in Canada (the first of over 20 programmes set up in the Sistema model) www.sjma.ca, Sistema Portugal (also known as Orquestra Geração) www.orquestra.geracao.aml.pt, and El Sistema USA (the first of many spin-off programmes in the USA) www.elsistemausa.org. Other models of using music to support young people from socially deprived backgrounds include Music Basti, an organization based in India running music workshops for children living in community homes or slum areas without access to quality education: www.musicbasti.org.

The growing interest in arts and public health is supported by a select number of training courses, such as the online Graduate Certificate in Arts in Public Health offered by the University of Florida: www.artsinmedicine.arts.ufl.edu/certificate-in-arts-in-public-health. There are also some helpful resources online including a guide to developing your own arts and public health project *Arts Organisations & Public Heath: Developing Relationships and Programs to Address Local Health Priorities* (2011) available through the US organization Partners for Liveable Communities: www.livable.org.

References

1. **Acheson ED.** On the state of the public health [the fourth Duncan lecture]. Public Health. 1988 Sep 1;**102**(5):431–7.

2. **Johansson SE, Konlaan BB, Bygren LO.** Sustaining habits of attending cultural events and maintenance of health: a longitudinal study. Health Promot Int. 2001 Sep;**16**(3):229–34.

3. **Wang H-X, Karp A, Winblad B, Fratiglioni L.** Late-life engagement in social and leisure activities is associated with a decreased risk of dementia: a longitudinal study from the Kungsholmen project. Am J Epidemiol. 2002 Jun 15;**155**(12):1081–7.

4. **Kouvonen A, Swift JA, Stafford M, Cox T, Vahtera J, Vaananen A,** et al. Social Participation and Maintaining Recommended Waist Circumference: Prospective Evidence From the English Longitudinal Study of Aging. J Aging Health. 2012 Mar 1;**24**(2):250–68.

5. **Cuypers K, De Ridder K, Kvaløy K, Knudtsen MS, Krokstad S, Holmen J,** et al. Leisure time activities in adolescence in the presence of susceptibility genes for obesity: risk or resilience against overweight in adulthood? The HUNT study. BMC Public Health. 2012;**12**:820.

6. **Bygren LO, Konlaan BB, Johansson SE.** Attendance at cultural events, reading books or periodicals, and making music or singing in a choir as determinants for survival: Swedish interview survey of living conditions. BMJ. 1996 Dec 21;**313**(7072):1577–80.

7. Väänänen A, Murray M, Koskinen A, Vahtera J, Kouvonen A, Kivimäki M. Engagement in cultural activities and cause-specific mortality: prospective cohort study. Prev Med. 2009 Sep;**49**(2–3):142–7.

8. Fancourt D, Perkins R. Associations between singing to babies and symptoms of postnatal depression, wellbeing, self-esteem and mother-infant bond. Public Health. 2017; in press.

9. Clift S, Camic PM, editors. Oxford Textbook of Creative Arts, Health, and Wellbeing: International perspectives on practice, policy and research. OUP Oxford; 2015. 368 pp.

Fact file 11: Psychiatry

Overview

Psychiatry is a branch of medicine dealing with mental health conditions, including anxiety and depression; disorders such as obsessive compulsive disorder, post-traumatic stress disorder, personality disorders, eating disorders, sleep disorders and bipolar disorder; phobias; paranoia; schizophrenia; and addictions such as drug and alcohol misuse. Diagnosis can involve case assessments, physical examinations, psychological tests, neuroimaging, and neurophysiological tests. Treatments encompass psychiatric medication and psychotherapy alongside other professional support from both health and social work professionals.

Key research findings

1. Drama therapy for sexually abused teenagers can reduce hostility, depression, and psychotic thinking (1)

2. The use of arts therapies in forensic psychiatry can reduce destructive aggression and promote self-expression, self-control, and empathy (2)

3. Group drumming can reduce anxiety, depression, and inflammatory immune response in mental health service users (3,4)

4. Rock and metal music are significantly associated with acts of deliberate self-harm, depression, delinquency, drug-taking, and family dysfunction (5,6)

5. Ballroom, tango, and Turkish folklore dancing classes have all been shown to reduce anxiety and depression (7–9)

Project ideas

- Could an arts-based app be used to monitor mental health among the general population and deliver targeted interventions to those who need them?

- How could a patient's room in an in-patient psychiatric facility be redesigned to enhance wellbeing?

- Could an arts therapy intervention be developed for patients recovering from substance abuse?

Q For further reading, *Mental Health, Psychiatry and the Arts* edited by Victoria Tischler (2010) explores how arts interventions from poetry to creative writing, art psychotherapy, drama, and blues music can support people with different mental health conditions.(10) For research and guidance on working with more specific conditions, the online magazine *Science of Eating Disorders* published a piece on 5 October 2013 by someone who has an eating disorder entitled 'The Art of Therapy: using arts-based therapies in eating disorder treatment': www.scienceofeds. org. *Music Therapy and Addictions* edited by David Aldridge (2010) contains case studies and practical advice for music therapists.(11) *Integrative Art Therapy and Depression* by Vibeke Skov (2015) looks at how different approaches to art therapy and creativity can support clinical outcomes.(12) And *Art Therapy and Anger* by Marian Liebmann and Annette Coulter (2008) explores the arts with varied populations from abused children to young offenders, to women who self-harm and returning war veterans.(13)

There are several powerful online films about art and psychiatry. Crazy Art has produced a short documentary exploring how three artists with schizophrenia, mania, and depression use art to help them cope. It also looks back at famous artists such as Van Gogh who have struggled with mental health issues: www.crazyartonline.com. Similarly, 'Art Therapy: A Documentary' by Lynn-Ellin Zeigler follows several young people who tell their story of how the arts have supported them in coping with mental illness: www. youtube.com/watch?v=9zuiDuNwre4. The topic is depicted in a number of popular films, including 'Shine' (1996) and 'The Soloist' (2009); both about musicians with mental health conditions.

There is a large body of organizations delivering arts programmes in psychiatry. As just a few examples, Castle Craig in Scotland, one of Europe's leading addiction clinics, uses art groups, dance, and drumming as part of its treatment programme: www. castlecraig.co.uk/treatment/complementary-therapies. In the USA, Art Therapy Connection in Chicago uses the arts to support the mental health of children and teenagers: www.atcchicago.com. For military veterans, 'Voices of Valor' uses music to help people transition back to military life, with a particular focus on people with posttraumatic stress disorder or self-medicating or engaging in substance abuse: www. voicesofvalor.org. Finally, CoolTan Arts, run by and for people with mental health issues, uses creativity to give adults training, support, and volunteering opportunities www.cooltanarts.org.uk.

References

1. **Mackay B, Gold M, Gold** E. A pilot study in drama therapy with adolescent girls who have been sexually abused. Arts Psychother. 1987;**14**(1):77–84.

2. **Smeijsters H, Cleven** G. The treatment of aggression using arts therapies in forensic psychiatry: Results of a qualitative inquiry. Arts Psychother. 2006;**33**(1):37–58.

3. **Fancourt D, Perkins R, Ascenso S, Atkins L, Kilfeather S, Carvalho LA,** et al. Group drumming modulates cytokine activity in mental health service users: a preliminary study. Psychother Psychosom. 2016;**85**(1):53–5.

4. Fancourt D, Perkins R, Ascenso S, Carvalho LA, Steptoe A, Williamon A. Effects of Group Drumming Interventions on Anxiety, Depression, Social Resilience and Inflammatory Immune Response among Mental Health Service Users. PLoS One. 2016 Mar 14;**11**(3):e0151136.

5. Baker F, Bor W. Can music preference indicate mental health status in young people? Australas Psychiatry. 2008 Jan 1;**16**(4):284–8.

6. Martin G, Clarke M, Pearce C. Adolescent Suicide: Music Preference as an Indicator of Vulnerability. J Am Acad Child Adolesc Psychiatry. 1993 May;**32**(3):530–5.

7. Eyigor S, Karapolat H, Durmaz B, Ibisoglu U, Cakir S. A randomized controlled trial of Turkish folklore dance on the physical performance, balance, depression and quality of life in older women. Arch Gerontol Geriatr. 2009 Feb;**48**(1):84–8.

8. Haboush A, Floyd M, Caron J, LaSota M, Alvarez K. Ballroom dance lessons for geriatric depression: An exploratory study. Arts Psychother. 2006;**33**(2):89–97.

9. Pinniger R, Brown RF, Thorsteinsson EB, McKinley P. Argentine tango dance compared to mindfulness meditation and a waiting-list control: a randomised trial for treating depression. Complement Ther Med. 2012 Dec;**20**(6):377–84.

10. Tischler V. Mental Health, Psychiatry and the Arts: A Teaching Handbook. 1 edition. Oxford, UK ; New York: CRC Press; 2010. 176 pp.

11. Aldridge D, editor. Music Therapy and Addictions. 1 edition. London: Jessica Kingsley Publishers; 2010. 176 pp.

12. Skov V, Robbins A. Integrative Art Therapy and Depression: A Transformative Approach. London ; Philadelphia: Jessica Kingsley Publishers; 2015. 360 pp.

13. Coulter A, Coyle T, Brosh H, Ambridge M, Knight S, Law S, et al. Art Therapy and Anger. Liebmann M, editor. London; Philadelphia: Jessica Kingsley Publishers; 2008. 272 pp.

Fact file 12: Rehabilitation medicine

Overview

Rehabilitation medicine involves the treatment and active management of disabilities and other disabling conditions. The four major clinical areas of work are neurological rehabilitation (including working with people with conditions such as multiple sclerosis and cerebral palsy or people recovering from acute brain injuries and strokes), musculoskeletal rehabilitation (including supporting rheumatological conditions such as arthritis and back pain), amputee rehabilitation (often working in partnership with orthotics clinics and wheelchair centres), and rehabilitation following spinal cord injury.

Key research findings

1. Music-based movement therapy can improve balance, stride length, and walking velocity in patients with Parkinson's disease (1)
2. Dance can lead to increased lumbar bone mineral density and markers of osteoblastic activity in osteoporotic older women (2)
3. Singing can improve lung function and mental health in adults with chronic obstructive pulmonary disease (3)
4. Magic tricks for children with hemiplegia can improve speed and performance of the affected hand and lead to an increase in its use (4)
5. Drama therapy can nurture self-esteem and empower patients recovering from neuro-trauma as well as helping them to find personal space while in a neuro-rehabilitation unit (5)

Project ideas

- Could an arts-based app be used to encourage people to practice therapy exercises and monitor their progress?
- How could the arts be used to reduce pain or discomfort while undertaking rehabilitation activities?

◆ Could community arts activities be designed to act preventatively and maintain mobility among at-risk population such as the elderly or people with
chronic conditions such as diabetes?

Q One of the most popular areas within rehabilitation and the arts is dance therapy.
For an introduction to dance therapy, *The Arts and Science of Dance/Movement
Therapy* edited by Sharon Chaiklin and Hilda Wengrower (2015) gives an accessible
insight.(6) As an example of a live project, Rambert Dance Company, a contemporary
dance company in the UK, established a project for amputees in 2012. People Dancing,
the foundation for community dance, has published a webpage and editorial piece on
how the project was established and its impact entitled 'Witness the Magic' available at
www.communitydance.org.uk.

There are also a number of organizations that offer wheelchair dancing, such as the
Wheelchair Dance Sport Association (WDSA) in the UK where it is used both for recre-
ation and rehabilitation purposes. Information about the development of this activity is
described by WDSA: www.wdsauk.co.uk/services/history-of-wheelchair-dance. Similar
societies exist in other countries, such as the American DanceWheels Foundation www.
americandancewheels.org.

Among other rehabilitation programmes, more information on the use of magic
tricks for occupational therapy including research findings, case studies, and videos
can be found at www.breatheahr.org/breathe-magic. And there are also a number of
resources available for establishing choirs for people affected by lung disease, such
as the guide for singers *Living with COPD: How to improve your breathing by singing*
from Baywater Healthcare in the UK: www.baywater.co.uk/healthcare/how-singing-
can-help-copd; and the guidance book *Singing and People with COPD* by Ian Morrison
and Stephen Clift produced by the Sidney De Haan Research Centre in the UK: www.
canterbury.ac.uk.

For more resources related to neurological rehabilitation, see Fact file 5: Neurology.

References

1. **de Dreu MJ, van der Wilk ASD, Poppe E, Kwakkel G, van Wegen EEH**. Rehabilitation,
exercise therapy and music in patients with Parkinson's disease: a meta-analysis of the
effects of music-based movement therapy on walking ability, balance and quality of life.
Parkinsonism Relat Disord. 2012 Jan;**18**, Supplement 1:S114–9.

2. **Kudlacek S, Pietschmann F, Bernecker P, Resch H, Willvonseder R**. The impact of a
senior dancing program on spinal and peripheral bone mass. Am J Phys Med Rehabil
Assoc Acad Physiatr. 1997 Dec;**76**(6):477–81.

3. **Bonilha AG, Onofre F, Vieira ML, Prado MYA, Martinez JAB**. Effects of singing classes
on pulmonary function and quality of life of COPD patients. Int J Chron Obstruct
Pulmon Dis. 2009;**4**:1–8.

4. **Green D, Schertz M, Gordon AM, Moore A, Schejter Margalit T, Farquharson Y**, et al.
A multi-site study of functional outcomes following a themed approach to hand-arm

bimanual intensive therapy for children with hemiplegia. Dev Med Child Neurol. 2013 Jun;**55**(6):527–33.

5. **McKenna P, Haste E**. Clinical effectiveness of dramatherapy in the recovery from neuro-trauma. Disabil Rehabil. 1999 Apr;**21**(4):162–74.

6. Chaiklin S, Wengrower H, editors. The Art and Science of Dance/Movement Therapy: Life Is Dance. 1 edition. New York: Routledge; 2009. 380 pp.

Fact file 13: Surgery

Overview

From the Greek 'χείρ' meaning hand and 'ἔργον' meaning work, surgery investigates and/or treats diseases and injuries either for functional or cosmetic purposes. Elective surgery is carried out for non-life-threatening conditions at the patient's request, whereas emergency surgery has to be carried out quickly; exploratory surgery is used to aid or confirm diagnoses, while therapeutic surgery is used to treat a diagnosed condition. Although 'surgery' is typically used to refer to the period in the operating room, there are important pre-operative stages, including phlebotomy (blood tests) and anaesthesia, and sometimes complex post-operative care.

Key research findings

1. Relaxing recorded music chosen by surgeons can improve their speed and accuracy in operating rooms (1–3)
2. Tablet devices using arts, music and games can reduce delirium and time-to-discharge in children undergoing anaesthetic (4)
3. Recorded music pre-surgery has been shown to lead to lower morphine requirements after surgery (5)
4. Music has been shown to be as effective as medication in reducing pre-operative anxiety (6)
5. Aromatherapy can lead to lower pain and nausea and fewer analgesic and antiemetic requests from patients post surgery (7,8)

Project ideas

- Could an arts-based app be used in the home to prepare children for what happens in surgery, reducing their anxiety when they come into hospital for operations?
- How could the arts be used in recovery areas immediately post surgery to help re-orientate patients and reduce discomfort?
- Could surgical waiting areas be redesigned to reduce boredom, frustration, and perceived waiting time among relatives?

Q The *British Medical Journal* has a podcast available online with a surgeon interviewed about his choice of music while operating (alongside a humorous Christmas article). There is also an associated Spotify playlist. http://www.bmj.com/content/349/bmj.g7436. Further interviews with surgeons about their listening habits are available online via the *Guardian* newspaper in an article entitled 'The surgeon's cut: what do doctors listen to in the operating theatre?': www.theguardian.com.

There is also a 'Best Practice: Evidence based information sheet for health professionals' on the use of music in surgical settings, which includes advice on how to integrate music into a patient's care process: http://connect.jbiconnectplus.org/viewsourcefile. aspx?0=493.

Chelsea and Westminster Hospital in London, UK, has also developed a tablet app to relax children and distract them during anaesthetics procedures prior to surgery. The app, which links children with suitable arts, games, and music, has won a number of awards. The story of the app is available in *Anaesthesia News* No.346 from May 2016.

References

1. Siu K-C, Suh IH, Mukherjee M, Oleynikov D, Stergiou N. The effect of music on robot-assisted laparoscopic surgical performance. Surg Innov. 2010 Dec;17(4):306–11.

2. Allen K, Blascovich J. Effects of music on cardiovascular reactivity among surgeons. JAMA. 1994 Sep 21;272(11):882–4.

3. Conrad C, Konuk Y, Werner P, Cao CG, Warshaw A, Rattner D, et al. The effect of defined auditory conditions versus mental loading on the laparoscopic motor skill performance of experts. Surg Endosc. 2010 Jun;24(6):1347–52.

4. Seiden SC, McMullan S, Sequera-Ramos L, De Oliveira GS, Roth A, Rosenblatt A, et al. Tablet-based Interactive Distraction (TBID) vs oral midazolam to minimize perioperative anxiety in pediatric patients: a noninferiority randomized trial. Pediatr Anesth. 2014;24(12):1217–23.

5. Cepeda MS, Carr DB, Lau J, Alvarez H. Music for pain relief. Cochrane Database Syst Rev. 2006;(2):CD004843.

6. Berbel P, Moix J, Quintana S. [Music versus diazepam to reduce preoperative anxiety: a randomized controlled clinical trial]. Rev Esp Anestesiol Reanim. 2007 Jun;54(6):355–8.

7. Kim JT, Ren CJ, Fielding GA, Pitti A, Kasumi T, Wajda M, et al. Treatment with lavender aromatherapy in the post-anesthesia care unit reduces opioid requirements of morbidly obese patients undergoing laparoscopic adjustable gastric banding. Obes Surg. 2007 Jul;17(7):920–5.

8. Hunt R, Dienemann J, Norton HJ, Hartley W, Hudgens A, Stern T, et al. Aromatherapy as treatment for postoperative nausea: a randomized trial. Anesth Analg. 2013 Sep;117(3):597–604.

Index

Note: Tables and figures are indicated by an italic *t* and *f* following the page number.
Names beginning with 'Mac' or 'Mc' are sorted as if spelled out as 'Mac'.